Health Reference Series Online Activation Code:

ik5947

To activate this title in your online database, go to "Settings" and enter the above Activation Code into the appropriate field.

To set up your online *Health Reference Series* database for the first time, go to www.online.omnigraphics.com/registration

Questions? Call (800) 234-1340, email help@omnigraphics.com or go to www.omnigraphics.com/health-reference-online

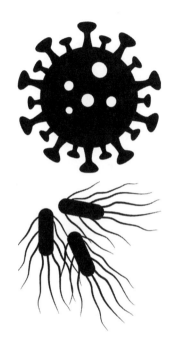

DISEASES AND ILLNESSES TRANSMITTED TO HUMANS BY ANIMALS, INSECTS AND CONTAMINATED FOOD AND WATER

First Edition

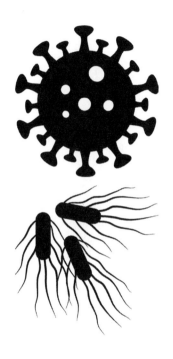

DISEASES AND ILLNESSES TRANSMITTED TO HUMANS BY ANIMALS, INSECTS AND CONTAMINATED FOOD AND WATER

First Edition

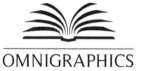

OMNIGRAPHICS
615 Griswold St., Ste. 520
Detroit, MI 48226

OMNIGRAPHICS

Kevin Hayes, *Managing Editor*

❀ ❀ ❀

Copyright © 2020 Omnigraphics

ISBN 978-0-7808-1792-0

E-ISBN 978-0-7808-1793-7

Library of Congress Cataloging-in-Publication Data

Title: Diseases and illnesses transmitted to humans by animals, insects and contaminated food and water

Description: First edition. | Detroit, MI: Omnigraphics, [2020] | Series: Health reference series: special edition | Summary: "Offers basic consumer health information about animal-, insect-, food-, and water-borne diseases, their outbreaks, tips to protect yourself and others, along with epidemiology of emerging and reemerging infectious diseases. Includes a directory of organizations for additional help and information"-- Provided by publisher.

Identifiers: LCCN 2019059730 (print) | LCCN 2019059731 (ebook) | ISBN 9780780817920 (library binding) | ISBN 9780780817937 (ebook)

Subjects: LCSH: Zoonoses--Popular works. | Foodborne diseases--Popular works. | Waterborne infection--Popular works. | Communicable diseases--Popular works. | Consumer education.

Classification: LCC RC113.5.A55 2020 (print) | LCC RC113.5 (ebook) | DDC 616.95/9--dc23

LC record available at https://lccn.loc.gov/2019059730
LC ebook record available at https://lccn.loc.gov/2019059731

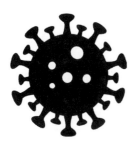

TABLE OF CONTENTS

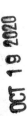

Part 5: How to Protect Yourself and Your Family from Diseases and Illnesses Transmitted to Humans by Animals, Insects, and Contaminated Water

Part 6: Resurgent and Emerging Diseases in a Changing World

Part 7: Additional Help and Information

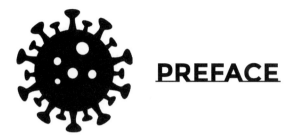 **PREFACE**

About This Book

According to statistics provided by the Centers for Disease Control and Prevention (CDC), it is estimated that every year in the United States around 3,000 people die from foodborne diseases and about 128,000 people are hospitalized. The CDC's estimate for the number of people affected by vector-borne diseases are around 640,000 cases between 2004 and 2016. Globally, malaria causes 400,000 deaths every year. Estimates show that more than 6 out of every 10 known infectious diseases in people are spread by animals, and 3 out of every 4 emerging infectious diseases in people are spread by animals. Every year, the United States registers an estimated 4 to 32 million cases of people affected with acute gastrointestinal illness (AGI) due to public drinking-water systems.

Diseases and Illnesses Transmitted to Humans from Animals, Insects and Contaminated Food and Water, First Edition explains the various diseases that are spread by animals, insects, and through the contamination of food and water, along with the processes used to identify and track these disease outbreaks. The book also provides tips and safety measures to protect yourself and your family, including information about the epidemiology of these emerging and reemerging infectious diseases, illnesses, and outbreaks. The book also includes a directory of organizations that provide additional help and information.

How to Use This Book

This book is divided into parts and chapters. Parts focus on broad areas of interest. Chapters are devoted to single topics within a part.

Part 1: Animal-Borne Illnesses and Diseases describes the animal-borne diseases, along with information about emerging and zoonotic and recent animal-borne diseases such as coronavirus, SARS, and hantavirus diseases including the risk of animal-borne infections among specific population.

Part 2: Insect-Borne Illnesses and Diseases explains the vector-borne diseases, along with other related diseases such as rickettsial zoonoses, Lyme disease, and leishmaniasis caused by bacterias, arbovirus, protozoan parasites, and pathogens.

Part 3: Food- and Water-Borne Illnesses and Diseases discusses the illnesses and diseases caused by the consumption of contaminated food and water. It provides information about the effects of water contamination and the major sources of water contamination and its impact on children, along with the magnitude and burden of waterborne diseases in the United States, and water safety for travelers.

Part 4: Diseases and Outbreaks Transmitted to Humans from Animals, Insects, and Contaminated Food and Water describes the identification and outbreaks of animal-, vector-, and food-borne diseases, along with information on the novel coronavirus and how to identify the animal-, insect-, food-, and water-borne illnesses and diseases.

Part 5: How to Protect Yourself and Your Family from Diseases and Illnesses Transmitted to Humans by Animals, Insects, and Contaminated Water provides tips on how to protect yourself and your family from illnesses and diseases transmitted to humans by animals, insects, and contaminated food and water, along with a guide to safe water systems.

Part 6: Resurgent and Emerging Diseases in a Changing World discusses major factors in the emergence of infectious disease. It describes countering bioterrorism and gives information about new approaches to the prevention of foodborne diseases and strengthening global health capacity against infectious disease threats. It also discusses the climate impacts on risk for waterborne pathogens, and the mitigation and adaptation for waterborne illness.

Part 7: Additional Help and Information consists of a directory of organizations that provide help and information regarding diseases and illnesses transmitted to humans by animals, insects, and contaminated food and water.

Bibliographic Note

This volume contains documents and excerpts from publications issued by the following U.S. government agencies: Centers for Disease Control and Prevention (CDC); National Institute of Environmental Health Sciences (NIEHS); Office of Disease Prevention and Health Promotion (ODPHP); U.S. Department of Agriculture (USDA); U.S. Department of Health and Human Services (HHS); U.S. Environmental Protection Agency (EPA); U.S. Food and Drug Administration (FDA); and U.S. Global Change Research Program (USGCRP).

The photograph on the front cover is © Dragon Images/Shutterstock.

About the *Health Reference Series*

The *Health Reference Series* is designed to provide basic medical information for patients, families, caregivers, and the general public. Each volume concentrates on a particular topic and provides comprehensive coverage. This is especially important for people who may be dealing with a newly diagnosed disease or a chronic disorder in themselves or a family member. People looking for preventive guidance, information about disease warning signs, medical statistics, and risk factors for health problems will also find answers to their questions in the *Health Reference Series*. The *Series*, however, is not intended to serve as a tool for diagnosing illness, in prescribing treatments, or as a substitute for the physician–patient relationship. All people concerned about medical symptoms or the possibility of disease are encouraged to seek professional care from an appropriate healthcare provider.

About *Health Reference Series* *Special Editions*

Omnigraphics' *Health Reference Series Special Editions* are designed for the general reader seeking to understand historical and current global health developments, threats, international initiatives, and population data, and why a public-health crisis across the globe affects them.

A Note about Spelling and Style

Health Reference Series editors use *Stedman's Medical Dictionary* as an authority for questions related to the spelling of medical terms and *The Chicago Manual of Style* for questions related to grammatical structures, punctuation, and other editorial concerns. Consistent adherence is not always possible, however, because the individual volumes within the *Series* include many documents from a wide variety of different producers, and the editor's primary goal is to present material from each source as accurately as is possible. This sometimes means that information in different chapters or sections may follow other guidelines and alternate spelling authorities. For example, occasionally a copyright holder may require that eponymous terms be shown in possessive forms (Crohn's disease vs. Crohn disease) or that British spelling norms be retained (leukaemia vs. leukemia).

Medical Review

Omnigraphics contracts with a team of qualified, senior medical professionals who serve as medical consultants for the *Health Reference Series*. As necessary, medical consultants review reprinted material for currency and accuracy. Citations including the phrase "Reviewed (month, year)" indicate material reviewed by this team. Medical consultation services are provided to the *Health Reference Series* editors by:

Dr. Vijayalakshmi, MBBS, DGO, MD
Dr. Senthil Selvan, MBBS, DCH, MD
Dr. K. Sivanandham, MBBS, DCH, MS (Research), PhD

Our Advisory Board

We would like to thank the following board members for providing initial guidance on the development of this series:

- Dr. Lynda Baker, Associate Professor of Library and Information Science, Wayne State University, Detroit, MI

- Nancy Bulgarelli, William Beaumont Hospital Library, Royal Oak, MI
- Karen Imarisio, Bloomfield Township Public Library, Bloomfield Township, MI
- Karen Morgan, Mardigian Library, University of Michigan-Dearborn, Dearborn, MI
- Rosemary Orlando, St. Clair Shores Public Library, St. Clair Shores, MI

Health Reference Series Update Policy

The inaugural book in the *Health Reference Series* was the first edition of *Cancer Sourcebook* published in 1989. Since then, the *Series* has been enthusiastically received by librarians and in the medical community. In order to maintain the standard of providing high-quality health information for the layperson the editorial staff at Omnigraphics felt it was necessary to implement a policy of updating volumes when warranted.

Medical researchers have been making tremendous strides, and it is the purpose of the *Health Reference Series* to stay current with the most recent advances. Each decision to update a volume is made on an individual basis. Some of the considerations include how much new information is available and the feedback we receive from people who use the books. If there is a topic you would like to see added to the update list, or an area of medical concern you feel has not been adequately addressed, please write to:

Managing Editor
Health Reference Series
Omnigraphics
615 Griswold St., Ste. 520
Detroit, MI 48226

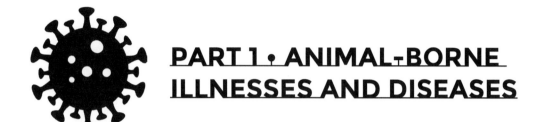

PART 1 • ANIMAL-BORNE ILLNESSES AND DISEASES

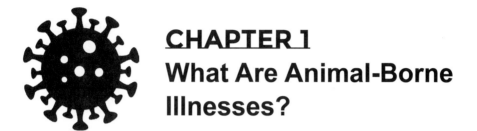

CHAPTER 1
What Are Animal-Borne Illnesses?

Zoonotic diseases (also known as "zoonoses") are caused by infections that spread between animals and people.

Every year, tens of thousands of Americans get sick from diseases and harmful germs spread between animals and people. These are known as "zoonotic diseases." "Zoonotic" means infectious diseases that are spread between animals and people. Because these diseases can cause sickness or death in people, the Centers for Disease Control and Prevention (CDC) works 24/7, tracking and reporting them.

Animals provide many benefits to people. Many people interact with animals in their daily lives, both at home and away from home. Pets offer companionship and entertainment, with millions of households having one or more pets. We might come into close contact with animals at a county fair or petting zoo, or encounter wildlife while enjoying outdoor activities. Also, animals are an important food source and provide meat, dairy, and eggs.

However, some animals can carry harmful germs that can be shared with people and cause illness—these are known as "zoonotic diseases" or "zoonoses." Zoonotic diseases are caused by harmful germs such as viruses, bacteria, parasites, and fungi. These germs can cause many different types of illnesses in people and animals that range from mild to serious illness and

This chapter includes text excerpted from "Zoonotic Diseases," Centers for Disease Control and Prevention (CDC), July 14, 2017.

even death. Some animals can appear healthy even when they are carrying germs that can make people sick.

Zoonotic diseases are very common, both in the United States and around the world. Scientists estimate that more than 6 out of every 10 known infectious diseases in people are spread from animals, and 3 out of every 4 new or emerging infectious diseases in people are spread from animals.

How Do Germs Spread between Animals and People?

Because of the close connection between people and animals, it is important to be aware of the common ways people can get infected with germs that can cause zoonotic diseases. These can include:

- **Direct contact.** Coming into contact with the saliva, blood, urine, mucous, feces, or other body fluids of an infected animal. Examples include petting or touching animals, and bites or scratches.
- **Indirect contact.** Coming into contact with areas where animals live and roam, or objects or surfaces that have been contaminated with germs. Examples include aquarium tank water, pet habitats, chicken coops, plants, and soil, as well as pet food and water dishes.
- **Vector-borne.** Being bitten by a tick, or an insect such as a mosquito or a flea.
- **Foodborne.** Each year, 1 in 6 Americans get sick from eating contaminated food. Eating or drinking something unsafe (such as unpasteurized milk, undercooked meat or eggs, or raw fruits and vegetables that are contaminated with feces from an infected animal).

Who Is at a Higher Risk of Serious Illness from Zoonotic Diseases?

Anyone can become sick from a zoonotic disease, including healthy people. However, some people may be more at risk than others and should take steps to protect themselves or family members. These people are more likely than others to get really sick, and even die, from infection with certain diseases.

These groups of people include:
- Children younger than 5
- Adults older than 65
- People with weakened immune systems

What Can You Do to Protect Yourself and Your Family from Zoonotic Diseases?

People come into contact with animals in many places. This includes at home and away from home, in places such as petting zoos, fairs, schools, stores, and parks. Insects, such as mosquitoes and fleas, and ticks bite people and animals day and night. Thankfully, there are things you can do to protect yourself and your family from zoonotic diseases.

- Keep your hands clean. Washing your hands right after being around animals, even if you did not touch any animals, is one of the most important steps you can take to avoid getting sick and spreading germs to others.
  - Always wash your hands after being around animals, even if you did not touch the animals.
  - Many germs are spread by not washing hands with soap and clean, running water.
  - If clean, running water is not accessible, use soap and available water.
  - If soap and water are unavailable, use an alcohol-based hand sanitizer that contains at least 60 percent alcohol to clean hands. Because hand sanitizers do not eliminate all types of germs, it is important to wash your hands as soon as soap and water are available.
- Know the simple things you can do to stay safe around your pets.
- Prevent bites from mosquitoes, ticks, and fleas.
- Learn more about ways to handle food safely—whether it is for yourself or your family, your pet, or other animals.
- Be aware of zoonotic diseases both at home, away from home (such as at petting zoos or other animal exhibits), in childcare settings or schools, and when you travel.
- Avoid bites and scratches from animals.

CHAPTER 2
Emerging and Zoonotic Infections in the United States

Chapter Contents

Section 2.1

U.S. Outbreaks of Zoonotic Diseases Spread between Animals and People

This section includes text excerpted from "U.S. Outbreaks of Zoonotic Diseases Spread between Animals and People," Centers for Disease Control and Prevention (CDC), January 28, 2020.

Below is a selected list from the Centers for Disease Control and Prevention (CDC) of outbreaks of human infections linked to contact with animals and animal products in the United States. This list is not comprehensive, and outbreaks may have occurred that are not included here.

Table 2.1. Outbreaks of Human Infections Linked to Contact with Animals and Animal Products in the United States

Year	Animal Products	Reptiles and Amphibians	Cattle	Dogs	Poultry	Small Mammals
2007	Dry Pet Food –*Salmonella* Schwarzengrund					
2010	Dry Dog Food – *Salmonella* Infantis					Frozen Rodents –*Salmonella*
2011	Pig Ear Dog Treats –Multidrug-resistant *Salmonella*	Water Frogs –*Salmonella* Typhimurium			Chicks and Ducklings– *Salmonella* Altona, *Salmonella* Johannesburg	
2012		Small Turtles –*Salmonella* Sandiego, *Salmonella* Pomona, *Salmonella* Poona			Live Poultry – *Salmonella* Hadar Live Poultry –*Salmonella* Montevideo Live Poultry –*Salmonella* Infantis, *Salmonella* Newport, *Salmonella* Lille	Hedgehogs –*Salmonella* Typhimurium Rodents – Hantavirus Infections Rodents – Lymphocytic choriomeningitis virus (LCMV

Table 2.1. Continued

Year	Animal Products	Reptiles and Amphibians	Cattle	Dogs	Poultry	Small Mammals
2013		Small Turtles –*Salmonella* Sandiego, *Salmonella* Pomona, *Salmonella* Poona				
2014		Pet Bearded Dragons– *Salmonella* Cotham			Live Poultry –*Salmonella* Typhimurium Live Poultry –*Salmonella* Infantis, *Salmonella* Lille, *Salmonella* Newport, *Salmonella* Mbandaka	Frozen Feeder Rodents– *Salmonella* Typhimurium
2015		Small Turtles –*Salmonella* Sandiego, *Salmonella* Poona Pet Crested Geckos– *Salmonella* Muenchen			Live Poultry –*Salmonella* Enteritidis, *Salmonella* Hadar, *Salmonella* Indiana, *Salmonella* Muenchen	
2016			Dairy Bull Calves– *Salmonella* Heidelberg		Live Poultry –*Salmonella* Enteritidis, *Salmonella* Muenster, *Salmonella* Hadar, *Salmonella* Indiana, *Salmonella* Mbandaka, *Salmonella* Infantis, *Salmonella* Braenderup	
2017		Pet Turtles– *Salmonella* Agbeni Infections		Pet Store Puppies– Campylo-bacter Infections	Live Poultry –*Salmonella* Infections	Pet Rats–Seoul Virus Infections

Table 2.1. Continued

Year	Animal Products	Reptiles and Amphibians	Cattle	Dogs	Poultry	Small Mammals
2018					Poultry at Poultry Slaughter Plants– Psittacosis Live Poultry –*Salmonella* Infections	Guinea Pigs –*Salmonella* Infections
2019		Pet Turtles– *Salmonella* Oranienburg infections		Pet Store Puppies– Campy-lobacter Infections	Backyard Poultry– *Salmonella* Infections	Pet Hedgehogs –*Salmonella* Infections
2020		Pet Turtles– *Salmonella* Typhimurium				

Section 2.2

Zoonoses of Most Concern in the United States

This section includes text excerpted from "8 Zoonotic Diseases Shared between Animals and People of Most Concern in the U.S.," Centers for Disease Control and Prevention (CDC), May 6, 2019.

The Centers for Disease Control and Prevention (CDC) and its U.S. government partners have released the first federal collaborative report listing the top zoonotic diseases of national concern for the United States. Zoonotic diseases are illnesses that spread between animals and people.

The CDC, the U.S. Department of the Interior (DOI), and the U.S. Department of Agriculture (USDA) developed the report after jointly hosting a One Health Zoonotic Disease Prioritization Workshop for the

United States. During the workshop, agencies agreed on a list of eight zoonotic diseases that are of greatest concern to the nation and made recommendations for next steps using a One Health approach.

"Every year, tens of thousands of Americans get sick from diseases spread between animals and people. The CDC's One Health Office is collaborating with DOI, USDA, and other partners across the government to bring together disease detectives, laboratorians, physicians, and veterinarians to prevent those illnesses and protect the health of people, animals, and our environment," said Casey Barton Behravesh, M.S., D.V.M., Dr.P.H., director, One Health Office, CDC.

The zoonotic diseases of most concerns in the United States are:

- Zoonotic influenza
- Salmonellosis
- West Nile virus
- Plague
- Emerging coronaviruses (e.g., severe acute respiratory syndrome and Middle East respiratory syndrome)
- Rabies
- Brucellosis
- Lyme disease

Six out of every 10 infectious diseases in people are zoonotic, which makes it crucial that the nation strengthen its capabilities to prevent and respond to these diseases using a One Health approach. One Health is an approach that recognizes the connection between people, animals, plants, and their shared environment and calls for experts in human, animal, and environmental health to work together to achieve the best health outcomes for all.

The one Health Zoonotic Disease Prioritization Workshop was the first time multiple government agencies in the United States worked together on this topic and is a critical step toward a coordinated U.S.-specific approach to One Health. The workshop report outlines the process, the resulting list of prioritized zoonotic diseases, and discussions and recommendations by the participants.

The One Health Zoonotic Disease Prioritization Workshop report is a resource for organizations that work on One Health issues, the media, and other stakeholders and includes recommendations on how to work together to address the prioritized diseases and strengthen One Health efforts in the United States. You can download a copy of the report at cdc.gov/onehealth/pdfs/us-ohzdp-report-508.pdf.

CHAPTER 3
Specific Populations at Risk of Animal-Borne Infections

Chapter Contents

Schools and Daycares

This section includes text excerpted from "Animals in Schools and Daycares," Centers for Disease Control and Prevention (CDC), August 7, 2019.

Some people are more likely to get sick from germs animals can carry. It is important for people at increased risk to know how to stay healthy around animals, and veterinarians and healthcare providers should also be aware of the risks for certain groups so they can counsel patients and clients.

Animals in Schools and Daycares

Animals can be entertaining and educational. But, children, especially children under 5 years of age, are more likely to get sick from germs that animals can sometimes carry. Children can learn a lot from animals, and it is important to make sure they stay safe and healthy while they are learning. Schools that have animals in classrooms, whether it is a class pet or for a hands-on learning experience, should be aware of the risks and understand how to prevent illness. This knowledge helps kids enjoy and learn from animals while staying healthy.

Animals Can Sometimes Spread Germs

Animals can sometimes carry germs that can make people sick, even if they look clean and healthy. You do not have to touch an animal to get sick — the germs can spread to cages, bedding, and wherever animals roam.

There have been disease outbreaks from hatching eggs and chicks in the classroom and from contaminated animal products used for hands-on learning, such as owl pellets for dissection. *Salmonella* and *E. coli* are common germs spread by animals.

How to Prevent Germs from Spreading in the Classroom

- Do not bring reptiles, amphibians, poultry, rodents, or ferrets into schools, daycare centers, or other settings that include children under 5 years of age.
- Adults should always supervise children's contact with animals. Never allow children to put their hands or objects (including pacifiers) in their mouth while around animals.
- Create specific areas for interaction with animals. Do not allow animals to roam freely around the classroom, especially in areas where food or drink is prepared, served, or eaten.
- Do not dissect animals or other animal products where food for people is prepared, served, or eaten. Thoroughly clean and disinfect surfaces used for dissection.
- Consult with parents to determine special considerations for children who have allergies, asthma, or other illnesses.
- Students should wash their hands with water and soap right after handling animals, their food, or their habitats (for example, cages, terrariums, aquariums, water bowls, and toys).
  - When around animals, also wash hands after removing dirty clothes or shoes, before eating and drinking, and before preparing food or drinks.
  - Adults, including teachers, should always supervise handwashing for young children.
  - Use hand sanitizer if running water and soap are not available. If you only use hand sanitizer, be sure to wash your hands with soap and water as soon as possible.
- Clean and disinfect all areas where animals have been.
- Do not clean tanks, feeders, water containers, and other equipment in sinks or areas where food is prepared, served, or eaten.

Check That Animals Are Healthy before Bringing Them into School

- Animals can look clean and healthy and still spread germs. Make sure all animals have appropriate and regular veterinary care, and proof of rabies vaccination for dogs and cats, according to local or state requirements.

- If the animal comes from a different state or country, it may need a health certificate issued by a veterinarian to travel across state lines or to enter the United States.
- Check local regulations, as well as school policies, before bringing animals into schools.
- If the animal becomes sick or dies:
  - Contact your veterinarian.
  - Take extra precaution when handling a sick animal because a sick or stressed animal is more likely to be shedding harmful germs that can make people sick or to bite, which can cause injury or spread germs.
  - Inform the pet store or breeder from whom the animal was purchased about the animal's illness or death as soon as possible. Consider waiting before purchasing another pet from the same source.
  - Clean and disinfect the cage before reusing with another animal.
- If the animal bites someone:
  - Wash wounds with warm soapy water immediately.
  - Seek medical attention if:
    - The animal appears sick.
    - You do not know if the animal has been vaccinated against rabies.
    - The wound is serious.
    - The wound becomes red, painful, warm, or swollen.
    - It has been more than 5 years since your last tetanus shot.

Animals Not Suitable for School or Childcare Settings

- Reptiles, amphibians, poultry, rodents, and ferrets are not suitable for settings that include children under 5 years of age.
- Nonhuman primates, such as monkeys and apes
- Wild animals more likely to spread rabies, such as bats, raccoons, skunks, foxes, and coyotes
- Stray animals and aggressive or unpredictable animals
- Venomous or toxin-producing spiders, insects, and reptiles. Frogs, snakes, lizards, and other amphibians also may be venomous.

Section 3.2
Infants and Young Children

This section includes text excerpted from "Infants and Young Children," Centers for Disease Control and Prevention (CDC), January 28, 2020.

How to Keep Children Healthy around Animals

Infants and children younger than 5 years of age are more likely to get sick from germs that animals can carry. This is because young children often touch surfaces that may be contaminated with animal feces (poop), and they like to put their hands in their mouths. Objects such as pacifiers may fall on dirty surfaces and then be placed in an infant's mouth. Young children are less likely to wash their hands well.

Infants and young children are more likely to get a serious illness from germs that animals can carry because their immune systems are still developing. But, there is good news. You can take steps to keep your kids healthy while still enjoying animals.

Steps to Keep Infants and Young Children Healthy around Animals

- Always supervise children around animals.
- Never allow children to kiss animals or to put their hands or other objects into their mouths after handling animals.
- Always wash children's hands thoroughly with soap and water right after touching, feeding, or caring for animals or cleaning their habitats. Adults should supervise handwashing for young children.
- Wash your hands before breastfeeding or preparing formula.
- Keep children away from animals while they are eating to prevent the risk of bites or other injuries.

Because young children are more likely to get sick from harmful germs that animals can carry, the CDC recommends that infants and children under 5 years of age avoid contact with the following animals, which are commonly associated with outbreaks of disease:

- Reptiles (lizards, snakes, and turtles)
- Amphibians (frogs, toads, newts, and salamanders)
- Backyard poultry, including baby chicks or ducklings

Additionally, children younger than 5 years of age should be extra cautious when visiting farms and when they are around areas with farm animals, including animals at petting zoos and fairs.

Section 3.3
Pregnant Women

This section includes text excerpted from "Pregnant Women," Centers for Disease Control and Prevention (CDC), January 26, 2019.

When Should You Be Concerned about Toxoplasmosis?

Generally, if you were infected with *Toxoplasma gondii* before becoming pregnant, your unborn child is protected by your immunity. Some experts suggest waiting for 6 months after a recent infection to become pregnant.

How Do You Know If You Have Been Infected with *Toxoplasma Gondii?*

Your healthcare provider may suggest one or more varieties of blood tests to check for antibodies to *Toxoplasma*.

How Can *Toxoplasma Gondii* Affect Your Unborn Child?

If you are newly infected with *Toxoplasma* while you are pregnant, or just before pregnancy, then you can pass the infection on to your unborn baby. You may not have any symptoms from the infection. Most infected infants do not have symptoms at birth, but can develop serious symptoms, such as blindness or a mental disability, later in life. Occasionally, infected newborns have serious eye or brain damage at birth.

How Is Toxoplasmosis Spread?

Cats play an important role in the spread of toxoplasmosis. They become infected by eating infected rodents, birds, or other small animals. The parasite is then passed in the cat's feces. Kittens and cats can shed millions of parasites in their feces for as long as 3 weeks after infection. Mature cats are less likely to shed *Toxoplasma* if they have been previously infected. Cats and kittens prefer litter boxes, garden soils, and sandboxes for elimination, and you may be exposed unintentionally by touching your mouth after changing a litter box, or after gardening without gloves. Fruits and vegetables may have contact with contaminated soil or water also, and you can be infected by eating fruits and vegetables if they are not cooked, washed, or peeled.

Is There Treatment Available for Toxoplasmosis?

If you are infected during pregnancy, medication is available. You and your unborn baby should be closely monitored during your pregnancy and after your baby is born.

What Are the Best Ways to Protect Yourself or Your Unborn Child against Toxoplasmosis?

Cat owners and women who are exposed to cats should follow these tips to reduce exposure to *Toxoplasma*.

- Avoid changing cat litter if possible. If no one else can perform the task, wear disposable gloves and wash your hands with soap and water afterwards.
- Ensure that the cat litter box is changed daily. The *Toxoplasma gondii* parasite does not become infectious until 1 to 5 days after it is shed in a cat's feces.
- Feed your cat commercial dry or canned food, not raw or undercooked meats.
- Keep cats indoors.
- Avoid stray cats, especially kittens. Do not get a new cat while you are pregnant.
- Keep outdoor sandboxes covered.
- Wear gloves when gardening and during contact with soil or sand because it might be contaminated with cat feces that contains *Toxoplasma*. Wash hands with soap and water after gardening or contact with soil or sand.

You should also:
- Cook food to safe temperatures. A food thermometer should be used to measure the internal temperature of cooked meat. Color is not a reliable indicator that meat has been cooked to a temperature high enough to kill harmful pathogens such as *Toxoplasma*. Do not sample meat until it is cooked.

The U.S. Department of Agriculture (USDA) recommends the following for meat preparation:

For Whole Cuts of Meat (Excluding Poultry)

Cook to at least 145°F (63°C) as measured with a food thermometer placed in the thickest part of the meat, then allow the meat to rest for three minutes before carving or consuming. According to the USDA, "A 'rest time' is the amount of time the product remains at the final temperature, after it has been removed from a grill, oven, or other heat source. During the three minutes after meat is removed from the heat source, its temperature remains constant or continues to rise, which destroys pathogens."

For Ground Meat (Excluding Poultry)

Cook to at least 160°F (71°C); ground meats do not require a rest time.

For All Poultry (Whole Cuts and Ground)

Cook to at least 165°F (74°C). The internal temperature should be checked in the innermost part of the thigh, innermost part of the wing, and the thickest part of the breast. Poultry do not require a rest time.

Safe Food Handling

- Freeze meat for several days at subzero (below 0°F) temperatures before cooking to greatly reduce your chances of infection. Freezing does not reliably kill other parasites that may be found in meat (such as certain species of *Trichinella*) or harmful bacteria. Cooking meat to USDA-recommended internal temperatures is the safest method to destroy all parasites and other pathogens.
- Peel or wash fruits and vegetables thoroughly before eating.
- Wash cutting boards, dishes, counters, utensils, and hands with soapy water after contact with raw meat, poultry, seafood, or unwashed fruits or vegetables.
- Avoid drinking untreated water.
- Do not drink unpasteurized goat's milk.
- Do not eat raw or undercooked oysters, mussels, or clams (as these may be contaminated with *Toxoplasma gondii* that has washed into seawater).

Should a Woman Breastfeed Her Infant If She Has Contracted a *Toxoplasma Gondii* Infection during Her Pregnancy?

Yes. Among healthy women, the possibility of breast-milk transmission of *Toxoplasma* infection is not likely. While *Toxoplasma* infection has been associated with infants who consumed unpasteurized goat's milk, there are no studies documenting breast milk transmission of *Toxoplasma gondii* in humans. In the event that a nursing woman experiences cracked and bleeding nipples or breast inflammation within several weeks immediately following an acute *Toxoplasma* infection (when the organism is still circulating in her bloodstream), it is theoretically possible that she could transmit *Toxoplasma gondii* to the infant through her breast milk. Immune-suppressed women could have circulating *Toxoplasma* for even longer periods of time. However, the likelihood of human milk transmission is very small.

Section 3.4
Organ-Transplant Patients

This section includes text excerpted from "Organ Transplant Patients," Centers for Disease Control and Prevention (CDC), April 30, 2014.
Reviewed March 2020.

Pet Safety Tips

Patients who have received organ transplants are more likely than most people to get diseases from animals. However, simple tips can be followed to reduce their risk of getting sick after contact with animals. These recommendations were originally made for bone-marrow transplant patients, but they also may be useful for other organ-transplant patients. Although this section focuses on how to protect organ-transplant patients from pet-related diseases, many groups support the health benefits of pets.

Keep Your Hands Clean

Wash your hands thoroughly with running water and soap after handling animals and their feces (stool). If possible, you should avoid direct contact with animal feces. Adults should supervise the handwashing of children.

Caring for Your Pet

If your pet is ill, seek veterinary care as soon as possible. Any cat or dog that has diarrhea should be checked by a veterinarian for infection with *Cryptosporidium*, *Giardia*, *Salmonella*, and *Campylobacter*.

Caring for Birds

Birdcage linings should be cleaned daily. Wear gloves whenever handling items contaminated with bird droppings. Routine screening of healthy birds for zoonotic diseases is not recommended.

Caring for Fish

Avoid cleaning fish tanks by yourself; ask a family member or friend for assistance. If this task cannot be avoided, you should wear disposable gloves during such activities. Wash your hands thoroughly with running water and soap afterwards.

Caring for Cats

If you have a cat, try to have another person clean out your litter box on a regular (daily) basis. Do not place litter boxes in kitchens, dining rooms, or other areas where food is prepared and eaten. Keep your cat indoors. Avoid handling stray cats. Pet cats do not need to be tested for toxoplasmosis.

Feeding Your Pet

Just like people, pets can get diseases from eating contaminated food. By protecting your pet from foodborne diseases, you can protect your own health as well. Pets should be fed only high-quality commercial pet foods. If eggs, poultry, or meat products are given to your pet as supplements, they should be well-cooked. Any dairy products given to your pets should be pasteurized. Additionally, pets should be prevented from drinking toilet-bowl water and from having access to garbage. Do not let your pet scavenge for food, hunt, or eat other animals' feces.

Getting a Pet

When getting a pet, avoid animals that are ill, stray, or young (cats and dogs less than 6 months old). These animals are more likely to carry diseases that can make you ill.

Animals to Avoid

The following animals are considered high-risk animals for immunocompromised people (including organ-transplant patients):

- Reptiles, including lizards, snakes, and turtles
- Baby chicks and ducklings
- Exotic pets, including monkeys

Note: All persons should avoid direct contact with wild animals. Do not adopt wild animals as pets or bring them into your home.

Contact with these animals and their environments should be avoided by people with compromised immune systems. If you do touch these animals or their environment (their food or cage, for example), wash your hands thoroughly with running water and soap. Additionally, organ transplant patients should be extra cautious when visiting farms and when in contact with farm animals, including animals at petting zoos and fairs.

Section 3.5

People Visiting Animal Exhibits

This section includes text excerpted from "Stay Healthy at Animal Exhibits," Centers for Disease Control and Prevention (CDC), June 11, 2019.

Interacting with animals at fairs, educational farms, petting zoos, summer camps, aquariums, schools, and other places can be educational and fun, and helps people learn about and experience animals they may not see in their daily lives. However, it is important to know that animals sometimes carry germs that can make people sick.

Every year, many people get sick after visiting an animal exhibit. From 2010 to 2015, about 100 outbreaks of illness in people linked to animals in public settings such as zoos, fairs, and educational farms were reported to public-health officials. Some of the most common harmful germs people get from animals at exhibits are *E. coli* O157:H7, *Cryptosporidium*, and *Salmonella* infections, but there are also many other types of germs that can spread between animals and people.

Children 5 years of age and younger, people with weakened immune systems, and adults over 65 years of age are more likely to get sick from the germs animals can carry, and should take extra precautions at animal exhibits. If you forget to wash your hands after petting an animal or bring food or drinks into an area with animals, you increase your chance of getting sick. Even animals that look clean and healthy can carry harmful germs, and areas, where animals live or roam, can be contaminated—you do not have to touch an animal to get sick.

How to Stay Healthy If You Visit an Animal Exhibit or Have Contact with Animals in a Public Setting

Animal encounters such as touching or petting, feeding, and holding animals are becoming more popular, especially at zoos and aquariums. An animal exhibit can be anything from a large zoo to a livestock show at the county fair. You might also encounter animals at schools, as part of local festivals, or just out and about. Wherever you are, it is important to know ways to stay healthy while enjoying animals.

Protect Yourself and Your Family
Wash Your Hands

- Find where the handwashing stations are located.
- Wash your hands right after touching animals or anything in the areas where they live, roam, or eat.
- Wash your hands when you leave animal areas, even if you did not touch the animals; hands should still be washed if you wore gloves.
- Running water and soap are best, but if they are not available, use an alcohol-based hand sanitizer that contains at least 60 percent alcohol and wash your hands with soap and running water as soon as you can.

Keep Food and Animals Separate

- Do not eat or drink around animals, and keep food and drinks away from animal areas.
- Do not share your food with the animals, even if you think the food is part of the animal's regular diet. Animals should eat the food provided for them by the animal exhibitors.
- Do not eat or drink raw (unpasteurized) products. Raw products made or sold at animal exhibits may include milk, cheese, cider, or juice.

Keep Children Safe around Animals

- Always supervise children around animals.
- Children 5 years of age and younger should not have contact with reptiles, amphibians, or live poultry because these animals are more likely to make them sick.
- Leave items such as strollers, pacifiers, cups, or toys outside the exhibit.
- Do not let children put their thumbs, fingers, or objects (such as pacifiers) in their mouths when they are around animals or in an animal area.

- Do not let children sit or play on the ground in animal areas.
- Teach children to approach animals with caution and to follow the rules. Do not let children put their fingers or objects near an animal's mouth, even if the animal seems friendly. Make sure to follow any rules provided on signs or verbally by the staff. For example, some contact exhibits have a "two-finger touch" rule.

If You Work at, Manage, or Design Animal Exhibits

The Compendium of Measures to Prevent Diseases Associated with Animals in Public Settings provides standardized recommendations for public-health officials, veterinarians, animal-venue operators, animal exhibitors, and others concerned with disease control and with minimizing risks associated with animals in public settings. The National Association of State Public Health Veterinarians (NASPHV) also provides a toolkit with examples of regulations on animal exhibitions, printable posters with messages on how to stay safe while enjoying animals, and a checklist of petting-zoo best practices.

Even healthy animals can carry germs that might make visitors sick. When designing an exhibit, you want to protect your animals and your visitors, while preserving the fun and education.

Design exhibits in ways that will help to prevent the spread of disease:

- Provide stations for handwashing at the exits of animal exhibits, including some that are low enough for children to reach.
- Educate staff and visitors on how to prevent illness after being around animals.
- Provide signs for guests on when and how to wash their hands, where people can eat, and areas for the animals. Use plain language and pictures.
- Keep dining and animal areas separate.
- Train staff and educate visitors on diseases animals may carry and how to prevent them.
- Educate your staff on the risks of working around animals. Encourage them to talk to visitors about safety around animals, such as handwashing.

- Provide your staff with resources on safety at animal exhibits, especially if your staff includes veterinarians or healthcare providers.

State public-health veterinarians are the local and state professionals who regularly work with physicians, emergency rooms, health departments, veterinarians, fair boards, local officials, schools, legislators, and communities on preventing and controlling diseases that people can get from animals and animal products. The CDC works closely with NASPHV to create guidance and recommendations for visitors to animal exhibits as well as people who manage or design exhibits.

Section 3.6
Veterinarians and Animal-Care Workers

This section includes text excerpted from "Veterinary Safety and Health—Veterinary Workers and Workplaces," Centers for Disease Control and Prevention (CDC), April 30, 2018.

Veterinary Safety and Health
Veterinary Workers and Workplaces

Veterinary medicine and animal care workers include:

- Veterinarians, veterinary technologists and technicians, veterinary assistants, and laboratory animal caretakers
- Zoo and aquarium workers, including animal caretakers and grounds keepers
- Animal shelter and animal control workers
- Stable and kennel workers
- Groomers
- Animal trainers

Other information about these workers:

- Many veterinary medical workers are female, including 62 percent of veterinarians, 95 percent of veterinary technicians, and 84 percent of veterinary assistants and laboratory animal workers (BLS 2017, NAVTA 2016).
- Small businesses often employ veterinarians, with up to 80 percent of veterinarians working in solo or group practices (AVMA 2017).
- Veterinary services ranks 2nd in incidence rates for nonfatal occupational injuries and illnesses (BLS 2016).

These workers are employed in many industries:

- Veterinary services
- Zoos and aquariums
- Nature parks
- Pet care (except veterinary) services
- Pet and pet supply stores

Veterinary work settings vary:

- Veterinary offices, clinics, and hospitals
- Animal shelters, rescue leagues, and humane societies
- Kennels, stables, and racetracks
- Grooming shops and pet stores
- Farms and ranches
- Animal facilities such as poultry houses, swine barns, feed lots, and sale barns
- Zoos, aquariums, and other captive and free-ranging wildlife settings
- Academic, private, and public clinical and research laboratories
- Slaughterhouses and meat-packing plants
- Disaster and emergency response shelters and facilities

Work can involve many animal species:

- Pets such as domestic dogs, cats, pocket pets, exotic animals, or fish
- Farm, ranch, or production agriculture animals such as cattle, swine, sheep, goats, poultry, ratites, horses, or farmed fish
- Laboratory animals from mice to nonhuman primates

- Captive and free-ranging wildlife such as amphibians, reptiles, birds, mammals, or aquatic species

Work tasks are diverse and variable:
- Facility management and maintenance
- Routine care and treatment of animals
- Emergency medical care of animals
- Medical, surgical, and necropsy procedures
- Laboratory testing or research
- Livestock and food inspection
- Disaster and emergency rescue and response

CHAPTER 4
Animals and the Germs They Spread

Chapter Contents

Backyard Poultry

This section includes text excerpted from "Backyard Poultry," Centers for Disease Control and Prevention (CDC), December 13, 2018.

Poultry includes any domesticated birds kept for producing eggs or meat, such as chickens, turkeys, ducks, and guinea fowl.

Diseases shared between people and poultry include:

Bird Flu, Avian Influenza

Avian influenza is a virus whose natural hosts include many species of waterfowl. Waterfowl, such as ducks, geese, and swans, do not always show signs of avian influenza infection, but poultry flocks can experience a range of illnesses, from decreased egg production to extremely high death rates. Strains of avian influenza that kill poultry will not necessarily make people sick, and strains of avian influenza that sicken people will not necessarily sicken or kill poultry.

No severe human illnesses caused by avian influenza have been reported in the United States. However, avian influenza has infected people in Africa, Asia, and Europe. In infected people, symptoms can range from fever, muscle aches, and conjunctivitis to severe respiratory distress, pneumonia, organ failure, and death.

Campylobacteriosis (*Campylobacter* spp.)

Campylobacter is a type of bacteria that spreads to people through contaminated food (meat and eggs) or water or from touching the stool of infected animals. It is difficult to predict the risk of *Campylobacter* from animals, because many animals, such as backyard poultry, can carry the bacteria without showing any signs of illness.

Most people who become ill with campylobacteriosis will have diarrhea, cramping, abdominal pain, and fever within two to five days after exposure to *Campylobacter*. *Campylobacter* can cause serious life-threatening infections such as Guillain-Barré syndrome (GBS) in infants, elderly people, and those with weakened immune systems.

Escherichia coli (*E. coli*)

Escherichia coli (*E. coli*) are bacteria found in the environment, foods, and intestines of people and animals, including poultry. *E. coli* are a large and diverse group of bacteria. Although most strains of *E. coli* are harmless, others can make people sick. Some kinds of *E. coli* can cause diarrhea, while others cause urinary-tract infections, respiratory illness and pneumonia, and other illnesses. The types of *E. coli* that can cause illness in people can be spread through contaminated water or food, or through contact with infected animals or their feces.

Salmonellosis (*Salmonella* spp.)

Salmonella spreads to people through contaminated food (eggs and meat) or contact with the stool of certain animals, including backyard poultry. Live poultry might acquire *Salmonella* from a contaminated environment or feed, or from carrier rodents, insects, wildlife, etc. Poultry may have *Salmonella* in their droppings and on their bodies (feathers, feet, beaks), even when they appear healthy and clean. While it usually does not make the birds sick, *Salmonella* can cause serious illness when it is passed to people.

People exposed to *Salmonella* might have diarrhea, vomiting, fever, and abdominal cramps. Infants, the elderly, and those with weakened immune systems are more likely than others to develop severe illness.

West Nile Virus

West Nile virus (WNV) is carried by birds and spread by mosquitoes. People, birds, and horses get WNV infection by being bitten by a carrier mosquito. Although many birds, such as poultry, show no signs of infection, the virus can kill some birds, such as crows.

People infected with WNV can have a wide variety of symptoms, ranging from flu-like illness to seizures or more serious disease. WNV infection can be fatal in people.

Section 4.2
Farm Animals

This section includes text excerpted from "Farm Animals," Centers for Disease Control and Prevention (CDC), October 15, 2019.

Anthrax (*Bacillus Anthracis*)

Anthrax can be found naturally in soil and commonly affects domestic and wild animals around the world. Although it is rare in the United States, people can get sick with anthrax if they come in contact with infected animals, including farm animals. People who live in areas where anthrax has been present should consider vaccinating their livestock against the disease every year.

How It Spreads

Farm animals can become infected with anthrax when they ingest spores in contaminated soil, plants, or water. People get infected by having contact with sick or dead animals or eating meat contaminated with spores. People can also get anthrax through a cut or scrape in the skin. Anthrax is not contagious, which means it is not spread from person to person.

Brucellosis (*Brucella* spp.)

Brucellosis is a bacterial disease caused by contact with infected animals and contaminated animal products like raw (unpasteurized) dairy products, such as milk or cheese.

How It Spreads

The most common way people get brucellosis is by eating or drinking raw dairy products. People can also get brucellosis by coming in contact with infected animals or contaminated animal tissues or fluids (such as blood) and/or getting the bacteria in skin wounds or mucus membranes.

Campylobacteriosis (*Campylobacter* spp.)

Campylobacter are bacteria that can make people and animals sick with a disease called "campylobacteriosis."

How It Spreads

Campylobacter bacteria are most often spread to animals and people through the feces (poop) of infected animals, contaminated food, or the environment. Many types of farm animals, including those found at zoos, petting zoos, and fairs, can carry *Campylobacter* and other germs that make people sick. People can get infected if they do not wash their hands after touching an animal or its poop, food, toys, habitats (including barns, pens, and cages) or equipment used around these animals (such as halters, chutes, and trailers).

Orf Virus (Sore Mouth Infection)

Orf virus causes infections in sheep and goats and can also spread to people. In animals, orf virus infection may be called "sore mouth," "scabby mouth," or "contagious echyma." Goats are typically more severely affected than sheep.

How It Spreads

Animals spread orf virus to each other through cuts or abrasions in the skin, typically during suckling. People get infected after touching an animal's sores or any piece of equipment, such as a harness, that has touched an infected animal's sores. Activities such as bottle or tube feeding, shearing animals, or petting animals can cause infection. Animal bites can also cause infection.

Cryptosporidiosis (*Cryptosporidium* spp.)

Cryptosporidiosis is a parasitic disease caused by the germ *Cryptosporidium* (or "Crypto" for short), which is spread by swallowing poop from an infected person or animal. The risk is greatest from contact with young calves, especially calves with diarrhea.

How It Spreads

Crypto spreads through swallowing poop containing the germ after contact with an infected person or animal, or through contaminated food or water.

Escherichia coli (*E. coli*)

E. coli are bacteria found in the environment, foods, and intestines of people and animals. Although most kinds of *E. coli* are harmless, others can make people—and newborn farm animals—sick.

How It Spreads

E. coli most often spreads to animals and people through the poop of infected animals, contaminated food, or the environment. Many types of healthy farm animals, including those found at zoos, petting zoos, and fairs, can carry *E. coli* and other germs that make people sick. People can get infected if they do not wash their hands after touching an animal or its poop, food, toys, habitats (including barns, pens, and cages) or equipment used around these animals (such as halters, chutes, and trailers).

Influenza

Influenza, or "flu," is a contagious respiratory illness caused by influenza viruses. Some influenza viruses that primarily circulate in animals have on rare occasion infected people. For example, some avian influenza (bird flu) viruses as well some swine influenza viruses can cause infections in people. When influenza viruses that normally circulate in animals cause an infection in people, this is called a "novel virus infection." Not all influenza viruses found in birds or pigs are known to cause human infections.

How It Spreads

Flu viruses are highly contagious. Most experts think that flu viruses spread mainly by droplets made when people with the flu cough, sneeze, or talk. These droplets can land in the mouths or noses of people who are nearby or possibly be inhaled into the lungs. People can also spread flu to each other. Avian and swine flu can spread to people through contact with the virus from saliva, nasal secretions, or poop from infected animals. A person can also get flu through contact with virus-contaminated surfaces, poultry coops, pig pens, and supplies. Less often, flu can also spread to people through touching infected animals and then touching your eyes, nose, or mouth.

Leptospirosis (*Leptospira* spp.)

Leptospirosis is a bacterial disease that can affect people and animals. Many kinds of animals can carry the bacteria in their urine, including farm animals. Cows, pigs, and horses can be vaccinated to protect against certain strains of leptospirosis.

How It Spreads

The bacteria that cause leptospirosis spread through the urine of infected animals, which can get into water or soil and survive there for weeks to months. People get infected through contact with urine or other body fluids (except saliva) from infected animals, or through contact with water, soil, or other materials (such as animal bedding) contaminated with urine from infected animals.

Listeriosis (*Listeria monocytogenes*)

Listeria monocytogenes are bacteria that cause people and animals to get sick with a disease called "listeriosis."

How It Spreads

Listeria most often spreads to people and animals through contaminated food, soil, or water. Some people have become infected after contact with an infected animal or its tissues, but most are infected by eating contaminated food.

MRSA (Methicillin-Resistant *Staphylococcus aureus*)

Staphylococcus aureus is a common type of bacteria normally found on the skin of people and animals. MRSA is *Staphylococcus aureus* bacteria that have become resistant to some antibiotics. MRSA can cause a variety of infections, including skin infections, pneumonia (lung infection), and other problems.

How It Spreads

MRSA can sometimes spread between people and animals through direct contact (touching). Even animals that are not sick can carry MRSA and spread it to people.

Q Fever (*Coxiella burnetii*)

Q fever is a disease caused by *Coxiella burnetii* bacteria. The bacteria naturally infect some animals, including goats, sheep, and cattle.

How It Spreads

People can get Q fever by breathing in dust that has been contaminated by infected animal feces, urine, milk, or birth products (such as the placenta and amniotic fluid) that contain *C. burnetii* bacteria. A person does not need to have direct contact with an animal to get infected. Wind can carry barnyard dust mixed with Q fever bacteria for miles. People can also get Q fever by eating or drinking contaminated unpasteurized (raw) dairy products.

Rabies

Rabies is a deadly neurologic disease caused by a virus that spreads primarily through the bites of infected animals. Though rabies in farm animals is rare, it is still a concern. Along with dogs and cats, cattle, horses, and sheep can get vaccinated against rabies.

How It Spreads

Rabies is spread through contact with saliva or brain/nervous-system tissue from an infected animal, usually through scratches or bites.

Ringworm

Ringworm is an infection caused by fungus that can infect the skin, hair, or nails of people and animals.

How It Spreads

Ringworm spreads through direct contact with an infected animal or person (touching), or from the environment. Ringworm affects pets such as dogs, cats, and rabbits, as well as farm animals, such as cows, sheep, goats, and pigs.

Salmonellosis (*Salmonella* spp.)

Salmonella are bacteria that can make people and animals sick with an illness called "salmonellosis."

How It Spreads

Salmonella most often spreads to animals and people through the poop of infected animals, contaminated food, or the environment. Many types of farm animals, including those found at zoos, petting zoos, and fairs (poultry, cows, pigs, sheep and goats, and horses), can carry *Salmonella* and other germs that make people sick. People can get infected if they do not wash their hands after touching an animal or its poop, food, toys, habitats (including barns, pens, and cages) or equipment used around these animals.

Section 4.3
Birds as Pets

This section includes text excerpted from "Birds Kept as Pets," Centers for Disease Control and Prevention (CDC), October 28, 2019.

Cryptococcosis (*Cryptococcus neoformans*)

Cryptococcosis is an infection caused by fungus found in the environment, particularly in soil, on decaying wood, in tree hollows, or in bird droppings.

How It Spreads

People can get cryptococcosis by breathing in the microscopic fungus from the environment.

Psittacosis (*Chlamydiophila psittaci*)

Psittacosis is a disease caused by bacteria (*Chlamydia psittaci*) spread through the droppings and respiratory secretions of infected birds. People most commonly get psittacosis after exposure to pet birds, such as parrots and cockatiels, and poultry, such as turkeys or ducks. When birds are infected, veterinarians call the disease "avian chlamydiosis."

How It Spreads

People most commonly get psittacosis by breathing in dust from droppings or respiratory secretions of infected birds. Less commonly, birds infect people through bites and beak-to-mouth contact.

Section 4.4

Cats as Pets

This section includes text excerpted from "Cats,"
Centers for Disease Control and
Prevention (CDC), April 1, 2019.

Campylobacteriosis (*Campylobacter* spp.)

Campylobacter are bacteria that can make people and animals sick with a disease called "campylobacteriosis."

How It Spreads

People get *Campylobacter* infection by coming into contact with feces (poop) of infected animals, including cats, or by consuming contaminated food or water. Typically, *Campylobacter* is spread when people do not wash their hands after touching animals or their food, poop, toys, or beds, but it can also sometimes infect you through an open wound. Cats commonly become infected by eating contaminated raw meat and shed the bacteria in their poop.

Cat Scratch Disease (*Bartonella henselae*)

Cat scratch disease (CSD) is an infection caused by the bacteria *Bartonella henselae*, and less commonly other *Bartonella* species.

How It Spreads

Cats become infected through flea bites, fights with other infected cats, or blood transfusions. People can be exposed to the bacteria through the scratch or lick of an infected cat.

Cat Tapeworm (*Dipylidium caninum*)

The cat tapeworm is a parasite spread to dogs, cats, and people through the ingestion of infected fleas. This parasite is common in cats, but rarely causes illness in other pets or people.

How It Spreads

The tapeworm is spread when a cat or person swallows an infected flea. Cats may swallow fleas when self-grooming. Treating pets for fleas can help prevent infection.

Cryptosporidiosis (*Cryptosporidium* spp.)

Cryptosporidiosis is a parasitic disease caused by the germ *Cryptosporidium* (or "Crypto" for short), which is spread by accidentally swallowing poop from an infected person or animal.

How It Spreads

Crypto spreads through swallowing poop containing the germ after contact with an infected person or animal, or through poop in contaminated food or water. For example, people can get Crypto after swallowing recreational water, drinking untreated water from a lake or river, or touching their mouth after handling an infected animal.

Giardiasis (*Giardia duodenalis*)

Giardiasis is a parasite that can be found on surfaces or in water, food, or soil that has been contaminated by poop from an infected person or animal.

How It Spreads

Giardia spreads through swallowing microscopic poop containing the parasite following contact with an infected person or animal, or by drinking water or eating food that has been contaminated with poop from infected people or animals.

Hookworm (*Ancylostoma tubaeforme, Ancylostoma braziliense, Uncinaria stenocephala*)

Hookworms are tiny worms that can spread through contact with contaminated soil or sand.

How It Spreads

People can get hookworm infection by walking barefoot, kneeling, or sitting on ground that is contaminated with poop from infected animals. Cats can become infected by ingesting the parasite from the environment or through their mother's milk or colostrum.

Rabies

Rabies is a deadly neurologic disease caused by a virus that spreads primarily through bites of infected animals. Cat owners should get cats vaccinated against rabies.

How It Spreads

Rabies spreads through contact with saliva or brain/nervous-system tissue from an infected animal, usually through scratches or bites.

Ringworm

Ringworm is an infection caused by fungus that can infect the skin, hair, or nails of people and animals.

How It Spreads

Ringworm spreads through direct contact with an infected animal or person (touching), or from the environment.

Roundworms (*Toxocara* spp.)

Roundworm is a parasite that can cause an infection called "toxocariasis." Roundworms are commonly found in the intestines of cats.

How It Spreads

Cats shed roundworm eggs in their poop. People and cats can get roundworms by swallowing roundworm eggs from the environment, such as dirt contaminated with cat poop.

Salmonellosis (*Salmonella* spp.)

Salmonellosis is caused by *Salmonella* bacteria, which are most commonly spread through contaminated food. *Salmonella* also spreads from animals, including cats, to people and from people to people.

How It Spreads

People can become infected by eating contaminated food or through contact with animal poop. Cats can become infected with *Salmonella* by eating infected birds, rodents, or contaminated pet food, especially raw pet food.

Sporotrichosis (*Sporothrix* spp.)

Sporotrichosis is an infection caused by fungus found in the environment.

How It Spreads

The fungus typically spreads from the environment through a cut or scrape in the skin, but has also been associated with scratches or bites from animals, particularly cats.

Tick-Borne Diseases

Pets are at risk for tick-borne infections, including Lyme disease, tularemia, ehrlichiosis, babesiosis, and others. Pet owners should consult with a veterinarian on appropriate products for their pets to prevent ticks. Treating pets for ticks can reduce the risk of tick-borne diseases for you and your pets.

How It Spreads

Tick-borne germs spread through the bite of an infected tick. During the feeding process, small amounts of saliva pass from the tick into the skin of the animal or person.

Toxoplasmosis (*Toxoplasma gondii*)

Toxoplasmosis is a disease caused by a parasite found in soil, water, meat, or poop from an infected animal, particularly cats.

How It Spreads

People can get toxoplasmosis through contact with cat poop or by eating undercooked meat or shellfish. Cats become infected by eating infected rodents, birds, or other small animals. The parasite then sheds in the cat's feces, contaminating the environment or the cat's litter box. People can get infected by consuming contaminated food or water. People can also become infected if they do not wash their hands after cleaning a cat's litter box or handling anything contaminated by cat poop.

Section 4.5

Dogs as Pets

This section includes text excerpted from "Dogs,"
Centers for Disease Control and
Prevention (CDC), February 21, 2020.

Campylobacteriosis (*Campylobacter* spp.)

Campylobacter spreads through contaminated food (meat and eggs), water, or through contact with the stool of infected animals. Dogs infected with *Campylobacter* might show no signs of illness at all or might have diarrhea and a slight fever.

Most people who become sick with campylobacteriosis will have diarrhea, cramping, abdominal pain, and fever within two to five days after exposure to the organism. *Campylobacter* can cause serious life-threatening infections in infants, older persons, and those with weakened immune systems.

Tapeworm (*Dipylidium caninum*)

The flea tapeworm is a parasite spread to dogs, cats, and people through the ingestion of infected fleas. This parasite is common in dogs, but rarely causes illness in other pets or people.

Hookworm (*Ancylostoma caninum, Ancylostoma braziliense, Uncinaria stenocephala*)

Dog hookworms are tiny worms that can spread through contact with contaminated soil or sand. Dogs can also become infected with hookworms through accidentally ingesting the parasite from the environment or through their mother's milk or colostrum. Young puppies are most often affected and might have dark, bloody stool and anemia. Severe infections in some puppies can lead to death.

People become infected with dog hookworms while walking barefoot, kneeling, or sitting on the ground contaminated with the stool of infected animals. Hookworm larvae enter the top layers of skin and cause an itchy reaction called "cutaneous larva migrans." A red squiggly line might appear where the larvae have migrated under the skin. Symptoms usually resolve without medical treatment in four to six weeks.

Rabies

Rabies, a fatal neurologic disease in animals and people, is caused by a virus. Animals and people are most commonly infected through bites from rabid animals. Infected dogs might have a variety of signs, but most often have a sudden behavioral change and progressive paralysis. Rabies is prevented by vaccination.

The first symptoms in people can start days to months after exposure and include generalized weakness, fever, and headache. Within a few days symptoms will progress to confusion, anxiety, behavioral changes, and delirium. If you have been bitten by a dog or other animal and feel that there is a risk for rabies, contact your healthcare provider right away. Once symptoms appear, it is almost always too late for treatment.

Roundworm (*Toxocara* spp.)

Toxocara roundworms cause a parasitic disease known as "toxocariasis." Dogs and people can become infected by accidentally swallowing roundworm eggs from the environment. In addition, larval worms can cross through the placenta, milk, or colostrum of a mother dog, passing the infection to her puppies. Infected puppies usually do not develop and grow well and might have a potbellied appearance.

In people, children are most often affected with roundworm. There are two forms of the disease in people. Ocular larva migrans happens when the larvae invade the retina and cause inflammation, scarring, and possibly blindness. Visceral larva migrans occurs when the larvae invade parts of the body, such as the liver, lung, or central nervous system.

Brucellosis (*Brucella* spp.)

Brucellosis is a bacterial disease that affects the ability of animals to reproduce. The disease can be transmitted to humans through contact with recently aborted tissue from infected animals or consumption of unpasteurized (raw) milk. Dogs that are infected might have decreased appetite, weight loss, behavioral changes, and lack of energy, but most dogs infected with brucellosis show no signs of illness. Brucellosis affects the reproductive organs and can cause early-term deaths of developing puppies.

People who are infected with brucellosis will usually become sick within six to eight weeks of exposure. Sick people will have flu-like symptoms that last two to four weeks. Sometimes brucellosis can become a chronic illness that can be difficult to treat.

Capnocytophaga spp.

Many species of *Capnocytophaga* bacteria live in the mouths of dogs and cats. These bacteria do not make dogs or cats sick.

Rarely, *Capnocytophaga* can spread to people through bites, scratches, or close contact from a dog or cat and cause illness. Most people who have contact with a dog or cat do not become sick. People with weakened immune systems who have difficulty fighting off infections (for example, people with cancer or those taking certain medications such as steroids) are at greater risk of becoming ill.

Cryptosporidiosis (*Cryptosporidium* spp.)

Cryptosporidiosis is a parasitic disease that is transmitted through contaminated food or water from an infected person or animal.

Cryptosporidium illness in dogs is rarely seen, but they can carry the germ without showing any signs of illness.

The Cryptosporidium parasite can cause profuse, watery diarrhea with cramping, abdominal pain, and nausea in both animals and people. Illness in people is usually self-limiting and lasts only two to four days, but can become severe in people with weakened immune systems.

Echinococcosis (*Echinococcus* spp.)

Echinococcosis is a parasitic disease caused by consuming food or water contaminated with a specific type of tapeworm eggs or through contact with an infected animal. Dogs become infected by eating the tissue of an infected animal. Dogs rarely show any signs of disease, but if they are infected with a large number of worms, dogs can have diarrhea and enteritis.

Although *Echinococcus* invades many different organs of the body, most people who are infected with the disease will not have any signs of illness for years. Symptoms start when the slow-growing cysts become large enough to press on the organs they have invaded. The tapeworms grow slowly in several different organs of the body, most commonly the liver and lungs.

Ehrlichiosis (*Ehrlichia* spp.)

Ehrlichiosis is a bacterial disease that affects animals and people and is transmitted by ticks. Dogs show variable signs that include depression, loss of stamina, stiffness and reluctance to walk, and coughing.

People show similar signs and symptoms, which include fever, headache, chills, muscle pain, nausea, vomiting, diarrhea, and rash.

Giardiasis (*Giardia* spp.)

Giardia is a parasite that causes diarrhea in animals and people. *Giardia* is transmitted to animals and people through food or water contaminated with stool.

Symptoms in animals and people include diarrhea, greasy stools, and dehydration. People can also have abdominal cramps, nausea, and vomiting. Symptoms can last one to two weeks.

Leishmaniasis (*Leishmania* spp.)

Leishmaniasis is a protozoan disease of people and animals. It is transmitted by sandflies and is uncommon in North America. The two forms of the disease are visceral and cutaneous. The cutaneous form of leishmaniasis is most common in people and appears as one or more painless ulcers on the skin. Visceral leishmaniasis is less common and is characterized by fever, weight loss, an enlarged spleen, and anemia. Dogs can develop both forms at the same time and have a variety of symptoms.

Leptospirosis (*Leptospira* spp.)

Leptospirosis is a bacterial disease of people and animals that is transmitted through contaminated water and urine or other body fluids from an infected animal. It is difficult to detect early stages of leptospirosis in animals, but the disease can lead to kidney and liver failure if left untreated.

People who become infected with leptospirosis might not have any signs of the disease. Others will have nonspecific flu-like signs within two to seven days after exposure. These symptoms usually resolve without medical treatment, but can reappear and lead to more severe disease.

Lyme Disease (*Borrelia burgdorferi*)

Lyme disease is a bacterial disease of people and animals that is transmitted by ticks. In dogs, the most common signs of illness from Lyme disease are lameness, fever, reluctance to eat, lack of energy, and enlarged lymph nodes, with or without swollen, painful joints.

Infected people will typically have a red "bull's eye" rash at the site of the tick bite that appears about seven days after being bitten. Flu-like symptoms quickly follow the rash. If not treated, this disease can spread to other parts of the body and cause symptoms such as arthritis and loss of facial muscle tone (Bell's palsy). Lyme disease can be fatal.

MRSA (Methicillin-Resistant *Staphylococcus aureus*)

Staphylococcus aureus is a common type of bacteria that is normally found on the skin of people and animals. Methicillin-resistant *Staphylococcus aureus* (MRSA) is the same bacterium that has become resistant to some antibiotics. Dogs and other animals often can carry MRSA without being sick, but MRSA can cause a variety of infections, including of the skin, respiratory tract, and urinary tract.

MRSA can be transmitted back and forth between people and animals through direct contact. In people, MRSA most often causes skin infections that can range from mild to severe. If left untreated, MRSA can spread to the bloodstream or lungs and cause life-threatening infections.

Pasteurellosis (*Pasteurella* spp.)

Pasteurellosis is a bacterial disease associated with animal bites and scratches. *Pasteurella* is a normal bacterium that lives in the mouths of healthy dogs. The bacteria do not typically make dogs sick; however, dogs can develop abscesses or skin infections in places where they were scratched or bitten by another animal.

Pasteurella is found in 50 percent of patients with infected dog-bite wounds. *Pasteurella* can cause painful wound and skin infections. In more severe cases, it can cause widespread infection and might even affect the nervous system.

Plague (*Yersinia pestis*)

Plague is a bacterial disease in animals and people that can lead to serious illness if left untreated. Dogs are unlikely to develop clinical disease if infected.

People most often become infected through flea bites or from contact with the body fluids of infected animals. An example is a hunter skinning an infected rabbit or other animal. Bubonic plague is the most common form; symptoms include sudden onset of high fever, chills, headache, malaise, and swollen lymph nodes. The other two forms of plague, septicemic and pneumonic, cause more severe disease.

Ringworm (*Microsporum canis*)

Ringworm is a condition caused by a fungus that can infect the skin, hair, and nails of both people and animals. Ringworm is transmitted from animals to people through direct contact with an infected animal's skin or hair. Puppies are most commonly affected and can have circular areas of hair loss anywhere on the body.

Ringworm infections in people can appear on almost any area of the body. These infections are usually itchy. Redness, scaling, cracking of the skin, or a ring-shaped rash may occur. If the infection involves the scalp or beard, hair may fall out. Infected nails become discolored or thick and may possibly crumble.

Salmonellosis (*Salmonella* spp.)

Salmonella spreads to people through contaminated food (eggs and meat) or from contact with the stool of certain animals, including dogs. *Salmonella* infections have been linked to some brands of dry dog food, treats, and chew toys such as pig ears and to "raw food" diets for dogs. While it usually does not make the dogs sick, *Salmonella* can cause serious illness when it is passed to people.

People exposed to *Salmonella* might have diarrhea, vomiting, fever, or abdominal cramps. Infants, elderly persons, and those with weakened immune systems are more likely than others to develop severe illness.

Sarcoptic Mange (*Sarcoptes scabeii*)

Sarcoptic mange, also known as "mange," is a parasitic skin disease that is caused by a tiny mite. Mange is transmitted between animals through close contact. In dogs, the mite causes severe itching and self-inflicted wounds from scratching.

People cannot become infested with the canine version of sarcoptic mange, but they can have a minor local reaction from the mites if they come into contact with an infested dog.

Section 4.6

Ferrets as Pets

This section includes text excerpted from "Ferrets,"
Centers for Disease Control and
Prevention (CDC), April 8, 2019.

Campylobacteriosis (*Campylobacter* spp.)

Campylobacter are bacteria that can make people and animals sick with a disease called "campylobacteriosis."

How It Spreads

Campylobacter most often spreads to animals and people through the feces (poop) of infected animals, contaminated food or water, or the environment. People can become infected if they do not wash their hands after touching a ferret or its poop, food, toys, or habitat.

Cheyletiellosis (*Cheyletiella* spp.)

Cheyletiellosis is a mild skin infection caused by parasitic mites feeding on skin cells.

How It Spreads

Cheyletiellosis is spread through contact with animals that have these mites (for example, ferrets, rabbits, cats, and other animals).

Giardiasis (*Giardia duodenalis*)

Giardia is a parasite that can be found on surfaces or in water, food, or soil that has been contaminated by the poop of an infected person or animal.

How It Spreads

Giardiasis spreads through swallowing microscopic poop containing the parasite after contact with an infected person or animal, or by drinking water or eating food that has been contaminated with poop from infected people or animals.

Influenza

Influenza, or "flu," is a contagious respiratory illness caused by influenza viruses that infect the nose, throat, and sometimes the lungs. Flu viruses that commonly spread among people (human seasonal flu) can also affect ferrets. Other (nonhuman) flu viruses are found in different animal species, such as chickens and pigs, but these flu viruses are not known to circulate among ferrets.

How It Spreads

Flu spreads through droplets released from coughing, sneezing, or talking. You can also get flu by touching a surface or object with the flu virus on it and then touching your mouth, nose, or possibly eyes. People can spread the flu to ferrets through droplets that spread through coughing, sneezing, or talking, or through direct contact (touching). Animals and people infected with flu viruses may be able to spread flu to others before they develop symptoms. There are no reports of flu spreading from ferrets to people, but because ferrets can get sick with human flu viruses, it may be possible for them to spread flu viruses to people.

Rabies

Rabies is a deadly neurologic disease caused by a virus that spreads primarily through the bites of infected animals. Ferret owners should get ferrets vaccinated against rabies.

How It Spreads

Rabies spreads through contact with saliva or brain/nervous-system tissue from an infected animal, usually through scratches or bites.

Who Is at Risk?

Rabies in people and domestic animals is rare in the United States because of successful animal control and vaccination programs, but the disease is still found in wild animals such as bats, foxes, raccoons, and skunks. You or your pet could be at risk for rabies if you come into contact with an infected animal.

Ringworm

Ringworm is an infection caused by fungus that can infect the skin, hair, or nails of people and animals.

How It Spreads

Ringworm spreads through direct contact with an infected animal or person (touching), or from the environment.

Salmonellosis (*Salmonella* spp.)

Salmonella are bacteria that can make people and animals sick with a disease called "salmonellosis."

How It Spreads

People can become infected with *Salmonella* by eating contaminated food or through contact with animal poop or an animal's food. *Salmonella* infection in ferrets is usually associated with feeding them raw or undercooked meat or unpasteurized milk.

Section 4.7

Fish, Reptiles, and Amphibians as Pets

This section includes text excerpted from "Fish,"
Centers for Disease Control and Prevention (CDC),
October 1, 2015. Reviewed March 2020.

Aeromonas spp.

Aeromonas is a type of bacteria that is commonly found in freshwater ponds and aquariums. This bacteria can cause disease in fish and amphibians, and cause discoloration in the limbs in amphibians and fins of fish. It can also cause internal bleeding in these aquatic animals.

People can become infected through open wounds or by drinking contaminated water. Young children and adults with weakened immune systems are most commonly affected and may develop diarrhea or blood infections as a result of the infection.

Maintaining good water quality in aquariums, promptly removing dead fish, and practicing healthy habits, including handwashing, will reduce the risk of an *Aeromonas* infection.

Mycobacterium marinum

Mycobacterium marinum is a type of bacteria that causes disease in fish, reptiles, and amphibians. This bacteria is found in fresh water ponds and aquariums. It is spread to people and animals through contaminated aquarium water. All fish are susceptible to mycobacteriosis. This disease is typically slow growing in fish, but can affect some fish more quickly. Affected fish may show no signs of illness or may stop eating, lose their fins or scales, develop sores, or appear deformed.

People can become infected with *Mycobacterium marinum* by having direct contact with infected animals or contaminated water (for example, contaminated ponds or aquariums). The most common sign of infection is development of a skin infection. In very rare cases, the bacteria can spread throughout the body's systems. Infections progress slowly and may get better on their own. In some instances, antibiotics and surgical wound treatments are required to prevent deep infection.

Salmonella spp.

Salmonella is a type of bacteria that spreads to people and animals through contaminated food or contact with the stool or habitat of certain animals, including fish. An animal's aquarium or terrarium may also be a source of *Salmonella*. Fish carrying *Salmonella* often do not show any signs of disease. Aquariums that contain reptiles or amphibians in addition to fish are at a higher risk for having *Salmonella*.

People infected with *Salmonella* might have diarrhea, vomiting, fever, or abdominal cramps. Infants, elderly people, and those with weakened immune systems are more likely than others to develop severe illness.

Streptococcus iniae

Streptococcus iniae is a type of bacteria that causes serious disease in fish. Fish dying from streptococcal disease often make disoriented, whirling motions at the water surface, hence the common disease name of "mad fish disease." Fish affected by this disease may have small red areas on their skin, and may develop a swollen abdomen and bulging eyes.

People, especially those with open skin abrasions or scrapes, could get infected by *Streptococcus iniae* bacteria while handling fish or cleaning aquariums. Affected people usually develop a skin infection at the site of open cuts or scrapes. Though rare, more serious illness can happen in people with weakened immune systems.

Section 4.8
Small Mammals

This section contains text excerpted from the following sources: Text in this section begins with excerpts from "Small Mammals," Centers for Disease Control and Prevention (CDC), October 28, 2019; Text under the heading "About Bats and Rabies" is excerpted from "Bats," July 5, 2017; Text beginning with the heading "Bats and Human Rabies in the United States" is excerpted from "Learning about Bats and Rabies," April 22, 2011. Reviewed March 2020.

Some of the diseases associated with small mammal pets that can cause human illnesses include:

Campylobacteriosis (*Campylobacter* spp.)

Campylobacter is a type of bacteria that spreads through contaminated food (meat and eggs), water, or contact with stool of infected animals. *Campylobacter* infections are rare in small mammals, but have been associated with rodents, such as hamsters, guinea pigs, and gerbils. Small mammals infected with *Campylobacter* may not show any signs of illness at all or may have diarrhea.

Most people who become sick with campylobacteriosis will have diarrhea, cramping, abdominal pain, and fever within two to five days after exposure. *Campylobacter* can cause serious life-threatening infections in infants, elderly persons, and other people with weakened immune systems.

Cheyletiellosis (*Cheyletiella* spp.)

Cheyletiella spp., also known as "rabbit fur mites" are tiny parasites that can be found on some healthy rabbits. These mites generally do not cause disease in people or animals. Adult mites may be easily seen on an affected animal. They are often white and may look like "walking dandruff," if they are observed moving. Affected rabbits may have hair loss, dandruff, and itching as a result of skin irritation from the mite.

People may get *Cheyletiella* mites when they pet or hold an infested rabbit. *Cheyletiella* can temporarily infest humans, causing skin irritation and itching. The best way to prevent infestation in rabbits is to use an insecticide approved by your veterinarian.

Giardiasis (*Giardia* spp.)

Giardia is a parasite that causes diarrheal illness in animals and people. *Giardia* is transmitted to animals and people through food or water contaminated with stool. This parasite is relatively uncommon in small mammals, but has been associated with chinchillas, rats, and mice.

Symptoms for animals and people include diarrhea, greasy stools, and dehydration. People can also have abdominal cramps, nausea, and vomiting. Symptoms can last one to two weeks.

Lymphocytic Choriomeningitis Virus (LCMV)

Lymphocytic choriomeningitis (LCM) is a rare viral disease that can be transmitted through the urine, droppings, saliva, or cage material of infected wild and domestic rodents, including hamsters, guinea pigs, rats, mice, and other small rodents. Infected small rodents often appear normal or have small decreases in activity and appetite. Later, these infected animals may show more significant signs of weight loss, hunched posture, and ultimately die.

Human infections with LCMV are rare, especially from pet rodents. If people are infected, they generally have symptoms similar to those of the common flu. These symptoms include fever, stiff neck, loss of appetite, muscle aches, headache, nausea, and vomiting and often occur one to two weeks after exposure. People with weakened immune systems, especially young children and pregnant women, are the most at risk.

Sarcoptic Mange (*Trixacarus caviae*)

Sarcoptic mange is a parasitic skin disease that is caused by a tiny mite and is transmitted between animals through close contact. Sarcoptic mange is rare, but has been associated with guinea pigs.

People cannot become infested with the animal versions of sarcoptic mange, but they can have a minor local reaction from the mites if they come in contact with an infested animal.

Monkeypox Virus

Monkeypox virus which is not currently in the United States is a rare viral disease that is usually found in central and western Africa, but can infect rats, mice, rabbits, and prairie dogs. Infected pets may appear healthy with no clinical signs of disease or may develop fever, cough, conjunctivitis, and lymphadenopathy, followed by a nodular rash.

Although the virus is not currently reported in the United States, people can become infected if they are bitten or come in contact with an affected animal's urine, blood, or rash. Signs and symptoms of monkeypox initially include fever, headache, muscle aches, and lymph nodes swelling. A rash that progresses to fluid-filled bumps may develop days later as the disease spreads.

Pasteurellosis (*Snuffles; Pasteurella multocida*)

Pasteurellosis is a bacterial disease often associated with animal bites and scratches. Hamsters, guinea pigs, rabbits, rats, and mice have all been associated with *Pasteurella*. Most small mammals show no signs of illness, but some rabbits can develop nose and eye discharge. This respiratory disease is called "snuffles." *Pasteurella* can also affect the lungs, skin, and reproductive tract of rabbits.

People rarely become sick with pasteurellosis from small mammal pets. Instead, people most commonly get *Pasteurella* through animal bites. *Pasteurella* can cause painful wound and skin infections. In more severe cases, it can cause widespread infection throughout the body and might even affect the nervous system. To prevent pasteurellosis, protect yourself from bites and seek veterinary care for pets that appear sick.

Rat-Bite Fever

Rat-bite fever is a rare bacterial disease transmitted by bites or scratches from infected rodents. It can also be spread by exposure to contaminated water, food, or rodent urine. The disease is typically seen in rats. Infected rats can carry the infection, but appear healthy. However, other animals may develop arthritis, skin infections, pneumonia, and swollen lymph nodes.

In people, clinical signs range from flu-like symptoms and a rash to more severe infections of the joints, liver, heart, lungs, brain, and blood if left untreated.

Ringworm (*Dermatophytosis*)

Ringworm is a condition caused by a fungus that can infect skin, hair, and nails of both people and animals. Ringworm is spread through direct contact with an infected animal's skin or hair. Affected animals, more commonly guinea pigs, may have circular areas of hair loss or crusts anywhere on their body. Symptoms in rodents and rabbits can vary from mild areas of hair loss to reddened, irritated, itchy, or flaky skin.

Ringworm infections in people can appear on almost any area of the body. These infections are usually itchy. Redness, scaling, cracking of the skin, or a ring-shaped rash may occur. If the infection involves the scalp or beard, hair may fall out. Infected nails become discolored or thick and may possibly crumble.

Salmonellosis (*Salmonella* spp.)

Salmonella spreads to people through contaminated food (eggs and meat) or contact with stool of certain animals, including small mammals. Although rare, *Salmonella* infections associated with small mammals have been linked to some outbreaks of human illness. While it usually does not make the animals sick, *Salmonella* can cause serious illness when it is passed to people.

People exposed to *Salmonella* might have diarrhea, vomiting, fever, or abdominal cramps. Infants, elderly persons, and people with weakened immune systems are more likely than others to develop severe illness.

About Bats and Rabies

Rabid bats have been documented in all 49 continental states. Hawaii is rabies-free. Bats are increasingly implicated as important wildlife reservoirs for variants of rabies virus transmitted to humans. The data suggest that transmission of rabies virus can occur from minor, seemingly unimportant, or unrecognized bites from bats. Human and domestic animal contact with bats should be minimized, and bats should never be handled by untrained and unvaccinated persons or be kept as pets.

In all instances of potential human exposures involving bats, the bat in question should be safely collected, if possible, and submitted for rabies diagnosis. Rabies postexposure prophylaxis (PEP) is recommended for all persons with bite, scratch, or mucous membrane exposure to a bat, unless the bat is available for testing and is negative for evidence of rabies.

Postexposure prophylaxis should be considered when direct contact between a human and a bat has occurred unless the exposed person can be certain a bite, scratch, or mucous membrane exposure did not occur.

In instances in which a bat is found indoors and there is no history of bat–human contact, the likely effectiveness of PEP must be balanced against the low risk such exposures appear to present. PEP can be considered for persons who were in the same room as a bat and who might be unaware that a bite or direct contact had occurred (e.g., a sleeping person awakens to find a bat in the room or an adult witnesses a bat in the room with a previously unattended child, mentally disabled person, or intoxicated person) and rabies cannot be ruled out by testing the bat. PEP would not be warranted for other household members.

Bats and Human Rabies in the United States

Rabies in humans is rare in the United States. There are usually only one or two human cases per year. But the most common source of human rabies in the United States is from bats. For example, among the 19 naturally acquired cases of rabies in humans in the United States from 1997–2006, 17 were associated with bats. Among these, 14 patients had known encounters with bats. Four people awoke because a bat landed on them and one person awoke because a bat bit him. In these cases, the bat was inside the home.

One person was reportedly bitten by a bat from outdoors while he was exiting from his residence. Six people had a history of handling a bat while removing it from their home. One person was bitten by a bat while releasing it outdoors after finding it on the floor inside a building. One person picked up and tried to care for a sick bat found on the ground outdoors. Three men ages 20, 29, and 64 had no reported encounters with bats but died of bat-associated rabies viruses.

Coming in Contact with Bats

People often know when they have been bitten by a bat, but most types of bats have very small teeth which may leave marks that disappear quickly.

If you are bitten by a bat—or if infectious material (such as saliva or brain material if it is killed) from a bat gets into your eyes, nose, mouth, or a wound—wash the affected area thoroughly with soap and water and get medical advice immediately. Whenever possible, the bat should be captured and sent to a laboratory for rabies testing.

People cannot get rabies just from seeing a bat in an attic, in a cave, at summer camp, or from a distance while it is flying. In addition, people cannot get rabies from having contact with bat guano (feces), blood, or urine, or from touching a bat on its fur.

If you think your pet has been bitten by a bat, contact a veterinarian or your health department for assistance immediately and have the bat tested for rabies. Remember to keep vaccinations current for cats, dogs, and other animals.

What If You Are Not Sure?

If you woke up because a bat landed on you while you were sleeping or if you awakened and found a bat in your room, you should try to safely capture the bat and have it tested. The same precautions should be used if you see a bat in a room with an unattended child, or see a bat near a mentally impaired or intoxicated person.

The small teeth of the bat can make a bite difficult to find. Be safe and in these situations, try to safely capture the bat, have the bat tested, and seek medical advice.

Coming in Contact with Bats Outdoors

More than 11 million persons enjoy camping each year in the United States. Few individuals will ever be exposed to a rabies-suspect animal or need medical intervention due a potential exposure while camping. To date, no human rabies cases due to bats in the United States have implicated camping as a risk factor for an unrecognized exposure.

The mere presence and sighting of bats outdoors and in camping situations is common and normal. Precautions such as avoiding intentional contact with a bat and using screens or mosquito netting are a good idea to prevent potential exposures to rabies.

If you or your family are camping or at summer camp and someone is bitten by a bat, postexposure vaccination is essential if the animal tests positive or is not available for testing.

If you re not sure if a contact has occurred, but a bat is found on or near you, then postexposure vaccination may be warranted. Infants, young children, and people with reduced mental function due to medication, alcohol, illness, or age should be considered to be at higher risk since they may not have known or be able to tell others if they were bitten.

Deciding Risk

If bats were present at a summer camp where campers were sleeping, local or state public-health professionals will make a careful assessment of the potential for rabies exposure on a case-by-case basis. Campers who may have been bitten by a bat, had direct contact with a bat, or were awakened by the presence of a bat near or on them need to be identified for appropriate evaluation, and, if needed, vaccinated to prevent rabies.

Public-health officials will consider many things in making this assessment. For example, if the child slept under mosquito netting or in an enclosure where bats were excluded by screening, this would reduce considerably any possibility of the child being bitten by a bat without knowing it.

Public-health professionals will also consider how many people saw bats, where and when the bats were seen, whether or not supervisory adults were present or made bed checks and how often. They'll look at the age of the campers, the number of persons present in a sleeping area, the mental function of persons in this situation, the type, size, age, and history of the structure in which the bats were found, the time of year, and, if it can be determined, the species of the bat.

Coming in Contact with Bats in Your Home
If You Are Certain No People or Pets Have Come in Contact with the Bat

Confine the bat to a room by closing all doors and windows leading out of the room except those to the outside. The bat will probably leave soon. If the bat does not leave, contact an animal control or public-health agency for assistance. If help is not available, follow the steps to capture a bat.

If There Has Been Contact between the Bat and People or Pets

If a bat is in your house and you have any questions about whether the bat has been in contact with people or pets, you will want to have the bat captured and tested. Call animal control or a wildlife conservation agency for assistance. If professional assistance is not available, follow the steps to safely capture the bat and save it for testing.

To Capture a Bat

- Find a small container such as a box or a large can, and a piece of cardboard large enough to cover the opening in the container. Punch small air holes in the cardboard.
- Put on leather work gloves. When the bat lands, approach it slowly and place the container over it. Slide the cardboard under the container to trap the bat inside.
- If you are certain there has been no contact between the bat and any people or pets, carefully hold the cardboard over the container and take the bat outdoors and release it away from people and pets.
- If there is any question about contact between the bat and people or pets, you want to save the bat for testing. Tape the cardboard to the container,

securing the bat inside, and then contact your health department to have the bat tested for rabies.

Keeping Bats Out of Your House

Some bats live in buildings, and there is no reason to evict them if there is little chance for contact with people.

Bats must not be allowed into your home. It is best to contact an animal-control or wildlife conservation agency for assistance with "bat-proofing" your home. If you choose to do the "bat-proofing" yourself, here are some suggestions.

Carefully examine your home for holes that might allow bats entry into your living quarters. Caulk any openings larger than a quarter-inch by a half-inch. Use window screens, chimney caps, and draft-guards beneath doors to attics, fill electrical and plumbing holes with stainless steel wool or caulking, and ensure that all doors to the outside close tightly.

Prevent bats from roosting in attics or buildings by covering outside entry points. Observe where the bats exit at dusk and keep them from coming back by loosely hanging clear plastic sheeting or bird netting over these areas. Bats can crawl out and leave, but cannot re-enter. When all the bats are gone, the openings can be permanently sealed.

Avoid doing this from May through August. If there are young bats in your attic, many of them cannot fly and keeping the adults out will trap the young who will die or try to make their way into your rooms.

Most bats leave in the fall or winter to hibernate, so these are the best times to "bat-proof" your home.

Section 4.9
Wildlife

This section includes text excerpted from "Wildlife,"
Centers for Disease Control and
Prevention (CDC), October 22, 2018.

Aeromoniasis (*Aeromonas* spp.)

Aeromonas is a type of bacteria that is commonly found in fresh and brackish water. This germ can cause disease in stressed fish and amphibians. *Aeromonas* spp. can cause discoloration of the limbs of amphibians and the fins of fish and can cause internal bleeding in these aquatic animals.

Though it very rarely happens, people can become infected when they handle infected fish or accidentally swallow contaminated food or water. If these germs are swallowed, *Aeromonas* infections can cause nausea, vomiting, and diarrhea. Skin infections can happen if the bacteria get into open wounds or scrapes. More severe disease can happen in children or people with weakened immune systems.

Practicing healthy habits, including handwashing, will reduce the risk of *Aeromonas* infection.

Anthrax (*Bacillus anthracis* spp.)

Anthrax is a naturally occurring disease of animals caused by a type of bacteria called "*Bacillus anthracis*." People and animals can get anthrax when they accidentally breathe in or swallow spores in contaminated soil, food, or water. The greatest risk is from contact with the bodily fluids of an animal that has anthrax or has recently died from anthrax. Anthrax can also get into open wounds. People who live in areas where anthrax has occurred should consider vaccinating their livestock against the disease.

Anthrax is a serious, but rare disease in the United States. The symptoms of anthrax depend on the route of infection and can take anywhere from one day to more than two months to appear. All types of anthrax have the potential, if untreated, to spread throughout the body and cause severe illness and even death. To prevent anthrax, be aware of areas where anthrax is present and wear gloves when handling animal carcasses from those regions. Use care when processing bloated or swollen carcasses so that accumulated gasses blow away from you when the carcass is opened.

Raccoon Roundworm (*Baylisascaris procyonis* spp.)

Raccoon Roundworm infection is caused by roundworm eggs found in raccoon, bear, and skunk droppings. The disease is passed to people and animals if they accidentally ingest contaminated food or soil.

If a person or dog ingests the eggs, the worm larvae then hatch inside them and can migrate through the body. Human infections are rare, but can be severe if the parasites invade the eye (ocular larva migrans), organs (visceral larva migrans), or brain (neural larva migrans).

Raccoon roundworm can be prevented by avoiding areas frequented by raccoons. If you need to clean raccoon droppings up, wear gloves and use caution so as not to kick up dust. Always wash your hands after working or playing in dirt.

Botulism (*Clostridium botulinum* spp.)

Clostridium botulinum produces a toxin that causes botulism—a rare, but serious condition in humans. *C. botulinum* is a type of bacteria that can be found in the intestines of many marine and freshwater species of fish worldwide. Though rare, outbreaks of botulism can be associated with fish, including aquatic game, canned foods, and smoked fish. Affected fish show few signs of illness, though some fish may have pale gill colorings or abdominal swelling.

A person with botulism can develop double vision, blurred vision, drooping eyelids, and paralysis, which can result in death. People are commonly exposed through the environment or contaminated food, such as smoked fish products. To protect yourself from botulism, avoid fishing in areas where there are dead fish or waterfowl and cook all fish thoroughly.

Anyone who thinks they may have botulism should seek emergency medical care.

Brucellosis (*Brucella* spp.)

Brucellosis is a bacterial disease that affects the ability of animals to reproduce. The disease can be spread to humans through contact with the birthing tissues from infected animals or through drinking unpasteurized (raw) milk. Among wildlife, bison, elk, caribou, moose, feral pigs, and some marine mammals can be infected with *Brucella*. Infected animals may have decreased appetite, weight loss, behavioral changes, and lack of energy, but most animals infected with brucellosis show no signs of illness. Brucellosis affects the reproductive organs and can cause miscarriage in animals and occasionally people.

People who hunt or eat fresh game meat are at highest risk for contracting brucellosis. They may be exposed through skin wounds while dressing a carcass or by eating undercooked meat. People who are infected with brucellosis will usually become sick within six to eight weeks of exposure. Sick people will have flu-like symptoms that last two to four weeks. Sometimes brucellosis can become a chronic illness that can be difficult to treat.

Prevent brucellosis by wearing gloves while handling fresh carcasses and thoroughly cooking any meat that will be eaten.

Cryptococcosis (*Cryptococcus neoformans* spp.)

Cryptococcosis is an infection that is caused by the fungus *Cryptococcus neoformans*. This fungus can be found in soil and bird droppings, especially droppings from pigeons. When dried bird droppings are disturbed, dust containing the fungus can be released into the air and be inhaled by people, cats, and dogs.

Most people do not become sick with cryptococcosis, but people with weakened immune systems may be at risk. Signs of disease include headaches, fever, cough, shortness of breath, and night sweats.

Prevent cryptococcosis by avoiding enclosed areas where pigeons or other wild birds roost.

Dermatophilosis (Lumpy Wool, Strawberry Footrot)

Dermatophilosis is a disease caused by a type of bacteria that can infect the skin and hair of both people and animals. The disease is spread from animals to people through touching an infected animal. Deer are the most common wildlife infected. Affected animals may have a "paintbrush" appearance of matted hair. The matted spots will often have scabs or crusts with pus. Other infected animals may show no symptoms at all.

This disease is most common among people who raise deer or who have contact with fawns. People who handle an infected animal may get pus-filled blisters on their hands and arms. These sores are usually not painful, but can develop into shallow, red ulcers that scar.

Wear gloves and protective clothing when working with any animals, especially those with the classic "paintbrush" matted hair appearance, to reduce the risk of getting this disease.

Hydatid Cyst Disease (*Echinococcosis* spp.)

Hydatid Cyst Disease is a parasitic disease caused by consuming food or water contaminated with tapeworm eggs or through contact with an infected animal. This parasite is a tapeworm that can form large fluid-filled cysts in the tissues of animals or people who accidentally eat the eggs. The adult tapeworm can be found in foxes, coyotes, cats, and other wild predators. Animals become infected by eating the tissue of an infected animal. Infected animals rarely show any signs of disease, but can have a large number of adult tapeworms.

Although the *Echinococcus* parasite invades many different organs of the body, most people who are infected with the disease will not have any signs of illness for years. Symptoms start when the slow-growing cysts become large enough to press on the organs they have invaded. The tapeworms grow slowly in several different organs of the body, but are most commonly found in the liver and lungs.

Prevent echinococcosis by avoiding the stool of wild canids, thoroughly cooking game meat, and practicing healthy habits, including handwashing.

Edwardsiellosis (*Edwardsiella tarda* spp.)

Edwardsiella tarda is a type of bacteria associated with fresh and saltwater animals, such as fish, amphibians, reptiles, and mammals. *E. tarda* is known to cause serious illness in fish. Affected fish may show abnormal swimming behavior, discoloration of the fins or skin, bulging or increased opacity of the eyes, and other complications.

People can become infected by accidentally swallowing contaminated water or through handling infected fish. Affected people commonly get nausea, vomiting, and/or diarrhea. People with weakened immune systems may also be at risk for more serious disease.

Wash your hands before and after handling fish to reduce the risk of edwardsiellosis.

Erysipeloid (*Erysipelothrix rhusiopathiae* spp.)

Erysipelothrix rhusiopathiae is a type of bacteria that causes erysipeloid, a skin condition that people can develop after contact with infected fish, poultry, or pork. Healthy fish often carry the bacteria on their scales with no signs of illness.

People, especially fish handlers, can become infected through open wounds on their hands. Affected people will usually develop a warm, raised, red, and intensely itchy area of skin at the site of the contaminated wound. If the infection spreads from the skin to deeper tissues, arthritis or more serious signs of illness (fever, weakness, muscle aches, headaches, etc.) may develop.

People who handle fish regularly should wear gloves and wash their hands often to reduce the risk of this disease.

Giardiasis (*Giardia* spp.)

Giardia is a parasite that causes diarrheal illness in animals and people. *Giardia* is transmitted to animals and people through food or water contaminated with stool. Though different types of *Giardia* affect humans and animals, both the human and animal types are carried by wildlife, including beavers, muskrats, deer, coyotes, and rodents. Pets may become infected after drinking from puddles or ponds or swallowing infected stool from other animals. Affected animals may have diarrhea, greasy stools, and dehydration.

In people, the symptoms of giardiasis may include diarrhea, gas, greasy stools, abdominal pain, nausea, and vomiting. Symptoms can last one to two weeks.

To avoid *Giardia* infection, hikers and backpackers should always treat water before offering it to their pets or drinking it themselves. People should also wash their hands often and use caution when swimming or wading in potentially contaminated ponds or lakes to avoid swallowing the water.

Hantavirus

Hantavirus is a virus that can cause severe respiratory disease. It is spread through accidentally breathing in virus particles in dust from dry rodent urine or through contact with rodents or their droppings or nests.

Early signs in people include fever, headache, muscle aches, vomiting, diarrhea, abdominal pain, dizziness, and chills.

Histoplasmosis (*Histoplasma capsulatum*)

Histoplasmosis is a fungal disease that is spread to people by breathing in dust from pigeon or bat droppings. Fungal spores are found in the environment, especially in areas with bird and bat droppings. Birds do not get sick from exposure to histoplasmosis.

Very few people become infected with histoplasmosis. People who do become sick tend to develop pneumonia-like symptoms (fever, chest pains, and a dry or nonproductive cough) within one to three weeks after exposure. Infants, older people, and those with weakened immune systems are more susceptible to the fungus and might develop more serious illness.

People with weakened immune systems should avoid activities such as disturbing material where there are bird or bat droppings, cleaning chicken coops, exploring caves, and cleaning, remodeling, or tearing down old buildings.

Leptospirosis (*Leptospira* spp.)

Leptospirosis is a bacterial disease of humans and animals that is transmitted through contaminated water and urine or other body fluids from an infected animal. The *Leptospira* spp. bacteria can infect raccoons, skunks, squirrels, opossums, deer, rodents, and other wild animals without any signs of disease. Though it is difficult to detect early stages of leptospirosis in animals, the disease can lead to kidney and liver failure if left untreated.

People who become infected with leptospirosis might not have any symptoms of the disease. Others will have nonspecific flu-like symptoms (fever, headache, chills, vomiting, rash) within two to seven days after exposure. These symptoms usually resolve without medical treatment, but can reappear and lead to more severe disease (yellow skin and eyes, rash, kidney or liver failure, meningitis).

Some ways to prevent leptospirosis from wildlife are to avoid contact with environments potentially contaminated with animal urine and to avoid swallowing water from lakes, rivers, or swamps while swimming.

Lyme Disease (*Borrelia burgdorferi*)

Lyme disease is a bacterial disease that affects humans and animals bitten by the Ixodes species of ticks. Rodents and other wildlife are reservoirs of the disease. Most infections occur from the nymphal-stage ticks, which are tiny and difficult to remove.

Infected people will typically have a red "bull's eye" rash (erythema migrans) at the site of the tick bite that appears about seven days after being bitten. Flu-like symptoms quickly follow the rash. If not treated, this disease can spread to other parts of the body and cause symptoms such as arthritis and loss of facial muscle tone (Bell's palsy).

Lyme disease can be prevented by avoiding exposure to ticks, using a tick repellent, and by finding and removing ticks from your pets and your family as soon as possible after returning from a tick-infested area.

Lymphocytic Choriomeningitis Virus (LCMV)

Lymphocytic choriomeningitis virus (LCMV) can be transmitted through the urine, droppings, saliva, or cage material of infected wild and domestic rodents, wild hogs, skunks, raccoons, and squirrels. Infected animals may appear normal or show more significant signs, including weight loss, hunched posture, and ultimately death.

Human infections with LCMV are rare. Symptoms are similar to those of the common flu (fever, stiff neck, loss of appetite, muscle aches, headache, nausea, and vomiting) and often occur one to two weeks after exposure.

Prevent LCMV infection by avoiding contact with wild rodents and their droppings.

Mycobacteriosis (*Mycobacterium marinum*)

Mycobacterium marinum is a type of bacteria that causes disease in fish, reptiles, and amphibians. It is spread to people and animals through contaminated aquarium water. All fish are susceptible to *mycobacterium*, but freshwater species seem to be most affected. This disease is slow growing in fish. Affected fish may stop eating, lose their fins or scales, develop sores, or appear deformed.

Though infection in humans is rare, people can become sick with mycobacteriosis after coming into contact with contaminated water through minor cuts and skin abrasions. People with this disease, commonly known as "fish tank granulomas," develop warm raised, red areas of the skin. Skin lesions can leave long-lasting scars.

Reduce the risk for *mycobacterium* by washing your hands after handling reptiles, amphibians, and fish.

Plague (*Yersinia pestis*)

Plague is a rare bacterial disease that affects animals and humans and is spread by infected fleas. Rodents such as mice, rats, prairie dogs, and squirrels can carry plague. Plague is found primarily in the western United States. People and animals can be infected when they are bitten by infected fleas or when they handle blood or tissues of infected animals. Wild and domestic carnivores (especially cats) can also become infected by eating infected rodents. Cats usually have fever, weight loss, and loss of energy with enlarged glands. Wild rodents may or may not have any signs of the disease.

People most often become infected with plague through flea bites or from contact with the body fluids of infected animals. Hunters may be at increased risk. Bubonic plague is the most common form of plague that affects people. Symptoms include a sudden onset of high fever, chills, headache, malaise, and swollen glands (lymph nodes). The other two forms of plague, septicemic and pneumonic, cause more severe disease.

Plague can be prevented by keeping fleas away from your pets and family and by wearing gloves while handling or skinning potentially infected animals.

Rabies

Rabies, a fatal neurologic disease in animals and humans, is caused by a virus. The rabies virus can infect most mammals, including bats, bears, beavers, deer, wild canids such as fox and coyotes, felids such as mountain lions and bobcats, raccoons, skunks, opossums, and other small mammals. Animals and people are most commonly infected through bites from rabid animals. Infected animals may have a variety of signs, but most often have sudden behavioral changes and progressive paralysis. Rabies can be prevented in some animals by vaccination.

The first symptoms in humans can start days to months after exposure and include generalized weakness, fever, and headache. Within a few days symptoms will progress to confusion, anxiety, behavioral changes, and delirium.

If you have been bitten by a wild animal that was not acting normal, contact your healthcare provider right away for treatment. Once symptoms appear, it is almost always too late for treatment.

Rat-Bite Fever (*Streptobacillus moniliformis*)

Rat-bite fever is a rare bacterial disease transmitted by bites or scratches from infected rodents. It can also be spread by exposure to contaminated water, food, or rodent urine. The disease is typically seen in rats. Infected rats can carry the infection, but appear healthy. However, other animals infected with rat-bite fever may develop arthritis, skin infections, pneumonia, and swollen lymph nodes.

In people infected with rat-bite fever, signs range from flu-like symptoms and a rash to more severe infections of the joints, liver, heart, lungs, brain, and blood, if left untreated.

Prevent rat-bite fever from wild rodents by avoiding contact with wild rodents and their urine.

Rocky Mountain Spotted Fever (RMSF, *Rickettsia rickettsii*)

Rocky Mountain spotted fever (RMSF) is a bacterial disease transmitted to dogs and humans by ticks. Dogs show a variety of symptoms similar to those in humans, including fever, lameness, coughing, vomiting, and diarrhea, and swelling of the face or extremities.

People who are infected with RMSF generally start getting sick 2 to 14 days after exposure. Symptoms may include fever, rash, headache, nausea, vomiting, abdominal pain, and muscle pain. RMSF can develop into a serious illness if not promptly treated.

Rocky Mountain spotted fever disease can be prevented by avoiding exposure to ticks, using a tick repellent, and by finding and removing ticks from your pets and your family as soon as possible after returning from a tick-infested area.

Salmonellosis (*Salmonella* spp.)

Salmonella spreads to people through contaminated food (eggs and meat) or contact with the stool of certain animals, including wildlife. In the wild, people usually become sick with *Salmonella* through direct contact with an infected animal's stool or by accidentally drinking contaminated water. While it usually does not make the animals sick, *Salmonella* can cause serious illness when it is passed to people.

People exposed to *Salmonella* might have diarrhea, vomiting, fever, or abdominal cramps. Infants, elderly persons, and people with weakened immune systems are more likely than others to develop severe illness.

Prevent salmonellosis by avoiding the stool of wild animals, thoroughly cooking game meat, and practicing healthy habits, including handwashing.

Trichinellosis or Trichinosis (*Trichinella spiralis*)

Trichinellosis is a parasitic disease caused by eating the raw or undercooked meat of animals infected with *Trichinella*. *Trichinella* infections are common in wild, meat-eating animals such as bears and cougars as well as some other meat and plant-eating animals such as wild hogs. People usually become infected by consuming raw or undercooked meat that is infected, especially from bear and wild hogs. Most animals infected with *Trichinella* do not show any signs of illness.

People infected with *Trichinella* can have a variety of symptoms depending on the amount of parasites ingested and how strong their immune system is. The first symptoms of trichinellosis include nausea, vomiting, diarrhea, and abdominal pain. Infected people may then develop facial swelling and flu-like symptoms, such as headache, fever, chills, and muscle pain. In very severe infections, people can lose control of their movements and have heart and breathing problems. *Trichinella* can cause death if severe infections are left untreated.

Prevent trichinellosis from wildlife by thoroughly cooking game meat.

Tuberculosis (Mycobacterium tuberculosis complex)

Mycobacterium tuberculosis complex is a group of bacteria that causes a disease called "tuberculosis." Bison, buffalo, opossums, badgers, and deer can all become infected.

People can get tuberculosis if they ingest undercooked meat, accidentally inhale the bacteria, or are infected through skin cuts or scrapes. Depending on the route of infection, people may have sores, swollen lymph nodes, difficulty breathing, weight loss, night sweats, fever, or intestinal upset.

Avoid tuberculosis from wildlife by thoroughly cooking meat and by washing your hands after handling wildlife.

Tularemia (*Francisella tularensis*)

Tularemia is a bacterial disease that can spread to people through bites from ticks or deer flies, handling or consuming infected animals, accidentally swallowing contaminated water, or inhaling contaminated dust. Though typically a wildlife disease, tularemia has been reported in all the U.S. states except Hawaii. Affected animals may have sudden onset of fever, weakness, decreased appetite, and reduced mobility. Within a few hours or days, the animal can become stiff and die.

People exposed to tularemia can have a variety of symptoms ranging from fever, chills, headache, and muscle aches to skin ulcers; swollen and painful lymph nodes; inflamed eyes; sore throat; mouth sores; and diarrhea. They may also develop pneumonia.

People exposed to an infected animal should be seen by their doctor immediately because treatment works best when started early. You can reduce your risk of tularemia by handling dead animals with gloves, cooking game meat thoroughly, wearing insect repellent, and when possible, avoiding mowing over dead animals during outside work.

Vesicular Stomatitis

Vesicular stomatitis is a disease caused by a virus. Vesicular stomatitis is primarily a disease of livestock, but people and several species of wildlife can become infected. Infected animals may have fluid-filled blisters, called "vesicles," around the mouth, on their feet, or under the belly.

It is very rare for people to get vesicular stomatitis. Infections can occur when people handle sick animals or contaminated tissues and blood from sick animals. Infected people may have a variety of symptoms ranging from no signs of illness to flu-like symptoms and blisters.

Reduce the risk for vesicular stomatitis by washing your hands after handling affected wildlife.

Vibriosis (*Vibrio* spp.)

Vibrio are bacteria that are mostly found in saltwater and cause serious disease in marine fish. People usually get sick with vibriosis after eating raw or undercooked fish or shellfish or after swallowing contaminated water. Fish affected by *Vibrio* can have symptoms ranging from deep skin ulcers to more widespread signs of skin darkening, scale loss, swelling of the abdomen, and loss of appetite.

In people, *Vibrio* can cause nausea, vomiting, and diarrhea. Some types of Vibrio can also cause skin infections from contact with contaminated water.

People can prevent vibriosis infections by eating cooked fish and shellfish and by avoiding exposure of open wounds or broken skin to warm salt or brackish water, and avoiding raw shellfish harvested from such waters.

West Nile Virus (WNV)

West Nile virus is carried by birds and transmitted by mosquitoes. People, birds, and horses get WNV by being bitten by an infected mosquito. Most animals infected with WNV will show no signs of illness. Some birds will die of the disease.

Most people who become infected with WNV do not have any signs of illness; however, people who do become ill usually have flu-like symptoms. A small percentage of people with WNV infection develop a more serious neurologic illness, such as encephalitis or meningitis (inflammation of the brain and surrounding tissues).

You can prevent WNV by using mosquito repellents, wearing long-sleeved shirts and long pants, and limiting outdoor exposure from dusk to dawn. Using air conditioning, installing window and door screens, and reducing mosquito breeding sites, can further decrease the risk for WNV exposure.

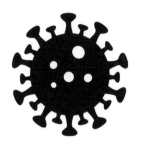

CHAPTER 5
Recent Animal-Borne Diseases

Chapter Contents

Middle East Respiratory Syndrome Coronavirus (MERS-CoV)

This section includes text excerpted from "Middle East Respiratory Syndrome (MERS)—About MERS," Centers for Disease Control and Prevention (CDC), October 28, 2019.

About Middle East Respiratory Syndrome

The Middle East respiratory syndrome (MERS) is an illness caused by a virus (more specifically, a coronavirus) called "Middle East respiratory syndrome coronavirus" (MERS-CoV). Most MERS patients developed severe respiratory illness with symptoms of fever, cough, and shortness of breath. About 3 or 4 out of every 10 patients reported with MERS have died.

All Cases Are Linked to the Arabian Peninsula

Health officials first reported the disease in Saudi Arabia in September 2012. Through retrospective (backward-looking) investigations, they later identified that the first known cases of MERS occurred in Jordan in April 2012. So far, all cases of MERS have been linked through travel to, or residence in, countries in and near the Arabian Peninsula. The largest known outbreak of MERS outside the Arabian Peninsula occurred in the Republic of Korea in 2015. The outbreak was associated with a traveler returning from the Arabian Peninsula.

People with MERS Can Spread It to Others

MERS-CoV has spread from ill people to others through close contact, such as caring for or living with an infected person.

MERS can affect anyone. MERS patients have ranged in age from younger than 1 to 99 years old.

The CDC continues to closely monitor the MERS situation globally. The CDC is working with partners to better understand the risks of this virus, including the source, how it spreads, and how to prevent infections. CDC recognizes the potential for MERS-CoV to spread further and cause more cases globally and in the United States. The CDC has provided information for travelers and are working with health departments, hospitals, and other partners to prepare for this.

Symptoms and Complications of Middle East Respiratory Syndrome

Most people confirmed to have MERS-CoV infection have had severe respiratory illness with symptoms of:

- Fever
- Cough
- Shortness of breath

Some people also had diarrhea and nausea/vomiting. For many people with MERS, more severe complications followed, such as pneumonia and kidney failure. About 3 or 4 out of every 10 people who reported with MERS have died. Most of the people who died had a preexisting medical condition that weakened their immune system, or an underlying medical condition that hadn't yet been discovered. Medical conditions sometimes weaken people's immune systems and make them more likely to get sick or have severe illness.

Preexisting conditions among people who got MERS have included:

- Diabetes
- Cancer
- Chronic lung disease
- Chronic heart disease
- Chronic kidney disease

Some infected people had mild symptoms (such as cold-like symptoms) or no symptoms at all.

The symptoms of MERS start to appear about 5 or 6 days after a person is exposed, but can range from 2 to 14 days.

Transmission of Middle East Respiratory Syndrome

MERS-CoV, like other coronaviruses, likely spreads from an infected person's respiratory secretions, such as through coughing. However, it is not fully understood the precise ways that it spreads.

MERS-CoV has spread from ill people to others through close contact, such as caring for or living with an infected person. Infected people have spread MERS-CoV to others in healthcare settings, such as hospitals. Researchers studying MERS have not seen any ongoing spreading of MERS-CoV in the community.

All reported cases have been linked to countries in and near the Arabian Peninsula. Most infected people either lived in the Arabian Peninsula or recently traveled from the Arabian Peninsula before they became ill. A few people have gotten MERS after having close contact with an infected person who had recently traveled from the Arabian Peninsula. The largest known outbreak of MERS outside the Arabian Peninsula occurred in the Republic of Korea in 2015 and was associated with a traveler returning from the Arabian Peninsula.

Public-health agencies continue to investigate clusters of cases in several countries to better understand how MERS-CoV spreads from person to person.

Prevention and Treatment of Middle East Respiratory Syndrome

Prevention

There is currently no vaccine to protect people against MERS. But scientists are working to develop one.

You can help reduce your risk of getting respiratory illnesses:

- Wash your hands often with soap and water for at least 20 seconds, and help young children do the same. If soap and water are not available, use an alcohol-based hand sanitizer.

- Cover your nose and mouth with a tissue when you cough or sneeze, then throw the tissue in the trash.
- Avoid touching your eyes, nose, and mouth with unwashed hands.
- Avoid personal contact, such as kissing, or sharing cups or eating utensils, with sick people.
- Clean and disinfect frequently touched surfaces and objects, such as doorknobs.

Treatment

There is no specific antiviral treatment recommended for MERS-CoV infection. Individuals with MERS often receive medical care to help relieve symptoms. For severe cases, current treatment includes care to support vital organ functions.

Section 5.2

Severe Acute Respiratory Syndrome Coronavirus (SARS-CoV)

This section includes text excerpted from "Severe Acute Respiratory Syndrome (SARS)—Fact Sheet for SARS Patients and Their Close Contacts," Centers for Disease Control and Prevention (CDC), December 6, 2017.

About Severe Acute Respiratory Syndrome

Severe acute respiratory syndrome (SARS) is a viral respiratory illness caused by a coronavirus, called "SARS-associated coronavirus" (SARS-CoV). SARS was recognized as a global threat in March 2003, after first appearing in Southern China in November 2002. Over the next few months, the illness spread to more than two dozen countries in North America, South America, Europe, and Asia. Although the 2003 global outbreak was contained, it is possible that person-to-person transmission of SARS-CoV might recur.

Symptoms of Severe Acute Respiratory Syndrome

The illness usually begins with a fever (measured temperature greater than 100.4°F [>38.0°C]). The fever is sometimes associated with chills or other symptoms, including headache, general feeling of discomfort, and body aches. Some people also have mild respiratory symptoms at the outset. About 10 percent to 20 percent of patients have diarrhea. After 2 to 7 days, SARS patients may develop a dry, nonproductive cough or feel short of breath. These symptoms might be accompanied by or progress to a condition in which the oxygen levels in the blood are low (hypoxia). Most patients develop pneumonia.

How Severe Acute Respiratory Syndrome Spreads

The main way that SARS appears to spread is by close person-to-person contact. The virus that causes SARS is thought to be transmitted most readily by respiratory droplets (droplet spread) produced when an infected person coughs or sneezes. Droplet spread can happen when droplets from the cough or sneeze of an infected person are propelled a short distance (generally up to 3 feet) through the air and deposited on the mucous membranes of the mouth, nose, or eyes of persons who are nearby. The virus also can spread when a person touches a surface or object contaminated with infectious droplets and then touches her or his mouth, nose, or eye(s). In addition, it is possible that SARS-CoV might be spread more broadly through the air (airborne spread) or by other ways that are not now known.

What Does "Close Contact" Mean?

In the context of SARS, "close contact" means having cared for or lived with someone with SARS or having a high likelihood of direct contact with the respiratory secretions and/or body fluids of a patient known to have SARS. Examples include kissing or embracing, sharing eating or drinking utensils, talking to someone within 3 feet, physical examination, and any other direct physical contact between people. Close contact does not include activities such as walking by a person or briefly sitting across a waiting room or office.

Steps to Protect Yourself and the People around You

If you have SARS, or you have close contact with someone who does, follow these instructions:

If You Think You (or Someone in Your Family) Might Have SARS, You Should:

- Call your healthcare provider as soon as possible. Call ahead and alert the healthcare provider before your visit so that precautions can be taken to keep from exposing other people.
- Cover your mouth and nose with a tissue when coughing or sneezing.
- Be careful not to expose others. If you have been exposed to SARS and become ill with any symptoms, limit your activities outside the home. Avoid public transportation (e.g., bus, taxi). Do not go to work, school, out-of-home child care, church, or activities in other public areas until after you are told that you do not have SARS.
- Follow any other instructions provided by local health authorities.

If You Have SARS and Are Being Cared for at Home, You Should:

- Follow the instructions given by your healthcare provider.
- Limit your activities outside the home except as necessary for medical care. For example, do not go to work, school, or public areas. If you

must leave the home, wear a mask, if tolerated. Do not use public transportation.

- Wash your hands often and well, especially after you blow your nose.
- Cover your mouth and nose with a tissue when you sneeze or cough.
- If possible, wear a surgical mask when around other people in your home. If you can't wear a mask, the members of your household should wear one when they are around you.
- Don't share silverware, towels, or bedding with anyone in your home until these items have been washed with soap and hot water.
- Be sure that surfaces (counters, tabletops, doorknobs, bathroom fixtures, etc.) that have been contaminated by your body fluids (sweat, saliva, mucous, or even vomit or urine) are cleaned with a household disinfectant used according to the manufacturer's instructions. Be sure that the person who cleans the surfaces wears disposable gloves during all cleaning activities. Disposable gloves should be thrown out after use and should not be reused.
- Follow these instructions for 10 days after your fever and respiratory symptoms have gone away or until the health department says you can return to normal activities.

If You Are Caring for Someone at Home Who Has SARS, You Should:

- Be sure that you understand and can help the SARS patient follow the healthcare provider's instructions for medication and care.
- Be sure that all members of your household are washing their hands frequently with soap and hot water or using an alcohol-based hand rub.
- Wear disposable gloves if you will have direct contact with body fluids of a SARS patient. However, wearing gloves is not a substitute for good hand hygiene. After contact with body fluids of a SARS patient, remove the gloves, throw them out, and wash your hands. Do not wash or reuse the gloves.
- Encourage the person with SARS to cover her or his mouth and nose with a tissue when coughing or sneezing. If possible, the person with SARS should wear a surgical mask during close contact with other

people in the home. If the person with SARS cannot wear a surgical mask, other members of the household should wear one when in the room with that person.

- Do not use silverware, towels, bedding, clothing, or other items that have been used by the person with SARS until these items have been washed with soap and hot water.

- Clean surfaces in the patient's room and the bathroom fixtures used by the patient daily, with a household disinfectant used according to the manufacturer's instructions. When cleaning, wear disposable gloves, and dispose of them after use. Or, use household utility gloves.

- Limit the number of persons in the household to those who are essential for patient support. Other household members should either be relocated or minimize contact with the patient in the home. This is particularly important for persons at risk of serious complications of SARS (e.g., persons with underlying heart or lung disease, diabetes mellitus, older age).

- Unexposed persons who do not have an essential need to be in the home should not visit.

- Follow these instructions for 10 days after the sick person's fever and respiratory symptoms have gone away or until the health department says the SARS patient can return to normal activities.

- For 10 days after your last exposure to the person with SARS, be vigilant for fever (i.e., measure your temperature twice daily), respiratory symptoms, and other early symptoms of SARS. Common early symptoms include chills, body aches, and headache. In some patients, body aches and headache may appear 12 to 24 hours before fever. Diarrhea, sore throat, and runny nose may also be early symptoms of SARS. If you do not have any of these symptoms, you do not need to limit your activities outside the home. You may go to work, school, out-of-home child care, church, or activities in other public areas.

- Follow any other instructions provided by local health authorities.

- If you start feeling sick, especially if you develop a fever, respiratory symptoms, or other early symptoms of SARS, contact your healthcare provider immediately, and tell the healthcare provider that you have had close contact with a SARS patient.

Section 5.3

Coronavirus Disease 2019 (COVID-19)

This section includes text excerpted from "What You Need to Know about Coronavirus Disease 2019 (COVID-19)," Centers for Disease Control and Prevention (CDC), March 20, 2020.

What Is Coronavirus Disease 2019 (COVID-19)?

Coronavirus disease 2019 (COVID-19) is a respiratory illness that can spread from person to person. The virus that causes COVID-19 is a novel coronavirus that was first identified during an investigation into an outbreak in Wuhan, China.

Can People in the United States Get COVID-19?

Yes. COVID-19 is spreading from person to person in parts of the United States. Risk of infection with COVID-19 is higher for people who are close contacts of someone known to have COVID-19, for example healthcare workers, or household members. Other people at higher risk for infection are those who live in or have recently been in an area with ongoing spread of COVID-19.

Have There Been Cases of COVID-19 in the United States?

Yes. The first case of COVID-19 in the United States was reported on January 21, 2020. The current count of cases of COVID-19 in the United States is available on CDC's webpage at www.cdc.gov/coronavirus/2019-ncov/cases-in-us.html.

How Does COVID-19 Spread?

The virus that causes COVID-19 probably emerged from an animal source, but is now spreading from person to person. The virus is thought to spread mainly between people who are in close contact with one another (within about 6 feet) through respiratory droplets produced when an infected person coughs or sneezes. It also may be possible that a person can get COVID-19 by touching a surface or object that has the virus on it and then touching their own mouth, nose, or possibly their eyes, but this is not thought to be the main way the virus spreads.

What Are the Symptoms of COVID-19?

Patients with COVID-19 have had mild to severe respiratory illness with symptoms of:

- Fever
- Cough
- Shortness of breath

What Are Severe Complications from This Virus?

Some patients have pneumonia in both lungs, multi-organ failure and in some cases death.

How Can I Help Protect Myself?

People can help protect themselves from respiratory illness with everyday preventive actions.

- Avoid close contact with people who are sick.
- Avoid touching your eyes, nose, and mouth with unwashed hands.
- Wash your hands often with soap and water for at least 20 seconds. Use an alcohol-based hand sanitizer that contains at least 60 percent alcohol if soap and water are not available.

If You Are Sick, to Keep from Spreading Respiratory Illness to Others, You Should

- Stay home when you are sick
- Cover your cough or sneeze with a tissue, then throw the tissue in the trash
- Clean and disinfect frequently touched objects and surfaces

What Should I Do If I Recently Traveled from an Area with Ongoing Spread of COVID-19?

If you have traveled from an affected area, there may be restrictions on your movements for up to 2 weeks. If you develop symptoms during that period (fever, cough, trouble breathing), seek medical advice. Call the office of your healthcare provider before you go, and tell them about your travel and your symptoms. They will give you instructions on how to get care without exposing other people to your illness. While sick, avoid contact with people, don't go out and delay any travel to reduce the possibility of spreading illness to others.

Is There a Vaccine?

There is currently no vaccine to protect against COVID-19. The best way to prevent infection is to take everyday preventive actions, like avoiding close contact with people who are sick and washing your hands often.

Is There a Treatment?

There is no specific antiviral treatment for COVID-19. People with COVID-19 can seek medical care to help relieve symptoms.

Section 5.4

Hantavirus Pulmonary Syndrome (HPS)

This section includes text excerpted from "Hantavirus,"
Centers for Disease Control and Prevention (CDC),
January 31, 2019.

Hantaviruses are a family of viruses spread mainly by rodents and can cause varied disease syndromes in people worldwide. Infection with any hantavirus can produce hantavirus disease in people. Hantaviruses in the Americas are known as "New World" hantaviruses and may cause hantavirus pulmonary syndrome (HPS). Other hantaviruses, known as "Old World" hantaviruses, are found mostly in Europe and Asia and may cause hemorrhagic fever with renal syndrome (HFRS).

Each hantavirus serotype has a specific rodent host species and is spread to people via aerosolized virus that is shed in urine, feces, and saliva, and less frequently by a bite from an infected host. The most important hantavirus in the United States that can cause HPS is the Sin Nombre virus, spread by the deer mouse.

About Hantavirus Pulmonary Syndrome

Hantavirus pulmonary syndrome is a severe, sometimes fatal, respiratory disease in humans caused by infection with hantaviruses.

Anyone who comes into contact with rodents that carry hantaviruses is at risk of HPS. Rodent infestation in and around the home remains the primary risk for hantavirus exposure. Even healthy individuals are at risk for HPS infection if exposed to the virus.

To date, no cases of HPS have been reported in the United States in which the virus was transmitted from one person to another. In fact, in a study of healthcare workers who were exposed to either patients or specimens infected with related types of hantaviruses (which cause a different disease in humans), none of the workers showed evidence of infection or illness.

In Chile and Argentina, rare cases of person-to-person transmission have occurred among close contacts of a person who was ill with a type of hantavirus called "Andes virus."

Transmission of Hantavirus Pulmonary Syndrome
How People Get Hantavirus Infection
Where Hantavirus Is Found

Cases of human hantavirus infection occur sporadically, usually in rural areas where forests, fields, and farms offer suitable habitat for the virus's rodent hosts. Areas around the home or work where rodents may live (for example, houses, barns, outbuildings, and sheds) are potential sites where people may be exposed to the virus. In the United States and Canada, the Sin Nombre hantavirus is responsible for the majority of cases of hantavirus infection. The host of the Sin Nombre virus is the deer mouse (*Peromyscus maniculatus*), present throughout the western and central U.S. and Canada.

Several other hantaviruses are capable of causing hantavirus infection in the United States. The New York hantavirus, carried by the white-footed mouse, is associated with HPS cases in the northeastern U.S. The Black Creek hantavirus, carried by the cotton rat, is found in the southeastern U.S. Cases of HPS have been confirmed elsewhere in the Americas, including Canada, Argentina, Bolivia, Brazil, Chile, Panama, Paraguay, and Uruguay.

How People Become Infected with Hantaviruses

In the United States, deer mice (along with cotton rats and rice rats in the southeastern states and the white-footed mouse in the Northeast) are reservoirs of the hantaviruses. The rodents shed the virus in their urine, droppings, and saliva. The virus is mainly transmitted to people when they breathe in air contaminated with the virus.

When fresh rodent urine, droppings, or nesting materials are stirred up, tiny droplets containing the virus get into the air. This process is known as "airborne transmission."

There are several other ways rodents may spread hantavirus to people:

- If a rodent with the virus bites someone, the virus may be spread to that person, but this type of transmission is rare.
- Scientists believe that people may be able to get the virus if they touch something that has been contaminated with rodent urine, droppings, or saliva, and then touch their nose or mouth.
- Scientists also suspect people can become sick if they eat food contaminated by urine, droppings, or saliva from an infected rodent.

The hantaviruses that cause human illness in the United States cannot be transmitted from one person to another. For example, you cannot get these viruses from touching or kissing a person who has HPS or from a healthcare worker who has treated someone with the disease.

In Chile and Argentina, rare cases of person-to-person transmission have occurred among close contacts of a person who was ill with a type of hantavirus called "Andes virus."

People at Risk for Hantavirus Infection

Anyone who comes into contact with rodents that carry hantavirus is at risk of HPS. Rodent infestation in and around the home remains the primary risk for hantavirus exposure. Even healthy individuals are at risk for HPS infection if exposed to the virus.

Any activity that puts you in contact with rodent droppings, urine, saliva, or nesting materials can place you at risk for infection. Hantavirus is spread when virus-containing particles from rodent urine, droppings, or saliva are stirred into the air. It is important to avoid actions that raise dust, such as sweeping or vacuuming. Infection occurs when you breathe in virus particles.

Potential Risk Activities for Hantavirus Infection
Opening and Cleaning Previously Unused Buildings

Opening or cleaning cabins, sheds, and outbuildings, including barns, garages and storage facilities, that have been closed during the winter is a potential risk for hantavirus infections, especially in rural settings.

Housecleaning Activities
Cleaning in and around your own home can put you at risk if rodents have made it their home too. Many homes can expect to shelter rodents, especially as the weather turns cold.

Work-Related Exposure
Construction, utility, and pest control workers can be exposed when they work in crawl spaces, under houses, or in vacant buildings that may have a rodent population.

Campers and Hikers
Campers and hikers can also be exposed when they use infested trail shelters or camp in other rodent habitats.

The chance of being exposed to hantavirus is greatest when people work, play, or live in closed spaces where rodents are actively living. However, recent research results show that many people who have become ill with HPS were infected with the disease after continued contact with rodents and/or their droppings. In addition, many people who have contracted HPS reported that they had not seen rodents or their droppings before becoming ill. Therefore, if you live in an area where the carrier rodents, such as the deer mouse, are known to live, take sensible precautions—even if you do not see rodents or their droppings.

Signs and Symptoms of Hantavirus Pulmonary Syndrome
Due to the small number of HPS cases, the "incubation time" is not positively known. However, on the basis of limited information, it appears that symptoms may develop between 1 and 8 weeks after exposure to fresh urine, droppings, or saliva of infected rodents.

Early Symptoms
Early symptoms include fatigue, fever, and muscle aches, especially in the large muscle groups—thighs, hips, back, and sometimes shoulders. These symptoms are universal.

There may also be headaches, dizziness, chills, and abdominal problems, such as nausea, vomiting, diarrhea, and abdominal pain. About half of all HPS patients experience these symptoms.

Late Symptoms

Four to 10 days after the initial phase of illness, the late symptoms of HPS appear. These include coughing and shortness of breath, with the sensation of, as one survivor put it, a "…tight band around my chest and a pillow over my face" as the lungs fill with fluid.

Is the Disease Fatal?

Yes. HPS can be fatal. It has a mortality rate of 38 percent.

Diagnosis and Treatment of Hantavirus Pulmonary Syndrome
Diagnosing Hantavirus Pulmonary Syndrome

Diagnosing HPS in an individual who has only been infected a few days is difficult, because early symptoms such as fever, muscle aches, and fatigue are easily confused with influenza. However, if the individual is experiencing fever and fatigue and has a history of potential rural rodent exposure, together with shortness of breath, would be strongly suggestive of HPS. If the individual is experiencing these symptoms they should see their physician immediately and mention their potential rodent exposure.

Treating Hantavirus Pulmonary Syndrome

There is no specific treatment, cure, or vaccine for hantavirus infection. However, it is known that if infected individuals are recognized early and receive medical care in an intensive care unit, they may do better. In intensive care, patients are intubated and given oxygen therapy to help them through the period of severe respiratory distress.

The earlier the patient is brought in to intensive care, the better. If a patient is experiencing full distress, it is less likely the treatment will be effective.

Therefore, if you have been around rodents and have symptoms of fever, deep muscle aches, and severe shortness of breath, see your doctor immediately. Be sure to tell your doctor that you have been around rodents—this will alert your physician to look closely for any rodent-carried disease, such as HPS.

Prevention of Hantavirus Pulmonary Syndrome

Eliminate or minimize contact with rodents in your home, workplace, or campsite. If rodents do not find that where you are is a good place for them to be, then you're less likely to come into contact with them. Seal up holes and gaps in your home or garage. Place traps in and around your home to decrease rodent infestation. Clean up any easy-to-get food.

Recent research results show that many people who became ill with HPS developed the disease after having been in frequent contact with rodents and/or their droppings around a home or a workplace. On the other hand, many people who became ill reported that they had not seen rodents or rodent droppings at all. Therefore, if you live in an area where the carrier rodents are known to live, try to keep your home, vacation place, workplace, or campsite clean.

Section 5.5

Ebola Virus Disease (EVD)

This section includes text excerpted from "Ebola
(Ebola Virus Disease)—What Is Ebola Virus Disease?"
Centers for Disease Control and Prevention (CDC),
October 28, 2019

What Is Ebola Virus Disease?

Ebola virus disease (EVD) is a deadly disease with occasional outbreaks that occur primarily on the African continent. EVD most commonly affects people and nonhuman primates (such as monkeys, gorillas, and chimpanzees). It is caused by an infection with a group of viruses within the genus *ebolavirus*.

- Ebola virus (species *Zaire ebolavirus*)
- Sudan virus (species *Sudan ebolavirus*)
- Taï Forest virus (species *Taï Forest ebolavirus*, formerly *Côte d'Ivoire ebolavirus*)
- Bundibugyo virus (species *Bundibugyo ebolavirus*)
- Reston virus (species *Reston ebolavirus*)
- Bombali virus (species *Bombali ebolavirus*)

Of these, only four (Ebola, Sudan, Taï Forest, and Bundibugyo viruses) are known to cause disease in people. Reston virus is known to cause disease in nonhuman primates and pigs, but not in people. It is unknown if Bombali virus, which was recently identified in bats, causes disease in either animals or people.

Ebola virus was first discovered in 1976 near the Ebola River in what is now the Democratic Republic of Congo. Since then, the virus has been infecting people from time to time, leading to outbreaks in several African countries. Scientists do not know where Ebola virus comes from. However, based on the nature of similar viruses, they believe the virus is animal-borne, with bats or nonhuman primates (chimpanzees, apes, monkeys, etc.) being the most likely source. Infected animals carrying the virus can transmit it to other animals, like apes, monkeys, duikers, and humans.

The virus spreads to people initially through direct contact with the blood, body fluids, and tissues of animals. Ebola virus then spreads to other people through direct contact with body fluids of a person who is sick with or has died from EVD. This can occur when a person touches these infected body fluids (or objects that are contaminated with them), and the virus gets in through broken skin or mucous membranes in the eyes, nose, or mouth. People can get the virus through sexual contact with someone who is sick with EVD, and also after recovery from EVD. The virus can persist in certain body fluids, like semen, after recovery from the illness.

Ebola survivors may experience side effects after their recovery, such as tiredness, muscle aches, eye and vision problems, and stomach pain.

Transmission of Ebola Virus Disease

Scientists think people are initially infected with Ebola virus through contact with an infected animal, such as a fruit bat or nonhuman primate. This is called a "spillover event." After that, the virus spreads from person to person, potentially affecting a large number of people.

The virus spreads through direct contact (such as through broken skin or mucous membranes in the eyes, nose, or mouth) with:

- Blood or body fluids (urine, saliva, sweat, feces, vomit, breast milk, and semen) of a person who is sick with or has died from Ebola virus disease (EVD)
- Objects (such as clothes, bedding, needles, and medical equipment) contaminated with body fluids from a person who is sick with or has died from EVD
- Infected fruit bats or nonhuman primates (such as apes and monkeys)
- Semen from a man who recovered from EVD (through oral, vaginal, or anal sex). The virus can remain in certain body fluids (including semen) of a patient who has recovered from EVD, even if they no longer have symptoms of severe illness. There is no evidence that

Ebola can be spread through sex or other contact with vaginal fluids from a woman who has had Ebola.

When people become infected with Ebola, they do not start developing signs or symptoms right away. This period between exposure to an illness and having symptoms is known as the "incubation period." A person can only spread Ebola to other people after they develop signs and symptoms of Ebola.

Additionally, Ebola virus is not known to be transmitted through food. However, in certain parts of the world, Ebola virus may spread through the handling and consumption of wild animal meat or hunted wild animals infected with Ebola. There is no evidence that mosquitoes or other insects can transmit Ebola virus.

Risk

- Health workers who do not use proper infection control while caring for Ebola patients, and family and friends in close contact with Ebola patients, are at the highest risk of getting sick. Ebola can spread when people come into contact with infected blood or body fluids.
- Ebola poses little risk to travelers or the general public who have not cared for or been in close contact (within 3 feet or 1 meter) with someone sick with Ebola.

Persistence of the Virus

The virus can remain in areas of the body that are immunologically privileged sites after acute infection. These are sites where viruses and pathogens, like the Ebola virus, are shielded from the survivor's immune system, even after being cleared elsewhere in the body. These areas include the testes, interior of the eyes, placenta, and central nervous system, particularly the cerebrospinal fluid. Whether the virus is present in these body parts and for how long varies by survivor. Scientists are now studying how long the virus stays in these body fluids among Ebola survivors.

During an Ebola outbreak, the virus can spread quickly within healthcare settings (such as clinics or hospitals). Clinicians and other healthcare personnel providing care should use dedicated, preferably disposable, medical equipment. Proper cleaning and disposal of instruments such as needles and syringes are important. If instruments are not disposable, they must be sterilized before using again.

Ebola virus can survive on dry surfaces, like doorknobs and countertops for several hours; in body fluids like blood, the virus can survive up to several days at room temperature. Cleaning and disinfection should be performed using a hospital-grade disinfectant.

Signs and Symptoms of Ebola Virus Disease

Symptoms may appear anywhere from 2 to 21 days after contact with the virus, with an average of 8 to 10 days. The course of the illness typically progresses from "dry" symptoms initially (such as fever, aches and pains, and fatigue), and then progresses to "wet" symptoms (such as diarrhea and vomiting) as the person becomes sicker.

Primary signs and symptoms of Ebola often include some or several of the following:

- Fever
- Aches and pains, such as severe headache, muscle and joint pain, and abdominal (stomach) pain
- Weakness and fatigue
- Gastrointestinal symptoms including diarrhea and vomiting
- Abdominal (stomach) pain
- Unexplained hemorrhaging, bleeding, or bruising

Other symptoms may include red eyes, skin rash, and hiccups (late stage).

Many common illnesses can have the same symptoms as EVD, including influenza (flu), malaria, or typhoid fever.

EVD is a rare but severe and often deadly disease. Recovery from EVD depends on good supportive clinical care and the patient's immune response. Studies show that survivors of Ebola virus infection have antibodies (proteins made by the immune system that identify and neutralize invading viruses) that can be detected in the blood up to 10 years after recovery.

Survivors are thought to have some protective immunity to the type of Ebola that sickened them.

Prevention and Vaccine of Ebola Virus Disease

In the United States, Ebola virus disease (EVD) is a very rare disease that has only occurred because of cases that were acquired in other countries, eventually followed by person-to-person transmission. EVD is most common in parts of sub-Saharan Africa, with occasional outbreaks occurring in people. In these areas, Ebola virus is believed to circulate at low rates in certain animal populations (enzootic). Occasionally, people become sick with Ebola after coming into contact with these infected animals, which can then lead to Ebola outbreaks where the virus spreads between people.

When living in or traveling to a region where Ebola virus is present, there are a number of ways to protect yourself and prevent the spread of EVD—

- Contact with blood and body fluids (such as urine, feces, saliva, sweat, vomit, breast milk, semen, and vaginal fluids) of persons who are ill.
- Contact with semen from a man who has recovered from EVD, until testing verifies the virus is gone from the semen.
- Items that may have come in contact with an infected person's blood or body fluids (such as clothes, bedding, needles, and medical equipment).
- Funeral or burial rituals that require handling the body of someone who died from EVD.
- Contact with bats and nonhuman primates' blood, fluids, or raw meat prepared from these animals (bushmeat).
- Contact with the raw meat of an unknown source.

These same prevention methods apply when living in or traveling to an area affected by an Ebola outbreak. After returning from an area affected by Ebola, monitor your health for 21 days and seek medical care immediately if you develop symptoms of EVD.

Ebola Vaccine

The U.S. Food and Drug Administration (FDA) approved the Ebola vaccine rVSV-ZEBOV (tradename "Ervebo") on December 19, 2019. The rVSV-ZEBOV vaccine is a single dose vaccine regimen that has been found to be safe and protective against only the *Zaire ebolavirus* species of ebolavirus. This is the first FDA approval of a vaccine for Ebola.

Another investigational vaccine was developed and introduced under a research protocol in 2019 to combat an Ebola outbreak in the Democratic Republic of the Congo. This vaccine leverages two different vaccine components (Ad26.ZEBOV and MVA-BN-Filo) and requires two doses with an initial dose followed by a second "booster" dose 56 days later. The second vaccine is also designed to protect against only the *Zaire ebolavirus* species of Ebola.

Diagnosis of Ebola Virus Disease

Diagnosing Ebola virus disease (EVD) shortly after infection can be difficult. Early symptoms of EVD such as fever, headache, and weakness are not specific to Ebola virus infection and often are seen in patients with other more common diseases, like malaria and typhoid fever.

To determine whether EVD is a possible diagnosis, there must be a combination of symptoms suggestive of EVD AND a possible exposure to EVD within 21 days before the onset of symptoms. An exposure may include contact with:

- Blood or body fluids from a person sick with or who died from EVD,
- Objects contaminated with blood or body fluids of a person sick with or who died from EVD,
- Infected fruit bats and nonhuman primates (apes or monkeys), or
- Semen from a man who has recovered from EVD.

If a person shows signs of EVD and has had a possible exposure, she or he should be isolated (separated from other people) and public-health authorities notified. Blood samples from the patient should be collected and tested to confirm infection. Ebola virus can be detected in blood after onset of symptoms. It may take up to three days after symptoms start for the virus to reach detectable levels.

Polymerase chain reaction (PCR) is one of the most commonly used diagnostic methods because of its ability to detect low levels of Ebola virus. PCR methods can detect the presence of a few virus particles in small amounts of blood, but the ability to detect the virus increases as the amount of virus increases during an active infection. When the virus is no longer present in great enough numbers in a patient's blood, PCR methods will no longer be effective. Other methods, based on the detection of antibodies an EVD case produces to an infection, can then be used to confirm a patient's exposure and infection by Ebola virus.

A positive laboratory test means that Ebola infection is confirmed. Public-health authorities will conduct a public-health investigation, including identifying and monitoring all possibly exposed contacts.

Treatment of Ebola Virus Disease

Symptoms of Ebola virus disease (EVD) are treated as they appear. When used early, basic interventions can significantly improve the chances of survival. These include:

- Providing fluids and electrolytes (body salts) through infusion into the vein (intravenously).
- Offering oxygen therapy to maintain oxygen status.
- Using medication to support blood pressure, reduce vomiting and diarrhea, and to manage fever and pain.
- Treating other infections, if they occur.

Antiviral Drugs

There is currently no antiviral drug licensed by the U.S. Food and Drug Administration (FDA) to treat EVD in people.

During the 2018 eastern Democratic Republic of the Congo outbreak, four investigational treatments were initially available to treat patients with confirmed Ebola. For two of those treatments, called "Regeneron"

(REGN-EB3) and "mAb114," overall survival rate was much higher. These two antiviral drugs currently remain in use for patients with confirmed Ebola.

Drugs that are being developed to treat EVD work by stopping the virus from making copies of itself.

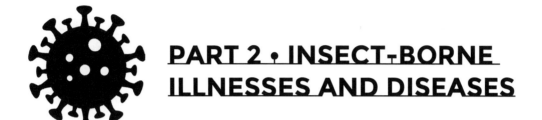

PART 2 • INSECT-BORNE ILLNESSES AND DISEASES

CHAPTER 6
What Are Vector-Borne Diseases?

Vector-borne diseases are illnesses that are transmitted by vectors, which include mosquitoes, ticks, and fleas. These vectors can carry infective pathogens, such as viruses, bacteria, and protozoa, which can be transferred from one host to another. In the United States, there are currently 14 vector-borne diseases that are of national public-health concern. These diseases account for a significant number of human illnesses and deaths each year and are required to be reported to the National Notifiable Diseases Surveillance System (NNDSS) at the Centers for Disease Control and Prevention (CDC). In 2013, state and local health departments reported 51,258 vector-borne disease cases to the CDC.

Vectors and hosts involved in the transmission of these infective pathogens are sensitive to climate change and other environmental factors which, together, affect vector-borne diseases by influencing one or more of the following: vector and host survival, reproduction, development, activity, distribution, and abundance; pathogen development, replication, maintenance, and transmission; geographic range of pathogens, vectors, and hosts; human behavior; and disease outbreak frequency, onset, and distribution.

This chapter includes text excerpted from "Vector-Borne Diseases," GlobalChange. gov, U.S. Global Change Research Program (USGCRP), December 15, 2005. Reviewed March 2020.

The seasonality, distribution, and prevalence of vector-borne diseases are influenced significantly by climate factors, primarily high- and low-temperature extremes and precipitation patterns. Climate change can result in modified weather patterns and an increase in extreme events that can affect disease outbreaks by altering biological variables, such as vector population size and density, vector survival rates, the relative abundance of disease-carrying animal-reservoir hosts, and pathogen reproduction rates. Collectively, these changes may contribute to an increase in the risk of the pathogen being transmitted to humans.

Climate change is likely to have both short- and long-term effects on vector-borne disease transmission and infection patterns, affecting both seasonal risk and broad geographic changes in disease occurrence over decades. However, models for predicting the effects of climate change on vector-borne diseases are subject to a high degree of uncertainty, largely due to two factors:

- Vector-borne diseases are maintained in nature in complex transmission cycles that involve vectors, other intermediate zoonotic hosts, and humans.
- There are a number of other significant social and environmental drivers of vector-borne disease transmission in addition to climate change.

For example, while climate variability and climate change both alter the transmission of vector-borne diseases, they will likely interact with many other factors, including how pathogens adapt and change, the availability of hosts, changing ecosystems and land use, demographics, human behavior, and adaptive capacity. These complex interactions make it difficult to predict the effects of climate change on vector-borne diseases.

The risk of introducing exotic pathogens and vectors not present in the United States, while likely to occur, is similarly difficult to project quantitatively. Several important vector-borne pathogens have been introduced or reintroduced into the United States. These include West Nile virus, dengue virus, and chikungunya virus. In the case of the 2009 dengue outbreak in southern Florida, climate change was not responsible for the reintroduction of the virus in this area, which arrived via infected travelers from disease-endemic regions of the Caribbean. In fact, vector populations capable of transmitting dengue have been present for many years throughout much of the southern United States, including Florida. Climate change has the potential to increase human exposure risk or disease transmission following shifts in extended spring and summer seasons as dengue becomes more established in the United States. Climate change effects, however, are difficult to quantify due to the adaptive capacity of a population that may reduce exposure to vector-borne pathogens through such means as air conditioning, screens on windows, vector control, and public-health practices.

The CDC completes case studies of Lyme disease and West Nile virus infection in relation to weather and climate. Although ticks and mosquitoes transmit multiple infectious pathogens to humans in the United States, Lyme disease and West Nile virus infection are the most commonly reported tick-borne and mosquito-borne diseases in this country. In addition, a substantial number of studies have been conducted to elucidate the role of climate in the transmission of these infectious pathogens. These broad findings, together with the areas of uncertainty from these case studies, are generalizable to other vector-borne diseases.

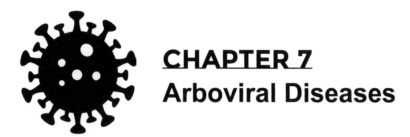

CHAPTER 7
Arboviral Diseases

Chapter Contents

Chikungunya Virus

This section includes text excerpted from
"Chikungunya Virus," Centers for Disease Control and
Prevention (CDC), September 19, 2019.

Chikungunya virus is spread to people by the bite of an infected mosquito. The most common symptoms of infection are fever and joint pain. Other symptoms may include headache, muscle pain, joint swelling, or rash. Outbreaks have occurred in countries, such as on the continents of Africa, Asia, Europe, and those bordering the Indian and Pacific Oceans. In late 2013, chikungunya virus was found for the first time in the Americas on islands in the Caribbean. There is a risk that the virus will be imported to new areas by infected travelers. There is no vaccine to prevent or medicine to treat chikungunya virus infection. Travelers can protect themselves by preventing mosquito bites. When traveling to countries with chikungunya virus, use insect repellent, wear long sleeves and pants, and stay in places with air conditioning or that use window and door screens.

Transmission of Chikungunya Virus
Through Mosquito Bites
- Chikungunya virus is transmitted to people through mosquito bites. Mosquitoes become infected when they feed on a person already infected with the virus. Infected mosquitoes can then spread the virus to other people through bites.
- Chikungunya virus is most often spread to people by *Aedes aegypti* and *Aedes albopictus* mosquitoes. These are the same mosquitoes that transmit dengue virus. They bite during the day and at night.

Rarely, from Mother to Child
- Chikungunya virus is transmitted rarely from mother to newborn around the time of birth.

- To date, no infants have been found to be infected with chikungunya virus through breastfeeding. Because of the benefits of breastfeeding, mothers are encouraged to breastfeed even in areas where chikungunya virus is circulating.

Rarely, through Infected Blood

- In theory, the virus could be spread through a blood transfusion. To date, there are no known reports of this happening.

Symptoms of Chikungunya Virus

Most people infected with chikungunya virus will develop some symptoms that usually begin three to seven days after being bitten by an infected mosquito.

- The most common symptoms are fever and joint pain.
- Other symptoms may include headache, muscle pain, joint swelling, or rash.
- Chikungunya disease does not often result in death, but the symptoms can be severe and disabling.
- Most patients feel better within a week. In some people, the joint pain may persist for months.
- People at risk for more severe disease include newborns infected around the time of birth, older adults ($\geq$65 years), and people with medical conditions such as high blood pressure, diabetes, or heart disease.
- Once a person has been infected, she or he is likely to be protected from future infections.

Diagnosis of Chikungunya Virus

- The symptoms of chikungunya are similar to those of dengue and Zika, diseases spread by the same mosquitoes that transmit chikungunya.
- See your healthcare provider if you develop the symptoms described above and have visited an area where chikungunya is found.
- If you have recently traveled, tell your healthcare provider when and where you traveled.

- Your healthcare provider may order blood tests to look for chikungunya or other similar viruses such as dengue and Zika.

Treatment of Chikungunya Virus

There is no vaccine to prevent or medicine to treat chikungunya virus. Ways to treat the symptoms include:

- Get plenty of rest.
- Drink fluids to prevent dehydration.
- Take medicine such as acetaminophen (Tylenol®) or paracetamol to reduce fever and pain.
- Do not take aspirin and other nonsteroidal anti-inflammatory drugs (NSAIDs) until dengue can be ruled out to reduce the risk of bleeding.
- If you are taking medicine for another medical condition, talk to your healthcare provider before taking additional medication.
- If you have chikungunya, prevent mosquito bites for the first week of your illness.
  - During the first week of infection, chikungunya virus can be found in the blood and passed from an infected person to a mosquito through mosquito bites.
  - An infected mosquito can then spread the virus to other people.

Section 7.2
West Nile Virus

This section includes text excerpted from "West Nile Virus," Centers for Disease Control and Prevention (CDC), November 12, 2019.

West Nile virus (WNV) is the leading cause of mosquito-borne disease in the continental United States. It is most commonly spread to people by the bite of an infected mosquito. Cases of WNV occur during mosquito season, which starts in the summer and continues through fall. There are no vaccines to prevent or medications to treat WNV in people. Fortunately, most people infected with WNV do not feel sick. About 1 in 5 people who are infected develop a fever and other symptoms. About 1 in 150 infected people develop a serious, and sometimes fatal, illness. You can reduce your risk of WNV by using insect repellent and wearing long-sleeved shirts and long pants to prevent mosquito bites.

Transmission of West Nile Virus

West Nile Virus is most commonly spread to people by the bite of an infected mosquito.

Mosquitoes become infected when they feed on infected birds. Infected mosquitoes then spread WNV to people and other animals by biting them.

In a very small number of cases, WNV has been spread through:
- Exposure in a laboratory setting
- Blood transfusion and organ donation
- Mother to baby, during pregnancy, delivery, or breastfeeding

West Nile virus is not spread:
- Through coughing, sneezing, or touching
- By touching live animals
- From handling live or dead infected birds. Avoid bare-handed contact when handling any dead animal. If you are disposing of a dead bird, use gloves or double plastic bags to place the carcass in a garbage can.

- Through eating infected birds or animals. Always follow instructions for fully cooking meat from either birds or mammals.

West Nile Virus and Dead Birds

West Nile virus has been detected in a variety of bird species. Some infected birds, especially crows and jays, are known to get sick and die from the infection. Reporting and testing of dead birds is one way to check for the presence of WNV in the environment. Some surveillance programs rely on citizens to report dead bird sightings to local authorities.

How Do Birds Get Infected with West Nile Virus?

West Nile virus is transmitted to birds through the bite of infected mosquitoes. Mosquitoes become infected by biting infected birds. Some birds that are predators (such as hawks and owls) or scavengers (such as crows) may become infected after eating sick or dead birds that were already infected with West Nile virus.

Do Birds Infected with West Nile Virus Die or Become Ill?

Yes. Since WNV was discovered in the United States in 1999, the virus has been detected in over 300 species of dead birds. Although some infected birds, especially crows and jays, frequently die of infection, most birds survive.

Can You Get West Nile Virus Directly from Birds?

There is no evidence that a person can get infected from handling live or dead infected birds. However, you should avoid bare-handed contact when handling any dead animal. If you must pick up a dead bird, use gloves or an inverted plastic bag to place the bird's carcass (body) in a garbage bag.

What Should You Do If You Find a Dead Bird?

State and local agencies have different policies for collecting and testing birds, so check with your state health department or state wildlife agency for information about reporting dead birds in your area. Wildlife agencies routinely investigate sick or dead bird events if large numbers are impacted. This type of reporting could help with the early detection of illnesses such as WNV or Avian influenza (bird flu), known to cause death in birds. If local authorities tell you to simply dispose of the bird's carcass (body), do not handle it with your bare hands. Use gloves or an inverted plastic bag to place the carcass in a garbage bag, which can then be disposed of in your regular trash.

Call or contact the U.S. Department of Agriculture's (USDA) Wildlife Services (WS) office at 866-4-USDA-WS (866-487-3297) for more information.

Symptoms of West Nile Virus

There are no symptoms in most people. Most people (8 in 10) infected with West Nile virus do not develop any symptoms.

Febrile illness (fever) in some people. About 1 in 5 people who are infected develop a fever with other symptoms, such as headache, body aches, joint pains, vomiting, diarrhea, or rash. Most people with this type of WNV disease recover completely, but fatigue and weakness can last for weeks or months.

Serious symptoms in a few people. About 1 in 150 people who are infected develop a severe illness affecting the central nervous system, such as encephalitis (inflammation of the brain) or meningitis (inflammation of the membranes that surround the brain and spinal cord).

- Symptoms of severe illness include high fever, headache, neck stiffness, stupor, disorientation, coma, tremors, convulsions, muscle weakness, vision loss, numbness, and paralysis.
- Severe illness can occur in people of any age; however, people over 60 years of age are at greater risk. People with certain medical conditions, such as cancer, diabetes, hypertension, kidney disease, and people who have received organ transplants, are also at greater risk.
- Recovery from severe illness might take several weeks or months. Some effects to the central nervous system might be permanent.
- About 1 out of 10 people who develop severe illness affecting the central nervous system die.

Diagnosis of West Nile Virus

- See your healthcare provider if you develop the symptoms described above.
- Your healthcare provider can order tests to look for WNV infection.

Treatment of West Nile Virus

- No vaccine or specific antiviral treatments for WNV infection are available.
- Over-the-counter (OTC) pain relievers can be used to reduce fever and relieve some symptoms.
- In severe cases, patients often need to be hospitalized to receive supportive treatment, such as intravenous (IV) fluids, pain medication, and medical care.
- If you think you or a family member might have WNV disease, talk with your healthcare provider.

Section 7.3

Yellow Fever Virus

This section includes text excerpted from
"Yellow Fever," Centers for Disease Control and
Prevention (CDC), January 15, 2019.

The yellow fever virus is found in tropical and subtropical areas of Africa and South America. The virus is spread to people by the bite of an infected mosquito. Yellow fever is a very rare cause of illness in U.S. travelers.

Illness ranges from a fever with aches and pains to severe liver disease with bleeding and yellowing skin (jaundice). Yellow fever infection is diagnosed based on laboratory testing, a person's symptoms, and travel history. There is no medicine to treat or cure infection. To prevent getting sick from yellow fever, use insect repellent, wear long-sleeved shirts and long pants, and get vaccinated.

Transmission of Yellow Fever Virus

Yellow fever virus is an RNA virus that belongs to the genus *Flavivirus*. It is related to West Nile virus, and to St. Louis and Japanese encephalitis viruses. Yellow fever virus is transmitted to people primarily through the bite of infected *Aedes* or *Haemagogus* species mosquitoes. Mosquitoes acquire the virus by feeding on infected primates (human or nonhuman) and then can transmit the virus to other primates (human or nonhuman). People infected with yellow fever virus are infectious to mosquitoes (referred to as being "viremic") shortly before the onset of fever and up to five days after onset.

Yellow fever virus has three transmission cycles: jungle (sylvatic), intermediate (savannah), and urban.

- The jungle (sylvatic) cycle involves transmission of the virus between nonhuman primates (e.g., monkeys) and mosquito species found in the forest canopy. The virus is transmitted by mosquitoes from monkeys to humans when humans are visiting or working in the jungle.
- In Africa, an intermediate (savannah) cycle exists that involves transmission of virus from mosquitoes to humans living or working in jungle border areas. In this cycle, the virus can be transmitted from monkey to human or from human to human via mosquitoes.
- The urban cycle involves transmission of the virus between humans and urban mosquitoes, primarily *Aedes aegypti*. The virus is usually brought to the urban setting by a viremic human who was infected in the jungle or savannah.

Symptoms of Yellow Fever Virus

The majority of people infected with yellow fever virus will either not have symptoms, or will have mild symptoms and completely recover.

For people who develop symptoms, the time from infection until illness is typically three to six days.

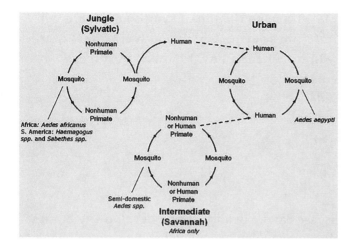

Figure 7.1. Transmission Cycle of Yellow Fever Virus

Because there is a risk of severe disease, all people who develop symptoms of yellow fever after traveling to or living in an area at risk for the virus should see their healthcare provider. Once you have been infected, you are likely to be protected from future infections.

- Most people will not have symptoms.
- Some people will develop yellow fever illness with initial symptoms including:
  - Sudden onset of fever
  - Chills
  - Severe headache
  - Back pain
  - General body aches
  - Nausea
  - Vomiting
  - Fatigue (feeling tired)
  - Weakness
  - Most people with the initial symptoms improve within one week.
  - For some people who recover, weakness and fatigue (feeling tired) might last several months.
- A few people will develop a more severe form of the disease.

- For 1 out of 7 people who have the initial symptoms, there will be a brief remission (a time during which you feel better) that may last only a few hours or for a day, followed by a more severe form of the disease.
- Severe symptoms include:
  - High fever
  - Yellow skin (jaundice)
  - Bleeding
  - Shock
  - Organ failure
- Severe yellow fever disease can be deadly. If you develop any of these symptoms, see a healthcare provider immediately.
- Among those who develop severe disease, 30 to 60 percent die.

Diagnosis of Yellow Fever Virus

Yellow fever infection is diagnosed based on laboratory testing, a person's symptoms, and travel history.

Treatment of Yellow Fever Virus

- There is no medicine to treat or cure infection from yellow fever.
- Rest, drink fluids, and use pain relievers and medication to reduce fever and relieve aching.
- Avoid certain medications, such as aspirin or other nonsteroidal anti-inflammatory drugs (NSAIDs), for example ibuprofen (Advil, Motrin), or naproxen (Aleve), which may increase the risk of bleeding.
- People with severe symptoms of yellow fever infection should be hospitalized for close observation and supportive care.
- If after returning from travel you have symptoms of yellow fever (usually about a week after being bitten by an infected mosquito), protect yourself from mosquito bites for up to five days after symptoms begin. This will help prevent spreading yellow fever to uninfected mosquitoes that can spread the virus to other people.

Yellow Fever Vaccine

A safe and effective yellow fever vaccine has been available for more than 80 years.

- A single dose provides lifelong protection for most people.
- The vaccine is a live, weakened form of the virus given as a single shot.
- Vaccine is recommended for people nine months of age or older and who are traveling to or living in areas at risk for yellow fever virus in Africa and South America.
- Yellow fever vaccine may be required for entry into certain countries.

Yellow Fever Vaccine Recommendations

Yellow fever vaccine is recommended for people who are nine months of age or older and who are traveling to or living in areas at risk for yellow fever virus in Africa and South America.

For most people, a single dose of yellow fever vaccine provides long-lasting protection and a booster dose of the vaccine is not needed. However, travelers going to areas with ongoing outbreaks may consider getting a booster dose of yellow fever vaccine if it has been 10 years or more since they were last vaccinated. Certain countries might also require a booster dose of the vaccine.

Talk to your healthcare provider to determine if you need a yellow fever vaccination or a booster shot before your trip to an area at risk for yellow fever.

Some people may have an increased risk of developing a reaction to the vaccine, but may still benefit from being vaccinated. These people, or their guardians, should talk to a healthcare provider about getting vaccinated:

- Between 6 and 8 months old
- Over 60 years old
- Pregnant
- Breastfeeding

A few people should not get vaccinated. Vaccine is not recommended for people who are:

- Allergic to a vaccine or something in the vaccine (such as eggs)
- 6 months of age or younger
- Organ-transplant recipients
- Diagnosed with a malignant tumor
- Diagnosed with thymus disorder associated with abnormal immune function
- Diagnosed with a primary immunodeficiency
- Using immunosuppressive and immunomodulatory therapies
- Showing symptoms of human immunodeficiency virus (HIV) infection or CD4+ T-lymphocytes less than $200/mm^3$ (less than 15% of total lymphocytes in children 6 years of age or younger)

It is important to remember that the Centers for Disease Control and Prevention's (CDC) vaccine recommendations are not the same as a country's entry requirements. Proof of yellow fever vaccine may be required for entry into certain countries.

Reactions to Yellow Fever Vaccine

Reactions to yellow fever vaccine are generally mild and include headaches, muscle aches, and low-grade fevers. Rarely, people develop severe and sometimes life-threatening reactions to the yellow fever vaccine, including:

- Allergic reaction, including difficulty breathing or swallowing (anaphylaxis)
- Swelling of the brain, spinal cord, or the surrounding tissues (encephalitis or meningitis)
- Guillain-Barré syndrome (GBS), an uncommon sickness of the nervous system in which a person's own immune system damages the nerve cells, causing muscle weakness, and sometimes, paralysis.
- Internal organ dysfunction or failure

If you recently received the yellow fever vaccination and develop fever, headache, tiredness, body aches, vomiting, or diarrhea, see your healthcare provider.

Yellow Fever Vaccine, Pregnancy, and Conception

Yellow fever vaccine has been given to many pregnant women without any apparent adverse effects on the fetus. However, since yellow fever vaccine is a live virus vaccine, it poses a theoretical risk.

Pregnant women should avoid or postpone travel to an area where there is risk of yellow fever. If travel cannot be avoided, discuss vaccination with your doctor.

While a two-week delay between yellow fever vaccination and conception is probably adequate, a one-month delay has been advocated as a more conservative approach.

If, for some reason, a woman is vaccinated during pregnancy, she is unlikely to have any problems from the vaccine and her baby is very likely to be born healthy.

Section 7.4

Zika Virus

This section includes text excerpted from
"About Zika," Centers for Disease Control and
Prevention (CDC), May 20, 2019.

Zika is spread mostly by the bite of an infected *Aedes* species mosquito (*Ae. aegypti* and *Ae. albopictus*). These mosquitoes bite during the day and night. Zika can be passed from a pregnant woman to her fetus. Infection during pregnancy can cause certain birth defects. There is no vaccine or medicine for Zika.

History of Zika

Zika virus was first discovered in 1947 and is named after the Zika Forest in Uganda. In 1952, the first human cases of Zika were detected and since then, outbreaks of Zika have been reported in tropical Africa, Southeast Asia, and the Pacific Islands. Zika outbreaks have probably occurred in many locations. Before 2007, at least 14 cases of Zika had been documented, although other cases were likely to have occurred and were not reported. Because the symptoms of Zika are similar to those of many other diseases, many cases may not have been recognized.

Zika Transmission
Through Mosquito Bites

Zika virus is transmitted to people primarily through the bite of an infected *Aedes* species mosquito (*Ae. aegypti* and *Ae. albopictus*). These are the same mosquitoes that spread dengue and chikungunya viruses.

- These mosquitoes typically lay eggs in or near standing water in things such as buckets, bowls, animal dishes, flower pots, and vases. They prefer to bite people, and live indoors and outdoors near people.
- Mosquitoes spread chikungunya, dengue, and Zika bite during the day and night.
- A mosquito gets infected with a virus when it bites an infected person during the period of time when the virus can be found in the person's blood, typically only through the first week of infection.
- Infected mosquitoes can then spread the virus to other people through bites.

From Mother to Child

- A pregnant woman can pass Zika virus to her fetus during pregnancy. Zika is a cause of microcephaly and other severe fetal brain defects. Researchers are studying the full range of other potential health problems that Zika virus infection may cause during pregnancy.
- A pregnant woman already infected with Zika virus can pass the virus to her fetus during the pregnancy or around the time of birth.
- Zika virus has been found in breast milk. Possible Zika virus infections have been identified in breastfeeding babies, but Zika virus transmission through breast milk has not been confirmed. Additionally, researchers do not yet know the long-term effects of Zika virus on young infants

infected after birth. Because current evidence suggests that the benefits of breastfeeding outweigh the risk of Zika virus spreading through breast milk, the Centers for Disease Control and Prevention (CDC) continues to encourage mothers to breastfeed, even if they were infected or lived in or traveled to an area with risk of Zika. The CDC continues to study Zika virus and the ways it can spread and will update recommendations as information becomes available.

Through Sex

- Zika can be passed through sex from a person who has Zika to her or his partners. Zika can be passed through sex, even if the infected person does not have symptoms at the time.
  - It can be passed from a person with Zika before their symptoms start, while they have symptoms, and after their symptoms end.
  - Though not well documented, the virus may also be passed by a person who carries the virus, but never develops symptoms.
- Studies are underway to find out how long Zika stays in the semen and vaginal fluids of people who have Zika, and how long it can be passed to sex partners. Zika can remain in semen longer than in other body fluids, including vaginal fluids, urine, and blood.

Through Blood Transfusion

- To date, there have not been any confirmed blood-transfusion transmission cases in the United States.
- There have been multiple reports of possible blood-transfusion transmission cases in Brazil.
- During the French Polynesian outbreak, 2.8 percent of blood donors tested positive for Zika and in previous outbreaks, the virus has been found in blood donors.

Through Laboratory and Healthcare-Setting Exposure

- There are reports of laboratory-acquired Zika virus infections, although the route of transmission was not clearly established in all cases.

- To date, no cases of Zika virus transmission in healthcare settings have been identified in the United States. Recommendations are available for healthcare providers to help prevent exposure to Zika virus in healthcare settings.

Risks

- Anyone who lives in or travels to an area with risk of Zika and has not already been infected with Zika virus can get it from mosquito bites. Once a person has been infected, she or he is likely to be protected from future infections.

Zika in Animals

Nonhuman primates (for example, apes and monkeys) can become infected with Zika. Zika was first discovered in a monkey with a mild fever in the Zika Forest of Uganda in the 1940s. The CDC does not know how often apes and monkeys are infected with Zika. A few studies suggest that apes and monkeys infected with Zika may have a fever or mild symptoms. More research is needed to better understand the role apes and monkeys play in spreading Zika to people.

Limited studies show that apes and monkeys infected with Zika during pregnancy can develop severe fetal brain defects.

One study done in Indonesia in the late 1970s showed that horses, cows, carabaos (water buffaloes), goats, ducks, and bats could become infected with Zika, but there is no evidence that they get sick or can spread Zika to people. There have not been any reports of pets or other types of animals becoming sick with Zika.

Risk to Monkeys and Apes in the United States

The risk of apes and monkeys in the United States becoming infected with Zika virus is low. All apes and monkeys imported into the United States undergo a mandatory 31-day quarantine period on arrival.

- The apes and monkeys are held indoors or in screened enclosures where it is unlikely they will have contact with mosquitoes.
- Any ape or monkey that may have entered quarantine while infected with Zika virus is not likely to pass it to others.
- If infected, apes and monkeys may be able to spread Zika for a limited time. This could occur if an uninfected mosquito bites a recently infected animal during the period of time when the virus is found in the ape or monkey's blood, typically during the first week of infection. All imported apes and monkeys should be free of Zika by the end of the quarantine period and pose no risk of infecting local mosquitoes.

Bringing Pets or Other Animals into the United States

Some animals, including apes and monkeys, are not allowed to be imported as pets under any circumstances. Each state and U.S. territory has its own rules for pet ownership.

Symptoms of Zika Virus

Many people infected with Zika virus will not have symptoms or will only have mild symptoms. The most common symptoms of Zika are:

- Fever
- Rash
- Headache
- Joint pain
- Conjunctivitis (red eyes)
- Muscle pain

How Long Symptoms Last

Zika is usually mild with symptoms lasting for several days to a week. People usually do not get sick enough to go to the hospital, and they very rarely die of Zika. For this reason, many people might not realize they have been infected. Symptoms of Zika are similar to other viruses that spread through mosquito bites, such as dengue and chikungunya.

How Soon You Should Be Tested

Zika virus usually remains in the blood of an infected person for about a week. See your doctor or other healthcare provider if you develop symptoms and you live in or have recently traveled to an area with risk of Zika. Your doctor or other healthcare provider may order blood or urine tests to help determine if you have Zika. Once a person has been infected, she or he is likely to be protected from future infections.

When to See a Doctor or Healthcare Provider

See your doctor or other healthcare provider if you have the symptoms described above and have visited an area with risk of Zika. This is especially important if you are pregnant. Be sure to tell your doctor or other healthcare provider where you traveled.

If You Think You Have Zika

- See your doctor or other healthcare provider for a diagnosis.
- Learn what you can do for treatment.
- Learn how you can protect others if you have Zika.

Testing for Zika

How Zika Is Diagnosed

- To diagnose Zika, a doctor or other healthcare provider will ask about any recent travel and any signs and symptoms.
- They may order blood or urine tests to help determine if you have Zika.

Remember to ask for your Zika test results even if you are feeling better.

Only Some People Need Zika Testing

Following the Zika virus outbreaks in 2016, the number of Zika cases reported from most parts of the world declined. The number is now very low. Therefore, very few people need Zika testing.

Testing is recommended if you have symptoms of Zika and have traveled to a country with a current Zika outbreak (red areas).

Note: There are no countries or U.S. territories currently reporting an outbreak of Zika.

- Testing should take place as soon as possible, while you still have symptoms.
- Testing may include a molecular test to look for the presence of the virus in the body or serological testing to look for antibodies your body makes to fight infection.
- If you have questions, talk to your healthcare provider.

Testing is recommended if you are a pregnant woman with symptoms of Zika and have traveled to an area with risk of Zika (purple areas) outside of the U.S. and its territories.

- Testing should take place as soon as possible, while you still have symptoms.
- Testing will be done using a molecular test to look for the presence of virus in the body.
- Serological testing is not recommended because antibodies against Zika persist for years and cross-react with other similar viruses, including dengue. For this reason, a positive lab result often cannot definitively tell you if you have a current or past infection or whether it is a Zika or dengue infection.
- If you have questions, talk to your healthcare provider.

Testing is no longer routinely recommended if you are a pregnant woman with no symptoms of Zika, but may be considered if you traveled to an area with risk of Zika (purple areas).

- Upon your return from travel, testing should take place as soon as possible.
- Testing will be done using a molecular test to look for the presence of virus in the body.
- Serological testing is not recommended because antibodies against Zika persist for years and cross-react with other similar viruses, including dengue. For this reason, a positive lab result often cannot definitively tell you if you have a current or past infection or whether it is a Zika or dengue infection.
- If you have questions, talk to your healthcare provider.

You should be tested for Zika if you are pregnant, traveled to an area with risk of Zika (purple areas) and your doctor sees Zika-associated abnormalities on an ultrasound, or you deliver a baby with birth defects that may be related to Zika.

- Testing may include a molecular test to look for the presence of virus in the body or serological testing to look for antibodies your body makes to fight infection.
- If you have questions, talk to your healthcare provider.

Preconception Zika testing is not recommended.

If You Have Tested Positive for Zika
- If you are pregnant, you can pass Zika to your fetus.
- You can pass Zika to your sex partner(s). Learn how you can prevent passing Zika to your partner.
- You can pass Zika to mosquitoes, which can bite you, get infected with Zika virus, and spread the virus to other people.

Sexual Transmission and Testing
- A blood or urine test can help determine if you have Zika from sexual transmission; however, testing blood, semen, vaginal fluids, or urine is not recommended to determine how likely a person is to pass Zika virus through sex.

If You Think You May Have or Have Had Zika
- Treat the symptoms
- Protect others from getting sick

Treatment of Zika Virus
- Treat the symptoms.
- Get plenty of rest.
- Drink fluids to prevent dehydration.
- Take medicine such as acetaminophen (Tylenol®) to reduce fever and pain.

- Do not take aspirin and other nonsteroidal anti-inflammatory drugs (NSAIDs) until dengue can be ruled out to reduce the risk of bleeding.
- If you are taking medicine for another medical condition, talk to your healthcare provider before taking additional medication.

If You Are Caring for a Person with Zika

Take steps to protect yourself from exposure to the person's blood and body fluids (urine, stool, or vomit, etc.). If you are pregnant, you can care for someone with Zika if you follow these steps:

- Do not touch blood or body fluids or surfaces with these fluids on them with your exposed skin.
- Wash hands with soap and water immediately after providing care.
- Immediately remove and wash clothes if they get blood or body fluids on them. Use laundry detergent and water temperature specified on the garment label. Using bleach is not necessary.
- Clean the sick person's environment daily using household cleaners according to label instructions.
- Immediately clean surfaces that have blood or other body fluids on them using household cleaners and disinfectants according to label instructions.

If you visit a family member or friend with Zika in a hospital, you should avoid contact with the person's blood and body fluids and surfaces with these fluids on them. Helping the person sit up or walk should not expose you. Make sure to wash your hands before and after touching the person.

Section 7.5

Dengue Viruses

This section includes text excerpted from "Dengue,"
Centers for Disease Control and Prevention (CDC),
September 26, 2019.

About Dengue

- Dengue viruses are spread to people through the bite of an infected *Aedes* species (*Ae. aegypti* or *Ae. albopictus*) mosquito. These mosquitoes also spread Zika, chikungunya, and other viruses.

- Dengue is common in more than 100 countries around the world.

- Forty percent of the world's population, about 3 billion people, live in areas with a risk of dengue. Dengue is often a leading cause of illness in areas with risk.

- Each year, up to 400 million people get infected with dengue. Approximately 100 million people get sick from infection, and 22,000 die from severe dengue.

- Dengue is caused by one of four related viruses: Dengue virus 1, 2, 3, and 4. For this reason, a person can be infected with a dengue virus as many as four times in her or his lifetime.

Transmission of Dengue Viruses
Through Mosquito Bites

Dengue viruses are spread to people through the bites of infected *Aedes* species mosquitoes (*Ae. aegypti* or *Ae. albopictus*). These are the same types of mosquitoes that spread Zika and chikungunya viruses.

- These mosquitoes typically lay eggs near standing water in containers that hold water, such as buckets, bowls, animal dishes, flower pots, and vases.

- These mosquitoes prefer to bite people, and live both indoors and outdoors near people.

- Mosquitoes that spread dengue, chikungunya, and Zika bite during the day and night.
- Mosquitoes become infected when they bite a person infected with the virus. Infected mosquitoes can then spread the virus to other people through bites.

From Mother to Child
- A pregnant woman already infected with dengue can pass the virus to her fetus during pregnancy or around the time of birth.
- To date, there has been one documented report of dengue spread through breast milk. Because of the benefits of breastfeeding, mothers are encouraged to breastfeed even in areas with risk of dengue.

Through Infected Blood, Laboratory, or Healthcare-Setting Exposures
Rarely, dengue can be spread through blood transfusion, organ transplant, or through a needle-stick injury.

Symptoms of Dengue Viruses
Mild symptoms of dengue can be confused with other illnesses that cause fever, aches and pains, or a rash.

The most common symptom of dengue is fever with any of the following:
- Nausea, vomiting
- Rash
- Aches and pains (eye pain, typically behind the eyes, muscle, joint, or bone pain)
- Any warning sign

Symptoms of dengue typically last two to seven days. Most people will recover after about a week.

Testing for Dengue Viruses
- See your healthcare provider if you have symptoms of dengue and live in or have recently traveled to an area with risk of dengue.

- If you have recently traveled to an area with risk of dengue, tell your healthcare provider.
- A blood test is the only way to confirm the diagnosis.
- Your healthcare provider may order blood tests to look for dengue or other similar viruses such as Zika or chikungunya.

Treatment of Dengue Viruses

- There is no specific medication to treat dengue.
- Treat the symptoms of dengue and see your healthcare provider.

If You Think You Have Dengue

- See a healthcare provider if you develop a fever or have symptoms of dengue. Tell him or her about your travel.
- Rest as much as possible.
- Take acetaminophen (also known as "paracetamol" outside of the United States) to control fever and relieve pain.
  - Do not take aspirin or ibuprofen!
- Drink plenty of fluids, such as water or drinks with added electrolytes, to stay hydrated.
- For mild symptoms, care for a sick infant, child, or family member at home.

Symptoms of dengue can become severe within a few hours. Severe dengue is a medical emergency.

Severe Dengue

- About 1 in 20 people who get sick with dengue will develop severe dengue.
- Severe dengue is a more serious form of disease that can result in shock, internal bleeding, and even death.
- You are more likely to develop severe dengue if you have had a dengue infection before.
- Infants and pregnant women are at increased risk for developing severe dengue.

Symptoms of Severe Dengue

Watch for signs and symptoms of severe dengue. Warning signs generally begin in the 24 to 48 hours after your fever has gone away.

If you or a family member develops any of the following symptoms, immediately go to a local clinic or emergency room:

- Stomach or belly pain, tenderness
- Vomiting (at least 3 times in 24 hours)
- Bleeding from the nose or gums
- Vomiting blood, or blood in the stool
- Feeling tired, restless, or irritable

Treatment of Severe Dengue

- If you develop any warning signs, see a healthcare provider or go to the emergency room immediately.
- Severe dengue is a medical emergency and requires immediate medical attention or hospitalization.
- If you are traveling, find healthcare abroad.

Section 7.6

Bourbon Virus

This section includes text excerpted from
"Bourbon Virus," Centers for Disease Control and
Prevention (CDC), January 24, 2019.

What Is Bourbon Virus?

Bourbon virus belongs to a group of viruses called "thogotoviruses." Viruses in this group are found all over the world. A few of these viruses can cause people to get sick.

How Do People Get Infected with Bourbon Virus?

The Centers for Disease Control and Prevention (CDC) does not yet fully know how people become infected with the Bourbon virus. However, based on what is known about similar viruses, it is likely that the Bourbon virus is spread through tick or other insect bites.

Where Have Cases of Bourbon Virus Disease Occurred?

As of June 2018, a limited number of Bourbon virus disease cases have been identified in the midwest and the southern United States. To date, the CDC does not know if the virus might be found in other areas of the United States.

What Are the Symptoms of Bourbon Virus?

Because there have been few cases identified thus far, scientists are still learning about possible symptoms caused by this virus. People diagnosed with Bourbon virus disease had symptoms including fever, tiredness, rash, headache, other body aches, nausea, and vomiting. They also had low blood counts for cells that fight infection and help prevent bleeding.

Who Is at Risk for Infection with Bourbon Virus?

People likely become infected with Bourbon virus when they are bitten by a tick or other insect. Therefore, people who do not take steps to protect themselves from tick or insect bites when they work or spend time outside may be more likely to be infected.

How Can People Reduce the Chance of Becoming Infected with Bourbon Virus?

There is no vaccine or drug to prevent or treat Bourbon virus disease. Therefore, preventing bites from ticks and other insects may be the best way to prevent infection. Here are ways to protect yourself from tick and other bug bites when you are outdoors:

- Use insect repellents
- Wear long sleeves and pants
- Avoid bushy and wooded areas
- Perform thorough tick checks after spending time outdoors

How Do You Know If You Have Been Infected with Bourbon Virus?

Tests that will help a doctor diagnose Bourbon virus infection are currently under development. See your healthcare provider if you have any symptoms that concern you.

What Is the Treatment for Bourbon Virus Disease?

Because there is no medicine to treat Bourbon virus disease, doctors can only treat the symptoms. For example, some patients may need to be hospitalized and given intravenous (IV) fluids and treatment for pain and fever. Antibiotics are not effective against viruses, including Bourbon virus.

What Should You Do If You Think Someone Might Be Infected with Bourbon Virus?

You should visit your healthcare provider if you have any symptoms that concern you.

Can Bourbon Virus Cause Animals to Become Ill?

Scientists do not yet know what animals can get infected or become sick from Bourbon virus. Studies are ongoing to determine the possibility of this. See your veterinarian if your pet or livestock have any symptoms that concern you.

Information about Bourbon Virus for Healthcare Providers

Bourbon virus is a novel ribonucleic acid (RNA) virus in the genus *Thogotovirus* (family *Orthomyxoviridae*) that was discovered in Bourbon County, Kansas, in 2014.

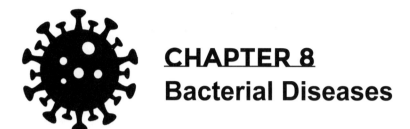

CHAPTER 8
Bacterial Diseases

Chapter Contents

Lyme Disease

This section includes text excerpted from "Lyme Disease," Centers for Disease Control and Prevention (CDC), December 16, 2019.

Lyme disease is the most common vector-borne disease in the United States. Lyme disease is caused by the bacterium *Borrelia burgdorferi* and rarely, *Borrelia mayonii*. It is transmitted to humans through the bite of infected black-legged ticks. Typical symptoms include fever, headache, fatigue, and a characteristic skin rash called "erythema migrans." If left untreated, infection can spread to joints, the heart, and the nervous system.

Lyme disease is diagnosed based on symptoms, physical findings (e.g., rash), and the possibility of exposure to infected ticks. Laboratory testing is helpful if used correctly and performed with validated methods. Most cases of Lyme disease can be treated successfully with a few weeks of antibiotics. Steps to prevent Lyme disease include using insect repellent, removing ticks promptly, applying environmental pesticides, and reducing tick habitat. The ticks that transmit Lyme disease can occasionally transmit other tick-borne diseases as well.

Transmission of Lyme Disease

The Lyme disease bacterium *Borrelia burgdorferi,* is spread through the bite of infected ticks. The black-legged tick (or deer tick, *Ixodes scapularis*) spreads the disease in the northeastern, mid-Atlantic, and north central United States. The western black-legged tick (*Ixodes pacificus*) spreads the disease on the Pacific Coast.

Ticks can attach to any part of the human body, but are often found in hard-to-see areas, such as the groin, armpits, and scalp. In most cases, the tick must be attached for 36 to 48 hours or more before the Lyme disease bacterium can be transmitted.

Most humans are infected through the bites of immature ticks called "nymphs." Nymphs are tiny (less than 2 mm) and difficult to see; they feed during the spring and summer months. Adult ticks can also transmit Lyme disease bacteria, but they are much larger and are more likely to be discovered and removed before they have had time to transmit the bacteria. Adult *Ixodes* ticks are most active during the cooler months of the year.

Are There Other Ways to Get Lyme Disease?

- There is no evidence that Lyme disease is transmitted from person to person. For example, a person cannot get infected from touching, kissing, or having sex with a person who has Lyme disease.
- Lyme disease acquired during pregnancy may lead to infection of the placenta and possible stillbirth. Therefore, early diagnosis and treatment is important. Fortunately, no negative effects on the fetus have been found when the mother receives appropriate antibiotic treatment. There are no reports of Lyme disease transmission from breast milk.
- Although no cases of Lyme disease have been linked to blood transfusions, scientists have found that the Lyme disease bacteria can live in blood that is stored for donation. Individuals being treated for Lyme disease with an antibiotic should not donate blood. Individuals who have completed antibiotic treatment for Lyme disease may be considered as potential blood donors.
- Although dogs and cats can get Lyme disease, there is no evidence that they spread the disease directly to their owners. However, pets can bring infected ticks into your home or yard. Protect your pet, and possibly yourself, through the use of tick-control products for animals.
- You will not get Lyme disease from eating venison or squirrel meat, but in keeping with general food-safety principles, always cook meat thoroughly. Note that hunting and dressing deer or squirrels may bring you into close contact with infected ticks.
- There is no credible evidence that Lyme disease can be transmitted through air, food, water, or from the bites of mosquitoes, flies, fleas, or lice.
- Ticks not known to transmit Lyme disease include lone star ticks (*Amblyomma americanum*), the American dog tick (*Dermacentor variabilis*),

the Rocky Mountain wood tick (*Dermacentor andersoni*), and the brown dog tick (*Rhipicephalus sanguineus*).

Preventing Tick Bites on People

Tick exposure can occur year-round, but ticks are most active during warmer months (April to September).

Before You Go Outdoors

- **Know where to expect ticks.** Ticks live in grassy, brushy, or wooded areas, or on animals. Spending time outside walking your dog, camping, gardening, or hunting could bring you in close contact with ticks. Many people get ticks in their own yard or neighborhood.
- **Treat clothing and gear** with products containing 0.5 percent permethrin. Permethrin can be used to treat boots, clothing, and camping gear, which remain protective through several washings. Alternatively, you can buy permethrin-treated clothing and gear.
- **Use U.S. Environmental Protection Agency (EPA)—registered insect repellents** containing N,N-Diethyl-meta-toluamide (DEET), picaridin, IR3535, oil of lemon eucalyptus (OLE), para-menthane-diol (PMD), or 2-undecanone. The EPA's helpful insect-repellent search tool can help you find the product that best suits your needs (see epa.gov/insect-repellents/find-repellent-right-you). Always follow product instructions. Do not use products containing OLE or PMD on children under three years old.
- Avoid wooded and brushy areas with high grass and leaf litter.
- Walk in the center of trails.

After You Come Indoors

Check your clothing for ticks. Ticks may be carried indoors on your clothing. Any ticks that are found should be removed. Tumble dry clothes in a dryer on high heat for 10 minutes to kill ticks on dry clothing after you come indoors. If the clothes are damp, additional time may be needed. If the clothes require washing first, hot water is recommended. Cold and medium temperature water will not kill ticks.

Examine gear and pets. Ticks can ride into the home on clothing and pets, then attach to a person later, so carefully examine pets, coats, and daypacks.

Shower soon after going outdoors. Showering within two hours of going indoors has been shown to reduce your risk of getting Lyme disease and may be effective in reducing the risk of other tick-borne diseases. Showering may help wash off unattached ticks and it is a good opportunity to do a tick check.

Check your body for ticks after going outdoors. Conduct a full body check upon return from potentially tick-infested areas, including your own backyard. Use a handheld or full-length mirror to view all parts of your body. Check these parts of your body and your child's body for ticks:

- Under the arms
- In and around the ears
- Inside the belly button
- Backs of the knees
- In and around the hair
- Between the legs
- Around the waist

Preventing Ticks on Your Pets

Dogs are very susceptible to tick bites and tick-borne diseases. Vaccines are not available for most of the tick-borne diseases that dogs can get, and they do not keep the dogs from bringing ticks into your home. For these reasons, it is important to use a tick preventive product on your dog.

Tick bites on dogs may be hard to detect. Signs of tick-borne disease may not appear for 7 to 21 days or longer after a tick bite, so watch your dog closely for changes in behavior or appetite if you suspect that your pet has been bitten by a tick.

Talk to your veterinarian about:

- The best tick prevention products for your dog
- Tick-borne diseases in your area

To further reduce the chances that a tick bite will make your dog sick:

- Check your pets for ticks daily, especially after they spend time outdoors.
- If you find a tick on your pet, remove it right away.
- Reduce tick habitat in your yard.

Preventing Ticks in the Yard
Create a Tick-Safe Zone through Landscaping

You can make your yard less attractive to ticks through strategic landscaping. Here are some simple landscaping techniques that can help reduce tick populations:

- Clear tall grasses and brush around homes and at the edge of lawns.
- Place a three-feet-wide barrier of wood chips or gravel between lawns and wooded areas and around patios and play equipment. This will restrict tick migration into recreational areas.
- Mow the lawn frequently and keep leaves raked.
- Stack wood neatly and in a dry area (to discourage rodents that ticks feed on).
- Keep playground equipment, decks, and patios away from yard edges and trees and place them in a sunny location, if possible.
- Remove any old furniture, mattresses, or trash from the yard that may give ticks a place to hide.

Apply Pesticides Outdoors to Control Ticks

Use of acaricides (tick pesticides) can reduce the number of ticks in treated areas of your yard. However, you should not rely on spraying to reduce your risk of infection.

If you have concerns about applying acaricides:

- Check with local health officials about the best time to apply acaricide in your area.
- Identify rules and regulations related to pesticide application on residential properties (the EPA and your state determine the availability of pesticides).
- Consider using a professional pesticide company to apply pesticides at your home.

Lyme Disease Vaccine

A Lyme disease vaccine is no longer available. The vaccine manufacturer discontinued production in 2002, citing insufficient consumer demand. Protection provided by this vaccine diminishes over time. Therefore, if you received the Lyme disease vaccine before 2002, you are probably no longer protected against Lyme disease.

Posttreatment Lyme Disease Syndrome

Lyme disease is caused by infection with the bacterium *Borrelia burgdorferi*. Although most cases of Lyme disease can be cured with a 2- to 4-week course of oral antibiotics, patients can sometimes have symptoms of pain, fatigue, or difficulty thinking that last for more than six months after they finish treatment. This condition is called "posttreatment Lyme disease syndrome" (PTLDS).

Why some patients experience PTLDS is not known. Some experts believe that *Borrelia burgdorferi* can trigger an "autoimmune" response causing symptoms that last well after the infection itself is gone. Autoimmune responses are known to occur following other infections, including campylobacter (Guillain-Barré syndrome), chlamydia (Reiter syndrome), and strep throat (rheumatic heart disease). Other experts hypothesize that PTLDS results from a persistent, but difficult to detect infection. Finally, some believe that the symptoms of PTLDS are due to other causes unrelated to the patient's *Borrelia burgdorferi* infection.

Unfortunately, there is no proven treatment for PTLDS. Although short-term antibiotic treatment is a proven treatment for early Lyme disease, studies funded by the U.S. National Institutes of Health (NIH) have found that long-term outcomes are no better for patients who received additional prolonged antibiotic treatment than for patients who received a placebo. Long-term antibiotic treatment for Lyme disease has been associated with serious and sometimes deadly complications.

Patients with PTLDS usually get better over time, but it can take many months to feel completely well. If you have been treated for Lyme disease and still feel unwell, see your healthcare provider to discuss additional options for managing your symptoms. If you are considering long-term antibiotic treatment for ongoing symptoms associated with a Lyme disease infection, please talk to your healthcare provider about the possible risks of such treatment.

Section 8.2
Plague

This section includes text excerpted from "Plague," Centers for Disease Control and Prevention (CDC), November 26, 2019.

Plague is a disease that affects humans and other mammals. It is caused by the bacterium *Yersinia pestis*. Humans usually get plague after being bitten by a rodent flea—such as the Oriental rat flea (*Xenopsylla cheopis*), also known as the tropical rat flea and primarily of the genus *Rattus*—that is carrying the plague bacterium or by handling an animal infected with plague. Plague is infamous for killing millions of people in Europe during the Middle Ages. Modern antibiotics are effective in treating plague, but without prompt treatment, the disease can cause serious illness or death. Presently, human plague infections continue to occur in rural areas in the western United States, but significantly more cases occur in parts of Africa and Asia.

Transmission of Plague

The plague bacteria can be transmitted to humans in the following ways:

- **Flea bites.** Plague bacteria are most often transmitted by the bite of an infected flea. During plague epizootics, many rodents die, causing hungry fleas to seek other sources of blood. People and animals that visit places where rodents have recently died from plague are at risk of being infected from flea bites. Dogs and cats may also bring plague-infected fleas into the home. Flea-bite exposure may result in primary bubonic plague or septicemic plague.

- **Contact with contaminated fluid or tissue.** Humans can become infected when handling tissue or body fluids of a plague-infected animal. For example, a hunter skinning a rabbit or other infected animal without using proper precautions could become infected with plague bacteria. This form of exposure most commonly results in bubonic plague or septicemic plague.
- **Infectious droplets.** When a person has plague pneumonia, they may cough droplets containing the plague bacteria into air. If these bacteria-containing droplets are breathed in by another person, they can cause pneumonic plague. Typically this requires direct and close contact with the person with pneumonic plague. Transmission of these droplets is the only way that plague can spread between people. This type of spread has not been documented in the United States since 1924, but still occurs with some frequency in developing countries. Cats are particularly susceptible to plague, and can be infected by eating infected rodents. Sick cats pose a risk of transmitting infectious plague droplets to their owners or to veterinarians. Several cases of human plague have occurred in the United States in recent decades as a result of contact with infected cats.

Symptoms of Plague

Plague symptoms depend on how the patient was exposed to the plague bacteria. Plague can take different clinical forms, but symptoms of the most common—bubonic, pneumonic, and septicemic—forms follow.

Bubonic Plague

Patients develop sudden onset of fever, headache, chills, and weakness, and one or more swollen, tender, and painful lymphgland (called a "bubo") or glands (called "buboes"). This form usually results from the bite of an infected flea. The bacteria multiply in the lymph node closest to where the bacteria entered the human body. If the patient is not treated with the appropriate antibiotics, the bacteria can spread to other parts of the body.

Septicemic Plague

Patients develop fever, chills, extreme weakness, abdominal pain, shock, and possibly bleeding into the skin and other organs. Skin and other tissues may turn black and die, especially on fingers, toes, and the nose. Septicemic plague can occur as the first symptom of plague, or may develop from untreated bubonic plague. This form results from bites of infected fleas or from handling an infected animal.

Pneumonic Plague

Patients develop fever, headache, weakness, and a rapidly developing pneumonia with shortness of breath, chest pain, cough, and sometimes bloody or watery mucous. Pneumonic plague may develop from inhaling infectious droplets or may develop from untreated bubonic or septicemic plague after the bacteria spread to the lungs. The pneumonia may cause respiratory failure and shock. Pneumonic plague is the most serious form of the disease and is the only form of plague that can be spread from person to person (by infectious droplets).

Plague is a serious illness. If you are experiencing symptoms such as those listed here, seek immediate medical attention. Prompt treatment with the correct medications is critical to prevent complications or death.

Diagnosis of Plague

Plague is a plausible diagnosis for people who are sick and live in, or have traveled to, the western United States or any other plague-endemic area. The most common sign of bubonic plague is the rapid development of a swollen and painful lymph gland (called a "buboes"). A known flea bite or the presence of a bubo may help a doctor to consider plague as a cause of the illness.

In many cases, particularly in septicemic and pneumonic plague, there are no obvious signs that indicate plague. Diagnosis is made by taking samples from the patient, especially blood or part of a swollen lymph gland, and submitting them for laboratory testing. Once plague has been identified as a possible cause of the illness, appropriate treatment should begin immediately.

Treatment of Plague

Plague is a very serious illness, but is treatable with commonly available antibiotics. The earlier a patient seeks medical care and receives treatment that is appropriate for plague, the better their chances are of a full recovery.

People in close contact with very sick pneumonic plague patients may be evaluated and possibly placed under observation. Preventive antibiotic therapy may also be given, depending on the type and timing of personal contact.

If you live or have traveled to the western United States or any other plague-endemic area and have symptoms suggestive of plague, seek medical care immediately.

Prevention of Plague

- Reduce rodent habitat around your home, workplace, and recreational areas. Remove brush, rock piles, junk, cluttered firewood, and possible rodent food supplies, such as pet and wild animal food. Make your home and outbuildings rodent-proof.
- Wear gloves if you are handling or skinning potentially infected animals to prevent contact between your skin and the plague bacteria. Contact your local health department if you have questions about the disposal of dead animals.
- Use repellent if you think you could be exposed to rodent fleas during activities such as camping, hiking, or working outdoors. Products containing DEET can be applied to the skin as well as clothing and products containing permethrin can be applied to clothing (always follow instructions on the label).
- Keep fleas off of your pets by applying flea-control products. Animals that roam freely are more likely to come in contact with plague-infected animals or fleas and could bring them into homes. If your pet becomes sick, seek care from a veterinarian as soon as possible.
- Do not allow dogs or cats that roam free in endemic areas to sleep on your bed.

Note: A plague vaccine is no longer available in the United States. New plague vaccines are in development, but are not expected to be commercially available in the immediate future.

Section 8.3

Tularemia

This section includes text excerpted from "Tularemia,"
Centers for Disease Control and Prevention (CDC),
December 13, 2018.

Tularemia is a disease that can infect animals and people. Rabbits, hares, and rodents are especially susceptible and often die in large numbers during outbreaks. People can become infected in several ways, including:

- Tick and deer-fly bites
- Skin contact with infected animals
- Drinking contaminated water
- Inhaling contaminated aerosols or agricultural and landscaping dust
- Laboratory exposure

In addition, people could be exposed as a result of bioterrorism.

Symptoms vary depending on how the person was infected. Tularemia can be life-threatening, but most infections can be treated successfully with antibiotics.

Steps to prevent tularemia include:

- Using insect repellent
- Wearing gloves when handling sick or dead animals
- Avoiding mowing over dead animals

In the United States, naturally occurring infections have been reported from all states except Hawaii.

Transmission of Tularemia

The bacterium that causes tularemia is highly infectious and can enter the human body through the skin, eyes, mouth, or lungs. Symptoms of infection vary depending on the route of entry. Usual sources of infection are described below. Transmission of tularemia from person to person has not been reported.

Tick or Deer-Fly Bites

In the United States, ticks that transmit tularemia to humans include the dog tick (*Dermacentor variabilis*), the wood tick (*Dermacentor andersoni*), and the lone star tick (*Amblyomma americanum*). Deer flies (*Chrysops* spp.) have been shown to transmit tularemia in the western United States. Infections due to tick and deer-fly bites usually take the form of ulceroglandular or glandular tularemia.

Handling Infected Animals

F. tularensis bacteria can be transmitted to humans via the skin when they are handling infected animal tissue. In particular, this can occur when hunting or skinning infected rabbits, muskrats, prairie dogs, and other rodents. Many other animals have also been known to become ill with tularemia. Domestic cats are very susceptible to tularemia and have been known to transmit the bacteria to humans. Care should be taken when handling any sick or dead animal. Outbreaks of tularemia have occurred among hamsters purchased from pet stores. At least one child in the United States developed tularemia after being bitten by a pet hamster. Infection due to handling wild or domesticated animals can result in glandular, ulceroglandular, and oculoglandular tularemia. Oropharyngeal tularemia can result from eating the undercooked meat of infected animals.

Other Exposures

Humans can acquire tularemia by inhaling dust or aerosols contaminated with *F. tularensis* bacteria. This can occur during farming or landscaping activities, especially when machinery (e.g., tractors or mowers) runs over infected animals or carcasses. Although rare, this type of exposure can result in pneumonic tularemia, one of the most severe forms of the disease. Water can also become contaminated with the bacteria through contact with infected animals. Humans who drink contaminated water that has not been treated may contract oropharyngeal tularemia. This mode of transmission appears to be much more common in Europe than in the United States.

Signs and Symptoms of Tularemia

The signs and symptoms of tularemia vary depending on how the bacteria enter the body. Illness ranges from mild to life-threatening. All forms are accompanied by fever, which can be as high as 104°F. Main forms of this disease are listed below:

- **Ulceroglandular.** This is the most common form of tularemia and usually occurs following a tick or deer-fly bite or after handling of an infected animal. A skin ulcer appears at the site where the bacteria entered the body. The ulcer is accompanied by swelling of regional lymph glands, usually in the armpit or groin.
- **Glandular.** Similar to ulceroglandular tularemia, but without an ulcer. Also generally acquired through the bite of an infected tick or deer fly or from handling sick or dead animals.
- **Oculoglandular.** This form occurs when the bacteria enter through the eye. This can occur when a person is butchering an infected animal and touches his or her eyes. Symptoms include irritation and inflammation of the eye and swelling of lymph glands in front of the ear.
- **Oropharyngeal.** This form results from eating or drinking contaminated food or water. Patients with oropharyngeal tularemia may have a sore throat, mouth ulcers, tonsillitis, and swelling of lymph glands in the neck.
- **Pneumonic.** This is the most serious form of tularemia. Symptoms include cough, chest pain, and difficulty breathing. This form results from breathing dusts or aerosols containing the organism. It can also occur when other forms of tularemia (e.g., ulceroglandular) are left untreated and the bacteria spread through the bloodstream to the lungs.
- **Typhoidal.** This form is characterized by any combination of the general symptoms (without the localizing symptoms of other syndromes).

Diagnosis and Treatment of Tularemia

Tularemia can be difficult to diagnose. It is a rare disease, and the symptoms can be mistaken for other, more common, illnesses. For this reason, it is important to share with your healthcare provider any likely exposures, such as tick and deer-fly bites, or contact with sick or dead animals.

Blood tests and cultures can help confirm the diagnosis. Antibiotics used to treat tularemia include streptomycin, gentamicin, doxycycline, and ciprofloxacin. Treatment usually lasts 10 to 21 days, depending on the stage of illness and the medication used. Although symptoms may last for several weeks, most patients completely recover.

Prevention of Tularemia
When Hiking, Camping, or Working Outdoors

- Use U.S. Environmental Protection Agency (EPA)-registered insect repellents containing N,N-Diethyl-meta-toluamide (DEET), picaridin, IR3535, oil of lemon eucalyptus (OLE), para-menthane-diol (PMD), or 2-undecanone. The EPA's helpful search tool can help you find the product that best suits your needs (see epa.gov/insect-repellents/find-repellent-right-you). Always follow product instructions.
- Wear long pants, long sleeves, and long socks to keep ticks and deer flies off your skin.
- Remove attached ticks promptly with fine-tipped tweezers.
- Do not drink untreated surface water.

When Mowing or Landscaping

- Do not mow over sick or dead animals. When possible, check the area for carcasses prior to mowing.
- Use of masks during mowing and other landscaping activities may reduce your risk of inhaling the bacteria, but this has not been studied.

If You Hunt, Trap, or Skin Animals

- Use gloves when handling animals, especially rabbits, muskrats, prairie dogs, and other rodents.
- Cook game meat thoroughly before eating.

A vaccine has been available to protect laboratorians routinely working with *Francisella tularensis*. This vaccine is currently under review by the U.S. Food and Drug Administration (FDA) and is not generally available in the United States.

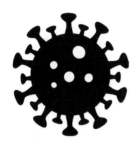

CHAPTER 9
Rickettsial Zoonoses

Chapter Contents

Q Fever

This section includes text excerpted from "Q Fever,"
Centers for Disease Control and Prevention (CDC),
January 15, 2019.

Q fever is a disease caused by the bacteria *Coxiella burnetii*. This bacteria naturally infects some animals, such as goats, sheep, and cattle. *C. burnetii* bacteria are found in the birth products (i.e., placenta, amniotic fluid), urine, feces, and milk of infected animals. People can get infected by breathing in dust that has been contaminated by infected animal feces, urine, milk, and birth products. Some people never get sick; however, those who do usually develop flu-like symptoms including fever, chills, fatigue, and muscle pain.

Transmission of Q Fever

People get infected by breathing in dust that has been contaminated by infected animal feces, urine, milk, and birth products that contain *Coxiella burnetii*. Direct contact (e.g., touching, being licked) with an animal is not required to become sick with Q fever. People may also get sick with Q fever by eating contaminated, unpasteurized dairy products. Rarely, Q fever has been spread through blood transfusion, from a pregnant woman to her fetus, or through sex.

People at Risk for Q Fever Infection

Certain professions are at increased risk for exposure to *C. burnetii*, including veterinarians, meat-processing plant workers, dairy workers, livestock farmers, and researchers at facilities housing sheep and goats. People working in these areas may need to take extra precautions.

Bioterrorism

- A biological attack, or bioterrorism, is the intentional release of viruses, bacteria, or other germs that can sicken or kill people, livestock, or crops.
- *C. burnetii*, the bacteria that causes Q fever, has been described as a potential bioterrorism agent.
- *C. burnetii* is a select agent subject to the select agent regulations found in the U.S. Code of Federal Regulations 42 CFR Part 73.
- *C. burnetii* is a highly infectious agent, in some cases requiring less than 10 bacteria to make you sick.
- *C. burnetii* is extremely resistant to heat, drying, and many common disinfectants.
- People get infected by breathing in contaminated dust.
- *C. burnetii* has been previously weaponized for use in biological warfare and is considered a potential terrorist threat.
- The Centers for Disease Control and Prevention (CDC) does not know if or when a bioterrorism attack might occur. However, federal agencies have worked for years with health departments across the country to plan and prepare for any such attack.

Signs and Symptoms of Q Fever

About 5 out of 10 people infected with *Coxiella burnetii* will get sick. Illness typically develops 2 to 3 weeks after beeing exposed to the bacteria. Signs and symptoms of Q fever may include:

- Fever
- Chills or sweats
- Fatigue (tiredness)
- Headache
- Muscle aches
- Nausea, vomiting, or diarrhea
- Chest pain
- Stomach pain
- Weight loss
- Nonproductive cough

Symptoms can be mild or severe. People who develop severe disease may experience infection of the lungs (pneumonia) or liver (hepatitis).

Women who are infected during pregnancy may be at risk for miscarriage, stillbirth, preterm delivery, or low infant birth weight.

Chronic Q Fever

A very small percentage of people (less than 5 out of 100) who become infected with *C. burnetii* bacteria develop a more serious infection called "chronic Q fever." Chronic Q fever develops months or years following initial Q fever infection. People with chronic Q fever often develop an infection of one or more heart valves (called "endocarditis"). People with endocarditis may experience night sweats, fatigue, shortness of breath, weight loss, or swelling of their limbs. A healthcare provider will need to perform a series of tests to diagnose endocarditis.

Chronic Q fever is serious and can be deadly if not treated correctly. Chronic Q fever infection requires months of antibiotic treatment. Chronic Q fever is more likely to occur in people with heart valve disease, blood vessel abnormalities, or in people with weakened immune systems. Women infected during pregnancy may also be at risk for developing chronic Q fever.

Diagnosis and Testing of Q Fever

The symptoms of Q fever are similar to many other diseases, often making diagnosis difficult. See your healthcare provider if you develop symptoms after spending time with or near animals—particularly sheep, goats, and cattle—or in areas where these animals may have been.

Your healthcare provider may order blood tests to look for Q fever or other diseases.

Laboratory testing and reporting of results can take several weeks, so your healthcare provider may start antibiotic treatment before results are available.

Treatment of Q Fever

- Most people who are sick with Q fever will recover without antibiotic treatment.
- However, for people who develop Q fever disease, treatment with two weeks of doxycycline antibiotic is recommended.

Chronic Q Fever Treatment

- A life-threatening infection, requiring several months of antibiotic treatment.
- Treated with a combination of antibiotics including doxycycline and hydroxychloroquine for several months.

Prevention of Q Fever

- Q fever vaccines are not available in the United States.
- Reduce your risk of getting Q fever by avoiding contact with animals, especially while animals are giving birth. Animals can be infected with *Coxiella burnetii* and appear healthy.
- Do not consume raw milk or raw milk products.
- If you have been diagnosed with Q fever and have a history of heart valve disease, blood vessel abnormalities, a weakened immune system, or are pregnant, talk to your healthcare provider about your risk for developing chronic Q fever.

Section 9.2

Rocky Mountain Spotted Fever

This section includes text excerpted from "Rocky Mountain Spotted Fever," Centers for Disease Control and Prevention (CDC), May 7, 2019.

Rocky Mountain spotted fever (RMSF) is a bacterial disease spread through the bite of an infected tick. Most people who get sick with RMSF will have a fever, headache, and rash. RMSF can be deadly if not treated early with the right antibiotic.

Transmission of Rocky Mountain Spotted Fever

Rocky Mountain spotted fever is a serious tick-borne illness which can be deadly if not treated early. It is spread by several species of ticks in the United States, including the American dog tick (*Dermacentor variabilis*), Rocky Mountain wood tick (*Dermacentor andersoni*), and, in parts of the southwestern United States and Mexico, the brown dog tick (*Rhipicephalus sanguineus*). RMSF cases occur throughout the United States, but are most commonly reported from North Carolina, Tennessee, Missouri, Arkansas, and Oklahoma.

Signs and Symptoms of Rocky Mountain Spotted Fever

Early signs and symptoms are not specific to RMSF (including fever and headache). However, the disease can rapidly progress to a serious and life-threatening illness. See your healthcare provider if you become ill after having been bitten by a tick or having been in the woods or in areas with high brush where ticks commonly live.

Signs and symptoms can include:
- Fever
- Headache
- Rash
- Nausea
- Vomiting
- Stomach pain
- Muscle pain
- Lack of appetite

Rash of Rocky Mountain Spotted Fever

Rash is a common sign in people who are sick with RMSF. Rash usually develops 2 to 4 days after fever begins. The look of the rash can vary widely over the course of illness. Some rashes can look like red splotches and some look like pinpoint dots. While almost all patients with RMSF will develop a rash, it often does not appear early in illness, which can make RMSF difficult to diagnose.

Long-Term Health Problems of Rocky Mountain Spotted Fever

- RMSF does not result in chronic or persistent infections.
- Some patients who recover from severe RMSF may be left with permanent damage, including amputation of arms, legs, fingers, or toes (from damage to blood vessels in these areas); hearing loss; paralysis; or mental disability. Any permanent damage is caused by the acute illness and does not result from a chronic infection.

Diagnosis and Testing of Rocky Mountain Spotted Fever

- The signs and symptoms of RMSF are similar to those of many other diseases. See your healthcare provider if you develop any of the signs or symptoms of RMSF.
- Be sure to tell your healthcare provider if you become ill and have recently been bitten by a tick or have spent time in areas where ticks may be found.
- Your healthcare provider may order certain blood tests to look for evidence of RMSF.
- The results of these tests can take weeks. If your healthcare provider thinks your illness might be RMSF, she or he should recommend antibiotic treatment before test results are available.

Treatment of Rocky Mountain Spotted Fever

- RMSF can be life-threatening.
- Early treatment with the antibiotic doxycycline can prevent death and severe illness.

Doxycycline is the recommended antibiotic treatment for RMSF in adults and children of all ages.

Section 9.3

Typhus Fevers

This section includes text excerpted from
"Typhus Fever," Centers for Disease Control and
Prevention (CDC), July 17, 2019.

Typhus fevers are a group of diseases caused by bacteria that are spread to humans by fleas, lice, and chiggers. Typhus fevers include scrub typhus, murine typhus, and epidemic typhus. Chiggers spread scrub typhus; fleas spread murine typhus; and body lice spread epidemic typhus. The most common symptoms are fever, headaches, and sometimes rash.

Scrub Typhus

Scrub typhus, also known as "bush typhus," is a disease caused by a bacteria called "*Orientia tsutsugamushi.*" Scrub typhus is spread to people through bites of infected chiggers (larval mites). The most common symptoms of scrub typhus include fever, headache, body aches, and sometimes rash. Most cases of scrub typhus occur in rural areas of Southeast Asia, Indonesia, China, Japan, India, and northern Australia. Anyone living in or traveling to areas where scrub typhus is found could get infected.

Signs and Symptoms

Symptoms of scrub typhus usually begin within 10 days of being bitten. Signs and symptoms may include:

- Fever and chills
- Headache
- Body aches and muscle pain
- A dark, scab-like region at the site of the chigger bite (also known as "eschar")
- Mental changes, ranging from confusion to coma

- Enlarged lymph nodes
- Rash

People with severe illness may develop organ failure and bleeding, which can be fatal if left untreated.

Diagnosis and Testing

- The symptoms of scrub typhus are similar to symptoms of many other diseases. See your healthcare provider if you develop the symptoms listed above after spending time in areas where scrub typhus is found.
- If you have recently traveled, tell your healthcare provider where and when you traveled.
- Your healthcare provider may order blood tests to look for scrub typhus or other diseases.
- Laboratory testing and reporting of results can take several weeks, so your healthcare provider may start treatment before results are available.

Treatment

- Scrub typhus should be treated with the antibiotic doxycycline. Doxycycline can be used in people of any age.
- Antibiotics are most effective if given soon after symptoms begin.
- People who are treated early with doxycycline usually recover quickly.

Prevention

- No vaccine is available to prevent scrub typhus.
- Reduce your risk of getting scrub typhus by avoiding contact with infected chiggers.
- When traveling to areas where scrub typhus is common, avoid areas with lots of vegetation and brush where chiggers may be found.

If you will be spending time outdoors:
- Use Environmental Protection Agency (EPA)-registered insect repellents containing N,N-Diethyl-meta-toluamide (DEET) or other active ingredients registered for use against chiggers, on exposed skin and clothing.

- Always follow product instructions.
- Reapply insect repellent as directed.
- Do not spray repellent on the skin under clothing.
- If you are also using sunscreen, apply sunscreen before applying insect repellent.
- If you have a baby or child:
  - Dress your child in clothing that covers arms and legs, or cover crib, stroller, and baby carrier with mosquito netting.
  - Do not apply insect repellent onto a child's hands, eyes, or mouth or on cuts or irritated skin.
  - Adults: Spray insect repellent onto your hands and then apply to child's face.
- Treat clothing and gear with permethrin or purchase permethrin-treated items.
- Permethrin kills chiggers and can be used to treat boots, clothing, and camping gear.
- Treated clothing remains protective after multiple washings. See product information to learn how long the protection will last.
- If treating items yourself, follow the product instructions carefully.
- Do not use permethrin products directly on skin. They are intended to treat clothing.

Flea-Borne (Murine) Typhus

Flea-borne (murine) typhus is a disease caused by a bacteria called "*Rickettsia typhi.*" Flea-borne typhus is spread to people through contact with infected fleas. Fleas become infected when they bite infected animals such as rats, cats, or opossums. When an infected flea bites a person or animal, the bite breaks the skin, causing a wound. Fleas poop when they feed. The poop (also called "flea dirt") can then be rubbed into the bite wound or other wounds, causing infection. People can also breathe in infected flea dirt or rub it into their eyes. This bacteria is not spread from person to person. Flea-borne typhus occurs in tropical and subtropical climates around the world, including areas of the United States (southern California, Hawaii, and Texas). Flea-borne typhus is a rare disease in the United States.

Signs and Symptoms

Symptoms of flea-borne typhus begin within 2 weeks after contact with infected fleas or flea dirt. However, people may not know they have been bitten by a flea or exposed to flea dirt, so tell your healthcare provider about time spent outdoors or contact with animals. Signs and symptoms may include:

- Fever and chills
- Body aches and muscle pain
- Loss of appetite
- Nausea
- Vomiting
- Stomach pain
- Cough
- Rash (typically occurs around day 5 of illness)

Severe illness is rare and most people recover completely, sometimes without treatment. Untreated disease can cause severe illness and damage to one or more organs, including the liver, kidneys, heart, lungs, and brain.

Diagnosis and Testing

- The symptoms of flea-borne typhus are similar to symptoms of many other diseases. See your healthcare provider if you develop the symptoms listed above, and be sure to mention contact with fleas, stray animals (such as cats), or wildlife (such as rats or opossums).
- Your healthcare provider may order a blood test to look for flea-borne typhus or other diseases.
- Laboratory testing and reporting of results can take several weeks, so your healthcare provider may start treatment before results are available.

Treatment

- Flea-borne typhus is treated with the antibiotic doxycycline. Doxycycline can be used in people of any age.
- Antibiotics are most effective when given soon after symptoms begin.

- People treated early with doxycycline usually recover quickly.
- There is no evidence that persistent or chronic infections occur.

Prevention

- There is no vaccine to prevent flea-borne typhus.
- Reduce your risk of getting flea-borne typhus by avoiding contact with fleas.
- Keep fleas off of your pets. Use veterinarian-approved flea-control products, such as flea collars, oral medication or spot-ons, for cats and dogs. Permethrin should not be used on cats. Animals that are allowed outside are more likely to come into contact with fleas and could bring them inside.
- Keep rodents and animals (e.g., opossums) away from your home, workplace, and recreational areas:
  - Store food, including pet food, in tight-sealing containers.
  - Remove brush, rock piles, junk, and cluttered firewood outside of your home.
  - Seal up holes in your home where rodents can enter.
  - Keep tight lids on compost and trash cans.
  - The Centers for Disease Control and Prevention (CDC)'s rodents website (cdc.gov/rodents/index.html) offers helpful suggestions on rodent control during and after a rodent infestation.
- Protect yourself from flea bites:
  - Do not feed or pet stray or wild animals.
  - Always wear gloves if you are handling sick or dead animals.
  - Use the EPA-registered insect repellents on your skin and clothing when spending time outside. Always follow instructions listed on the product label.

Epidemic Typhus

Epidemic typhus, also called "louse-borne typhus," is an uncommon disease caused by a bacteria called *"Rickettsia prowazekii."* Epidemic typhus is spread to people through contact with infected body lice. Though epidemic typhus was responsible for millions of deaths in previous centuries, it is now considered a rare disease. Occasionally, cases continue to occur, in areas where extreme overcrowding is common and body lice can travel from one person to another. In the United States, rare cases of epidemic typhus, called "sylvatic typhus," can occur. These cases occur when people are exposed to flying squirrels and their nests.

Signs and Symptoms

Symptoms of epidemic typhus begin within 2 weeks after contact with infected body lice. Signs and symptoms may include:

- Fever and chills
- Headache
- Rapid breathing
- Body and muscle aches
- Rash
- Cough
- Nausea
- Vomiting
- Confusion

Brill-Zinsser Disease

Some people can remain infected, without symptoms, for years after they first get sick. Rarely, these individuals can have a relapse in disease, called "Brill-Zinsser disease," months or years following their first illness. When this happens, it often occurs when the body's immune system is weakened due to certain medications, old age, or illness. The symptoms of Brill-Zinsser disease are similar to the original infection, but are usually milder than the initial illness.

Diagnosis and Testing

- The symptoms of epidemic typhus are similar to symptoms of many other diseases. See your healthcare provider if you develop the symptoms listed above following travel or contact with animals.
- Tell your healthcare provider if you have had contact with flying squirrels or their nests.

- Your healthcare provider will order a blood test to look for epidemic typhus and other diseases.
- Laboratory testing and reporting of results can take several weeks. Your healthcare provider may start treatment before results are available.

Treatment

- Epidemic typhus should be treated with the antibiotic doxycycline. Doxycycline can be used in people of any age.
- Antibiotics are most effective when given soon after symptoms begin.
- People who are treated early with doxycycline usually recover quickly.

Prevention

- There is no vaccine to prevent epidemic typhus.
- Reduce your risk of getting epidemic typhus by avoiding overcrowded areas.
- Body lice thrive in areas that are overcrowded and where people are not able to bathe or change clothes regularly. To avoid body louse infestations:
  - Bathe regularly and change into clean clothes at least once a week.
  - Wash louse-infested clothing at least once a week. Machine wash and dry infested clothing and bedding using hot water (at least 130°F), and dry on high heat when possible. Clothing and items that are not washable can be dry-cleaned OR sealed in a plastic bag and stored for 2 weeks.
  - Do not share clothing, beds, bedding, or towels used by a person who has body lice or is infected with typhus.
  - Treat bedding, uniforms, and other clothing with permethrin. Permethrin kills lice and may provide long-lasting protection for clothing for many washings. See product information to learn how long the protection will last. If treating items yourself, follow the product instructions carefully. Do NOT use permethrin products directly on skin. They are intended to treat clothing.
  - People should avoid contact with flying squirrels and their nests.

Section 9.4

Anaplasmosis

This section includes text excerpted from
"Anaplasmosis," Centers for Disease Control and
Prevention (CDC), January 11, 2019.

Anaplasmosis is a disease caused by the bacterium *Anaplasma phagocytophilum*. These bacteria are spread to people by tick bites primarily from the black-legged tick (Ixodes scapularis) and the western black-legged tick (*Ixodes pacificus*).

People with anaplasmosis will often have fever, headache, chills, and muscle aches. Doxycycline is the drug of choice for adults and children of all ages with anaplasmosis.

Transmission of Anaplasmosis

Anaplasmosis is a tick-borne disease caused by the bacterium *Anaplasma phagocytophilum*.

- Tick bites
  - *A. phagocytophilum* is primarily spread to people by the bite of an infected tick.
  - In the United States, the bacteria is carried by the black-legged tick (*Ixodes scapularis*) in the northeast and midwestern United States and the western black-legged tick (Ixodes pacificus) along the West Coast.
- Blood transfusion
  - In rare cases, *A. phagocytophilum* has been spread by blood transfusion.

Anaplasmosis is most commonly reported in the northeastern and upper midwestern states.

Signs and Symptoms of Anaplasmosis

- Signs and symptoms of anaplasmosis typically begin within one to two weeks after the bite of an infected tick.

- Tick bites are usually painless, and many people do not remember being bitten.
- See your healthcare provider if you become ill after having been bitten by a tick or having been in the woods or in areas with high brush where ticks commonly live.

Early Illness

Early signs and symptoms (days 1 to 5) are usually mild or moderate and may include:

- Fever, chills
- Severe headache
- Muscle aches
- Nausea, vomiting, diarrhea, and loss of appetite

Late Stage Illness

Rarely, if treatment is delayed or if there are other medical conditions present, anaplasmosis can cause severe illness. Prompt treatment can reduce your risk of developing severe illness.

Signs and symptoms of severe late-stage illness can include:

- Respiratory failure
- Bleeding problems
- Organ failure
- Death

Risk factors for severe illness:

- **Delayed treatment**
- **Age:** being older puts you at risk
- **Weakened immune system:** People with weakened immune systems (such as those receiving some cancer treatments, individuals with advanced HIV infection, prior organ transplants, or people taking some medications) are at risk for severe illness

Diagnosis and Testing of Anaplasmosis

- Your healthcare provider can order certain blood tests to look for evidence of anaplasmosis or other illnesses that cause similar symptoms.

- Test results may take several weeks.
- If your healthcare provider thinks you have anaplasmosis, or another tick-borne infection, she or he may prescribe antibiotics while you wait for test results.

Treatment of Anaplasmosis

- Early treatment with the antibiotic doxycycline can prevent death and severe illness.

Doxycycline is the recommended antibiotic treatment for anaplasmosis in adults and children of all ages.

Section 9.5

Ehrlichiosis

This section includes text excerpted from "Ehrlichiosis,"
Centers for Disease Control and Prevention (CDC),
January 17, 2019.

"Ehrlichiosis" is the general name used to describe diseases caused by the bacteria *Ehrlichia chaffeensis*, *E. ewingii*, or *E. muris eauclairensis* in the United States. These bacteria are spread to people primarily through the bite of infected ticks, including the lone star tick (*Amblyomma americanum*) and the black-legged tick (*Ixodes scapularis*).

People with ehrlichiosis will often have fever, chills, headache, muscle aches, and sometimes an upset stomach. Doxycycline is the treatment of choice for adults and children of all ages with ehrlichiosis.

Transmission of Ehrlichiosis

The majority of reported cases are due to infection with *E. chaffeensis*.

- Tick bites
  - Most people get ehrlichiosis from the bite of an infected tick.
  - In the United States, *E. chaffeensis* and *E. ewingii* are carried by the lone star tick (*A. americanum*), found primarily in the south central and eastern United States.
  - *E. muris eauclairensis* is carried by the black-legged tick (*I. scapularis*). While the black-legged tick is widely distributed in the eastern United States, *E. muris eauclairensis* has only been found in Wisconsin and Minnesota.
- Blood transfusion and organ transplant
  - In rare cases, *Ehrlichia* species have been spread through blood transfusion and organ transplant.

Ehrlichiosis caused by *E. chaffeensis* and *E. ewingii* is most frequently reported from the southeastern and south central United States, from the East Coast extending westward to Texas.

Signs and Symptoms of Ehrlichiosis

- Signs and symptoms of ehrlichiosis typically begin within 1 to 2 weeks after the bite of an infected tick.
  - Tick bites are usually painless, and many people do not remember being bitten.
- See your healthcare provider if you become ill after being bitten by a tick or spending time in grassy, brushy, wooded areas.

Early Illness

Early signs and symptoms (the first five days of illness) are usually mild or moderate and may include:

- Fever, chills
- Severe headache
- Muscle aches
- Nausea, vomiting, diarrhea, loss of appetite
- Confusion
- Rash (more common in children)

Rash

Up to 1 in 3 people with ehrlichiosis report a rash; rash is more common in people with *E. chaffeensis* ehrlichiosis and generally occurs more often in children than adults. Rash usually develops 5 days after a fever begins. If a person develops a rash, it can look like red splotches or pinpoint dots.

Late Stage Illness

If antibiotic treatment is delayed, ehrlichiosis can sometimes cause severe illness. Early treatment can reduce your risk of developing severe illness.

Signs and symptoms of severe late-stage illness can include:

- Damage to the brain or nervous system (e.g., inflammation of the brain and surrounding tissue, called "meningoencephalitis")
- Respiratory failure
- Uncontrolled bleeding
- Organ failure
- Death

Risk factors for severe illness:

- **Delayed antibiotic treatment**
- **Age:** being very young or very old
- **Weakened immune system:** such as those receiving some cancer treatments, individuals with advanced HIV infection, people who have received organ transplants, or people taking certain medications

Diagnosis and Testing of Ehrlichiosis

Your healthcare provider can order certain blood tests to look for evidence of ehrlichiosis or other illnesses that can cause similar symptoms.

Test results may take several weeks.

If your healthcare provider thinks you have ehrlichiosis or another tick-borne infection, she or he may prescribe antibiotics while you wait for test results.

Treatment of Ehrlichiosis

- Early treatment with the antibiotic doxycycline can prevent death and severe illness.

Doxycycline is the recommended antibiotic treatment for ehrlichiosis in adults and children of all ages.

Section 9.6
Other Spotted Fever

This section includes text excerpted from "Other Spotted Fever Group Rickettsioses," Centers for Disease Control and Prevention (CDC), January 18, 2019.

Spotted fever group rickettsioses (spotted fevers) are a group of diseases caused by closely related bacteria. These bacteria are spread to people through the bite of infected mites and ticks. The most serious and commonly reported spotted fever group rickettsiosis in the United States is Rocky Mountain spotted fever (RMSF).

Other causes of spotted fever group rickettsioses (spotted fevers) in the United States include:

- *Rickettsia parkeri* rickettsiosis, caused by *R. parkeri*
- Pacific Coast tick fever, caused by *Rickettsia* species 364D
- Rickettsialpox, caused by *Rickettsia akari*

Spotted fevers can range from mild to life-threatening. Most people who get sick with a spotted fever other than RMSF will have an eschar (dark scab at the site of the tick or mite bite), fever, headache, and rash. Doxycycline is the treatment of choice for all spotted fever infections.

Transmission of Spotted Fevers

Rickettsia parkeri rickettsiosis, caused by infection with *R. parkeri*, is spread by the Gulf Coast tick *Amblyomma maculatum*, which is found in the southeastern United States.

Pacific Coast tick fever is caused by the bacteria *R. philipii* (known previously as *Rickettsia sp. 364D*). Pacific Coast tick fever is spread by the bite of the infected Pacific Coast tick *Dermacentor occidentalis*, which can be found along the western coastline in California, Oregon, and Washington.

Rickettsialpox is caused by *R. akari*. Unlike the other spotted fevers described here, *R. akari* is spread through the bite of infected mouse mites (*Liponyssoides sanguineus*). Cases occur occasionally throughout the United States, and are most often reported out of the northeastern United States, particularly New York City.

Signs and Symptoms of Spotted Fevers

The first sign of many spotted fevers (including *Rickettsia parkeri rickettsiosis*, Pacific Coast tick fever, or rickettsialpox) is generally a dark scab at the site of tick or mite bite, known as an "eschar." Eschars usually develop a few days to a week following the bite of an infected tick or mite.

Several days after an eschar develops, patients can develop other signs and symptoms.

Signs and symptoms can include:

- Fever
- Headache
- Rash
- Muscle aches

R. parkeri rickettsiosis, Pacific Coast tick fever, and rickettsialpox are less severe than RMSF; however, it can be difficult to distinguish between RMSF and other spotted fevers, especially during early stages of these diseases. Ticks are typically found in grassy or wooded environments. See your healthcare provider if you become ill after having been bitten by a tick, or having spent time in areas where ticks may live. Rickettsialpox is spread by mites carried by the common house mouse. Be sure to mention any time spent in areas where mice may be found.

Diagnosis and Testing of Spotted Fevers

- The signs and symptoms of spotted fevers are similar to those of many other diseases. See your healthcare provider if you develop the signs or symptoms of spotted fevers.

- Be sure to tell your healthcare provider if you become ill and have recently been bitten by a tick, exposed to mice, or have spent time in areas where ticks or mice may be found.
- Your healthcare provider may order certain blood tests to look for evidence of spotted fever infection.
- The results of these tests can take weeks. If your healthcare provider thinks your illness might be a spotted fever, she or he should recommend antibiotic treatment before results are available.

Treatment of Spotted Fevers

Some spotted fevers are not life-threatening and can resolve over time, even without treatment. For others, especially RMSF, early treatment with the antibiotic doxycycline can be lifesaving.

Doxycycline is the recommended antibiotic treatment for all spotted fevers, including RMSF in adults and children of all ages.

Doxycycline saves lives. Doxycycline is the number one recommended treatment for suspected rickettsial infections in patients of all ages.

Imported Spotted Fevers

Spotted fever group rickettsioses (spotted fevers) occur worldwide and result in a broad range of illnesses, from relatively mild to life-threatening. People may become exposed to these tick-borne bacteria when traveling outside of the United States, and healthcare providers should be aware of these illnesses in patients who have signs and symptoms common to other spotted fevers and history of travel within two weeks of illness onset.

The most commonly reported spotted fever reported among United States patients following international travel is African tick bite fever, caused by *Rickettsia africae*. Almost 90 percent of imported spotted fevers occur among travelers to sub-Saharan Africa. Another frequently identified spotted fever group rickettsiosis is Mediterranean spotted fever, caused by *Rickettsia conorii*.

Commercial antibody tests for RMSF can be used to confirm any spotted fever infection. However, most commercial tests are unable to distinguish among the different species of spotted fever group *Rickettsia*. More specialized tests can be performed at the Centers for Disease Control and Prevention (CDC) laboratories. Spotted fever infections can range from mild to life-threatening. Doxycycline is the treatment of choice for all spotted fever infections.

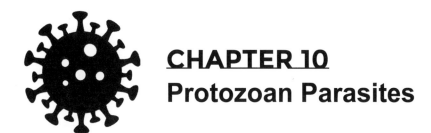

CHAPTER 10
Protozoan Parasites

Chapter Contents

Malaria

This section includes text excerpted from "Malaria," Centers for Disease Control and Prevention (CDC), November 14, 2018.

Malaria Parasites

Malaria parasites are microorganisms that belong to the genus *Plasmodium*. There are more than 100 species of *Plasmodium*, which can infect many animal species such as reptiles, birds, and various mammals. Four species of *Plasmodium* have long been recognized to infect humans in nature. In addition, is one species that naturally infects macaques has recently been recognized as a cause of zoonotic malaria in humans. (There are some additional species which can exceptionally or under experimental conditions, infect humans.)

The species infecting humans are the following:

- ***P. falciparum,*** which is found worldwide in tropical and subtropical areas, and especially in Africa where this species predominates. *P. falciparum* can cause severe malaria because it multiples rapidly in the blood, and can thus cause severe blood loss (anemia). In addition, infected parasites can clog small blood vessels. When this occurs in the brain, cerebral malaria results, a complication that can be fatal.
- ***P. vivax,*** which is found mostly in Asia, Latin America, and in some parts of Africa. Because of the density of populations, especially in Asia, it is probably the most prevalent human malaria parasite. *P. vivax* (as well as *P. ovale*) has dormant liver stages ("hypnozoites") that can activate and invade the blood ("relapse") several months or years after the infecting mosquito bite.
- ***P. ovale,*** which is found mostly in Africa (especially West Africa) and the islands of the western Pacific. It is biologically and morphologically very similar to *P. vivax*. However, unlike *P. vivax*, *P. ovale* can infect individuals who are negative for the Duffy blood group, which is the case for many residents of sub-Saharan Africa.

This explains the greater prevalence of *P. ovale* (rather than *P. vivax*) in most of Africa.

- **P. malariae,** found worldwide, is the only human malaria parasite species that have a quartan (three-day) cycle. (The three other species have a tertian, or two-day, cycle.) If untreated, *P. malariae* causes a long-lasting, chronic infection that in some cases can last a lifetime. In some chronically infected patients *P. malariae* can cause serious complications such as nephrotic syndrome.

- **P. knowlesi,** found throughout Southeast Asia, is a natural pathogen of long- and pig-tailed macaques. It was recently shown to be a significant cause of zoonotic malaria in that region, particularly in Malaysia. *P. knowlesi* has a 24-hour replication cycle and so can rapidly progress from an uncomplicated to a severe infection; fatal cases have been reported.

Human Factors and Malaria
Genetic Factors

Biologic characteristics present from birth can protect against certain types of malaria. Two genetic factors, both associated with human red blood cells (RBCs), have been shown to be epidemiologically important. People who have the sickle cell trait (heterozygotes for the abnormal hemoglobin gene HbS) are relatively protected against *P. falciparum* malaria and thus enjoy a biologic advantage. Because *P. falciparum* malaria has been a leading cause of death in Africa since remote times, the sickle cell trait is now more frequently found in Africa and in persons of African ancestry than in other population groups. In general, the prevalence of hemoglobin-related disorders and other blood cell dyscrasias, such as Hemoglobin C, the thalassemias and G6PD deficiency, are more prevalent in malaria-endemic areas and are thought to provide protection from malarial disease.

People who are negative for the Duffy blood group have RBCs that are resistant to infection by *P. vivax*. Since the majority of Africans are Duffy negative, *P. vivax* is rare in Africa south of the Sahara, especially in West Africa. In that area, the niche of *P. vivax* has been taken over by *P. ovale*, a very similar parasite that does infect Duffy-negative people.

Other genetic factors related to RBCs also influence malaria, but to a lesser extent. Various genetic determinants (such as the "HLA complex," which plays a role in the control of immune responses) may equally influence an individual's risk of developing severe malaria.

Acquired Immunity

Acquired immunity greatly influences how malaria affects an individual and a community. After repeated attacks of malaria, a people may develop a partially protective immunity. Such "semi-immune" people often can still be infected by malaria parasites, but may not develop severe disease, and, in fact, frequently lack any typical malaria symptoms.

In areas with high *P. falciparum* transmission (most of Africa south of the Sahara), newborns will be protected during the first few months of life, presumably by maternal antibodies transferred to them through the placenta. As these antibodies decrease with time, these young children become vulnerable to disease and death by malaria. If they survive repeated infections to an older age (2 to 5 years) they will have reached a protective semi-immune status. Thus, in high-transmission areas, young children are a major risk group and are targeted preferentially by malaria control interventions.

In areas with lower transmission (such as Asia and Latin America), infections are less frequent and a larger proportion of the older children and adults have no protective immunity. In such areas, malaria disease can be found in all age groups, and epidemics can occur.

In Asembo Bay, a highly endemic area in western Kenya, anemia occurs most in young children between the ages of 6 and 24 months. After 24 months, it decreases because the children have built up their acquired immunity against malaria (and its consequence, anemia).

Pregnancy and Malaria

Pregnancy decreases immunity against many infectious diseases. Women who have developed protective immunity against *P. falciparum* tend to lose this protection when they become pregnant (especially during their first and second pregnancies). Malaria during pregnancy is harmful not only to the mothers, but also to the unborn children. The latter are at greater risk of being delivered prematurely or with low birth weight, with consequently decreased chances of survival during the early months of life. For this reason pregnant women are also targeted (in addition to young children) for protection by malaria control programs in endemic countries.

Behavioral Factors

Human behavior, often dictated by social and economic reasons, can influence the risk of malaria for individuals and communities. For example:

- Poor rural populations in malaria-endemic areas often cannot afford the housing and bed nets that would protect them from exposure to mosquitoes. These people often lack the knowledge to recognize malaria and to treat it promptly and correctly. Often, cultural beliefs result in the use of traditional, ineffective methods of treatment.
- Travelers from nonendemic areas may choose not to use insect repellent or medicines to prevent malaria. Reasons may include cost, inconvenience, or a lack of knowledge.
- Human activities can create breeding sites for larvae (standing water in irrigation ditches, burrow pits, etc.).
- Agricultural work such as harvesting (also influenced by climate) may force increased nighttime exposure to mosquito bites.
- Raising domestic animals near the household may provide alternate sources of blood meals for *Anopheles* mosquitoes and thus decrease human exposure.
- War, migrations (voluntary or forced), and tourism may expose nonimmune individuals to an environment with high malaria transmission.

Human behavior in endemic countries also determines in part how successful malaria control activities will be in their efforts to decrease transmission. The governments of malaria-endemic countries often lack financial resources. As a consequence, health workers in the public sector are often underpaid and overworked. They lack equipment, drugs, training, and supervision. The local populations are aware of such situations when they occur, and cease relying on public-sector health facilities. Conversely, the private sector suffers from its own problems. Regulatory measures often do not exist or are not enforced. This encourages private consultations by unlicensed, costly health providers, and the anarchic prescription and sale of drugs (some of which are counterfeit products). Correcting this situation is a tremendous challenge that must be addressed if malaria control and, ultimately, elimination is to be successful.

Section 10.2
Leishmaniasis

This section includes text excerpted from
"Leishmaniasis—Biology," Centers for Disease Control
and Prevention (CDC), July 17, 2019.

Causal Agent

Leishmaniasis is a vector-borne disease that is transmitted by sand flies and caused by obligate intracellular protozoa of the genus *Leishmania*. Human infection is caused by more than 20 species. These include the *L. donovani* complex with 2 species (*L. donovani*, *L. infantum* [also known as "*L. chagasi*"]); the *L. mexicana* complex with 3 main species (*L. mexicana*, *L. amazonensis*, and *L. venezuelensis*); *L. tropica*; *L. major*; *L. aethiopica*; and the subgenus Viannia with 4 main species (*L.* [*V.*] *braziliensis*, *L.* [*V.*] *guyanensis*, *L.* [*V.*] *panamensis*, and *L.* [*V.*] *peruviana*). The different species are morphologically indistinguishable, but they can be differentiated by isoenzyme analysis, molecular methods, or monoclonal antibodies.

Disease

There are several different forms of leishmaniasis in people. Some people have a silent infection, without any symptoms or signs.

The most common form is **cutaneous leishmaniasis**, which causes skin sores. The sores typically develop within a few weeks or months of the sand fly bite. The sores can change in size and appearance over time. The sores may start out as papules (bumps) or nodules (lumps) and may end up as ulcers (like a volcano, with a raised edge and central crater); skin ulcers might be covered by a scab or crust. The sores usually are painless, but can be painful. Some people have swollen glands near the sores (for example, under the arm, if the sores are on the arm or hand).

The other main form is **visceral leishmaniasis**, which affects several internal organs (usually the spleen, liver, and bone marrow) and can be life-threatening. The illness typically develops within months (sometimes as long as years) of the sand fly bite. Affected people usually have fever, weight loss, enlargement (swelling) of the spleen and liver, and low blood counts—a low red blood cell count (anemia), a low white blood cell count (leukopenia), and a low platelet count (thrombocytopenia).

Mucosal leishmaniasis is an example of one of the less common forms of leishmaniasis. This form can be a sequela (consequence) of infection with some of the species (types) of the parasite that cause cutaneous leishmaniasis in parts of Latin America: certain types of the parasite might spread from the skin and cause sores in the mucous membranes of the nose (most common location), mouth, or throat.

Diagnosis of Leishmaniasis

Various laboratory methods can be used to diagnose leishmaniasis—to detect the parasite as well as to identify the *Leishmania* species (type). Some of the methods are available only in reference laboratories. In the United States, the Centers for Disease Control and Prevention (CDC) staff can assist with the testing for leishmaniasis.

Tissue specimens—such as from skin sores (for cutaneous leishmaniasis) or from bone marrow (for visceral leishmaniasis)—can be examined for the parasite under a microscope, in special cultures, and by molecular tests. Blood tests that detect antibodies (an immune response) to the parasite can be helpful for cases of visceral leishmaniasis; tests to look for the parasite (or its deoxyribonucleic acid (DNA)) itself usually also are done.

Treatment of Leishmaniasis

Before considering treatment, the first step is to make sure the diagnosis is correct.

Treatment decisions should be individualized. Healthcare providers may consult CDC staff about the relative merits of various approaches. Examples of factors to consider include the form of leishmaniasis, the *Leishmania* species that caused it, the potential severity of the case, and the patient's underlying health.

The skin sores of cutaneous leishmaniasis usually heal on their own, even without treatment. But, this can take months or even years, and the sores can leave ugly scars. Another potential concern applies to some (not all) types of the parasite found in parts of Latin America: certain types might spread from the skin and cause sores in the mucous membranes of the nose (most common location), mouth, or throat (mucosal leishmaniasis). Mucosal leishmaniasis might not be noticed until years after the original sores healed. Ensuring adequate treatment of the cutaneous infection may help prevent mucosal leishmaniasis.

If not treated, severe (advanced) cases of visceral leishmaniasis typically are fatal.

Section 10.3

Chagas Disease/American Trypanosomiasis

This section includes text excerpted from "Chagas Disease," Centers for Disease Control and Prevention (CDC), March 6, 2019.

Causal Agent

The protozoan parasite *Trypanosoma cruzi* causes Chagas disease, a zoonotic disease that can be transmitted to humans by bloodsucking triatomine bugs.

Disease

Chagas disease has an acute and a chronic phase. If untreated, infection is lifelong.

Acute Chagas disease occurs immediately after infection and can last up to a few weeks or months. During the acute phase, parasites may be found in the circulating blood. This phase of infection is usually mild or asymptomatic. There may be fever or swelling around the site of inoculation (where the parasite entered into the skin or mucous membrane). Rarely, acute infection may result in severe inflammation of the heart muscle or the brain and lining around the brain.

Following the acute phase, most infected people enter into a prolonged asymptomatic form of disease (called "chronic indeterminate"), during which few or no parasites are found in the blood. During this time, most people are unaware of their infection. Many people may remain asymptomatic for life and never develop Chagas-related symptoms. However, an estimated 20 to 30 percent of infected people will develop severe and sometimes life-threatening medical problems over the course of their lives.

Complications of chronic Chagas disease may include:

- Heart rhythm abnormalities that can cause sudden death
- A dilated heart that does not pump blood well

- A dilated esophagus or colon, leading to difficulties with eating or passing stool

In people who have suppressed immune systems (for example, due to AIDS or chemotherapy), Chagas disease can reactivate with parasites found in the circulating blood. Reactivation can potentially cause severe disease.

Diagnosis

During the acute phase of infection, parasites may be seen circulating in the blood. The diagnosis of Chagas disease can be made by observation of the parasite in a blood smear by microscopic examination. A thick and thin blood smear are made and stained for visualization of parasites.

Diagnosis of chronic Chagas disease is made after consideration of the patient's clinical findings, as well as by the likelihood of being infected, such as having lived in a country where Chagas disease is common. Diagnosis is generally made by testing for parasite-specific antibodies.

Treatment

Treatment for Chagas disease is recommended for people diagnosed early in the course of infection (acute phase), babies with congenital infection, and for those with suppressed immune systems. Many patients with chronic infection may also benefit from treatment.

Patients should consult with their primary healthcare provider. Some patients may be referred to a specialist, such as a cardiologist, gastroenterologist, or infectious-disease specialist.

Prevention and Control

In areas of Mexico, Central America, and South America, where the *Trypanosoma cruzi* parasite is present in triatomine bugs, improved housing and spraying insecticide inside housing to eliminate the bugs has significantly decreased the spread of Chagas disease. Screening of blood donations for Chagas is another important public-health tool to help prevent spreading the disease through blood transfusions. Early detection and treatment of new cases, including mother-to-baby (congenital) cases, will also help reduce the burden of disease.

In the United States and other regions where Chagas disease is now found but is not widespread, control strategies are focused on preventing transmission from blood transfusion, organ transplantation, and mother to baby.

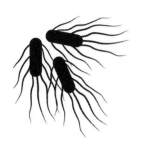

PART 3 • FOOD- AND WATER-BORNE ILLNESSES AND DISEASES

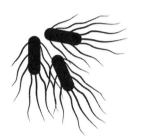

CHAPTER 11
The Burden of Foodborne Illness

Surveillance systems and surveys provide vital information about the burden of foodborne illness in the United States, but they do not capture every illness. Because only a fraction of illnesses are diagnosed and reported, the Centers for Disease Control and Prevention (CDC) needs periodic assessments of the total burden of illness in order to set public-health goals, allocate resources, and measure the economic impact of the disease. The CDC uses the best data available and makes reasonable adjustments—based on surveys, study results, and statistical methods—to account for shortcomings and missing pieces of information.

Foodborne Illness Estimates Help the CDC Understand Important Public-Health Problems

The CDC estimates that 48 million people get sick, 128,000 are hospitalized, and 3,000 die from foodborne diseases each year in the United States.

The 2011 estimates provide the most accurate picture yet of which foodborne pathogens (bacteria, viruses, and parasites) are causing the most illnesses in the United States, and also document the number of foodborne illnesses without a known cause. These estimates are the first

This chapter includes text excerpted from "Burden of Foodborne Illness: Overview," Centers for Disease Control and Prevention (CDC), November 5, 2018.

comprehensive estimates since 1999 and are the first ever to estimate illnesses caused solely by foods eaten in the United States.

Trends Let the CDC Know If Foodborne Illness Infections Are Increasing or Decreasing

Foodborne illness estimates provide the most accurate count of illness at a specific point in time, but they do not show disease trends—whether illnesses are increasing or decreasing. Yet documenting trends is essential for monitoring how well state and federal government organizations are doing in reducing foodborne illness.

Surveillance systems, such as the Foodborne Diseases Active Surveillance Network (FoodNet), are better at showing disease trends. FoodNet conducts surveillance for several important enteric pathogens, accomplishing its work through active surveillance; surveys of laboratories, physicians, and the general population; and through population-based epidemiologic studies.

Attribution of Foodborne Illness to Sources Tells Which Foods Are Most Important as Causes of Disease

By determining the sources of foodborne illness, the CDC can identify opportunities to improve foodsafety. Contamination can occur anywhere along the food production chain—from fields where food is grown to cutting boards in kitchens. Attribution estimates can help in deciding what new prevention strategies are needed to safeguard our food.

Attributing illness to foods is a challenge for several reasons. There are thousands of different foods, and humans eat many categories of food in a single meal. The CDC does not know what food is responsible for the vast majority of foodborne illnesses. However, the CDC gathers data to help bridge some gaps. Data collected during foodborne outbreak investigations can be used in attribution analyses. Outbreak investigations provide direct links between illnesses and the foods responsible for them. Other data and analyses are also used for attribution analyses.

Major Findings of Foodborne Illnesses

The CDC estimates that each year roughly 1 in 6 Americans (or 48 million people) gets sick, 128,000 are hospitalized, and 3,000 die of foodborne diseases.

These estimates provide the most accurate estimates yet of which known foodborne pathogens (bacteria, viruses, and parasites) are causing the most illnesses in the United States, and how many foodborne illnesses are caused by unspecified agents. The estimates also show that much work remains to be done—specifically in focusing efforts on the top known pathogens and identifying the additional causes of foodborne illness and death.

The CDC provides estimates for two major groups of foodborne illnesses. They are:

- **Known foodborne pathogens**—31 pathogens known to cause foodborne illness. Many of these pathogens are tracked by public-health systems that track diseases and outbreaks.
- **Unspecified agents**—Agents with insufficient data to estimate agent-specific burden; known agents not yet identified as causing foodborne illness; microbes, chemicals, or other substances known to be in food whose ability to cause illness is unproven; and agents not yet identified. Because you cannot "track" what is not yet identified, estimates for this group of agents started with the health effects or symptoms that are most likely to cause acute gastroenteritis.

Total Number of Foodborne Illnesses Each Year

The CDC estimates the number of illnesses, hospitalizations, and deaths caused by both known and unspecified agents and then estimates what proportion of each were foodborne. Table 11.1 provides estimates for domestically acquired foodborne illnesses and Table 11.2 provides estimates for domestically acquired illnesses caused by all transmission routes (foodborne, waterborne, person-to-person contact, animal contact, environmental contamination, and others).

Table 11.1. Estimated Annual Number of Domestically Acquired, Foodborne Illnesses, Hospitalizations, and Deaths Due to 31 Pathogens and the Unspecified Agents Transmitted through Food, United States

Foodborne Agents	Estimated Annual Number of Illnesses		Estimated Annual Number of Hospitalizations		Estimated Annual Number of Deaths	
	Number (90% Credible Interval)	%	Number (90% Credible Interval)	%	Number (90% Credible Interval)	%
31 known pathogens	9.4 million (6.6–12.7 million)	20	55,961 (39,534–75,741)	44	1,351 (712–2,268)	44
Unspecified agents	38.4 million (19.8–61.2 million)	80	71,878 (9,924–157,340)	56	1,686 (369–3,338)	56
Total	47.8 million (28.7–71.1 million)	100	127,839 (62,529–215,562)	100	3,037 (1,492–4,983)	100

Table 11.2. Estimated Annual Number of Illnesses, Hospitalizations, and Deaths Due to 31 Pathogens and the Unspecified Agents, United States

Foodborne Agents	Estimated Annual Number of Illnesses		Estimated Annual Number of Hospitalizations		Estimated Annual Number of Deaths	
	Number (90% Credible Interval)	%	Number (90% Credible Interval)	%	Number (90% Credible Interval)	%
31 known pathogens	37.2 million (28.4–47.6 million)	21	228,744 (188,326–275,601)	47	2,612 (1,723–3,819)	42
Unspecified agents	141.8 million	79	258,033	53	3,574	58
Total	179 million	100	486,777	100	6,186	100

Pathogens Causing the Most Foodborne Illnesses, Hospitalizations, and Deaths Each Year

Table 11.3. Top Five Pathogens Contributing to Domestically Acquired Foodborne Illnesses

Pathogen	Estimated Number of Illnesses	90% Credible Interval	%
Norovirus	5,461,731	3,227,078 to 8,309,480	58
Salmonella, nontyphoidal	1,027,561	644,786 to 1,679,667	11
Clostridium perfringens	965,958	192,316 to 2,483,309	10
Campylobacter spp.	845,024	337,031 to 1,611,083	9
Staphylococcus aureus	241,148	72,341 to 529,417	3
Subtotal			91

Table 11.4. Top Five Pathogens Contributing to Domestically Acquired Foodborne Illnesses Resulting in Hospitalization

Pathogen	Estimated Number of Hospitalizations	90% Credible Interval	%
Salmonella, nontyphoidal	19,336	8,545 to 37,490	35
Norovirus	14,663	8,097 to 23,323	26
Campylobacter spp.	8,463	4,300 to 15,227	15
Toxoplasma gondii	4,428	2,634 to 6,674	8
E. coli (STEC) O157	2,138	549 to 4,614	4
Subtotal			88

Table 11.5. Top Five Pathogens Contributing to Domestically Acquired Foodborne Illnesses Resulting in Death

Pathogen	Estimated Number of Deaths	90% Credible Interval	%
Salmonella, nontyphoidal	378	0 to 1,011	28
Toxoplasma gondii	327	200 to 482	24
Listeria monocytogenes	255	0 to 733	19
Norovirus	149	84 to 237	11
Campylobacter spp.	76	0 to 332	6
Subtotal			88

Improvements in Data and Methodology
Five Key Improvements in the Current Estimates
1. Increased (Larger) Sample Size Used to Estimate Acute Gastroenteritis

Because of investments in the FoodNet Population Survey (FNPS), three surveys were available for current estimates for 2000–2001, 2002–2003, and 2006–2007. The combined sample size from these surveys was more than 48,000 households—five times that for the previous estimates. Larger sample sizes typically result in more precise data.

2. Focus on Illnesses in the United States

Some illnesses reported in the United States are caused by contaminated food or water or other sources encountered in other countries during travel. The current estimates focus on foodborne illnesses that occurred from food consumed in the United States. This is important because efforts to improve food safety in the United States can only affect the burden of illness caused by food consumed here.

3. Improved Data on the Fraction of Norovirus That Is Foodborne

In the current estimates, the fraction of norovirus illnesses estimated to be foodborne was 26 percent, based on data from recently reported outbreaks. In previous estimates, this fraction was estimated to be 40 percent, but it was based on data that had substantial limitations.

Because norovirus causes millions of illnesses, the reduction in the proportion considered to be foodborne means a sizeable reduction in the estimated proportion of foodborne illnesses from the 24 known pathogens that cause acute gastroenteritis illness—from 36 percent to 25 percent.

4. Developed Specific Multipliers for the 31 Known Pathogens

For previous estimates, researchers assumed that infections with similar symptoms (such as *Salmonella* and *Yersinia*) had similar levels of underdiagnosis. Therefore, a general multiplier was applied to estimates of similar illnesses, even though there could be differences. For the 2011 estimates, specific multipliers were developed for the 31 major known pathogens transmitted through food. These multipliers were based on several factors, including:

- The proportion of severe illnesses for a given pathogen (people with severe stomach symptoms) that is likely to seek medical care, as only those seeking medical care can be captured in surveillance data.
- The frequency with which persons with mild and severe illness seek medical care and submit a stool sample for laboratory testing.
- The frequency with which laboratories test for that pathogen. Not all laboratories test for all the pathogens.
- The sensitivity of laboratory tests for that pathogen (i.e., the likelihood that the test correctly identifies the pathogen when it is actually present in a specimen).

Developing specific multipliers for the 31 known pathogens yielded more accurate estimates for each known pathogen and, ultimately, greater accuracy in the overall estimate of foodborne illness.

5. Accounting for Uncertainty

The CDC used many data sources, with varying degrees of reliability, to estimate foodborne illnesses, hospitalizations, and deaths. For each estimate, the CDC used a formula to account for the cumulative effect of all uncertainties in the data inputs. The results were upper and lower 90 percent credible limits, or a 90 percent credible interval. This means there is a 90 percent confidence level that the actual number fell within the range of that lower and upper limit. In previous estimates, this was not calculated.

Need for Improvements and Innovations Remains

Future investments and innovations in surveillance and data analysis could help increase the accuracy of estimates. Future efforts can also be directed toward quantifying the illnesses caused by long-term effects of foodborne infections and toxins and to estimate the economic costs associated with foodborne illness.

Future Refinement of Estimates of Foodborne Illness

Although investments made during the decade before the most recent estimates resulted in improvements and innovations and more accurate estimates, limitations remain that need to be addressed. For example:

- More detailed information on norovirus from improved surveillance and special studies in the United States will better inform future estimates. Most of the data underlying the norovirus estimates are from other countries.
- Improved information on the cases of acute gastroenteritis that are reported during FoodNet survey telephone interviews will be needed to help discern whether they might be caused by noninfectious conditions.
- Better methods may be devised to estimate the degree of underreporting of hospitalizations and deaths.
- Methods to estimate illnesses that do not result in gastroenteritis may be improved.

Methods and Data Sources for Estimating Foodborne Illnesses

Estimating U.S. Foodborne Illnesses for 31 Known Foodborne Pathogens

For each pathogen, the CDC gathered data from surveillance systems and corrected for underreporting and underdiagnosis and then multiplied the adjusted number by the proportion of illnesses that was acquired in the United States (i.e., not during international travel) and the proportion transmitted by food to yield an estimated number of illnesses that are domestically acquired and foodborne. Then, they added the estimates for each of the pathogens to arrive at a total, and used an uncertainty model to generate a point estimate and 90 percent credible interval (upper and lower limits) (Figure 11.1).

Estimating U.S. Foodborne Illnesses for Unspecified Agents

Unspecified agents fall into four general categories:

- Agents with insufficient data to estimate the agent-specific burden

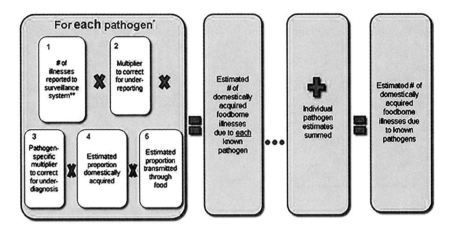

Figure 11.1. Estimating Illnesses for Pathogens Known to Cause Foodborne Illness, 2011*
*Probability distributions were used to model uncertainty in each of the data inputs. Point estimates were bounded by a 90 percent credible interval.
**For six of the 31 pathogens, no routine surveillance data were available so alternative approaches were used to estimate illnesses.

- Known agents not yet recognized as causing foodborne illness
- Microbes, chemicals, or other substances known to be in food whose pathogenicity is unproven
- Agents not yet described

To estimate foodborne illnesses from unspecified agents, they used symptom-based data from surveys to estimate the total number of acute gastroenteritis illnesses (AGI) and then subtracted the number of illnesses accounted for by known gastroenteritis pathogens. The CDC then multiplied this number by the proportion of domestically acquired illnesses and of illnesses attributable to food, just as they did for the known agents. Finally, again as with the known-pathogens estimate, they used an uncertainty model to generate a point estimate and 90 percent credible interval (upper and lower limits) (Figure 11.2).

Foodborne illnesses due to chemicals that cause acute gastroenteritis are included in the estimate of illnesses due to unspecified agents. However,

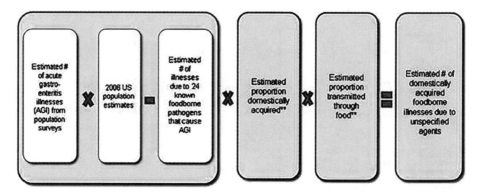

Figure 11.2. Estimating Foodborne Illnesses Due to Unspecified Agents, 2011**
Probability distributions were used to model uncertainty in each of the data inputs. Point estimates were bounded by a 90 percent credible interval.
**Estimated proportions were based on the 24 known pathogens that cause acute gastroenteritis illnesses.*

chemicals or unspecified agents that do not cause acute gastroenteritis are not included in the estimates.

Estimating Hospitalizations and Deaths from U.S. Foodborne Illnesses Due to Known Pathogens

For each known pathogen with surveillance data available, the CDC multiplied the estimated number of reported illnesses (after correcting for underreporting) by the pathogen-specific hospitalization and death rate from surveillance data, surveys, or outbreak data. Because some people with illnesses that were not laboratory-confirmed would also have been hospitalized and died, the CDC doubled the estimates to correct for underdiagnosis. The CDC multiplied the adjusted hospitalization and death estimates by the proportion of illnesses that were acquired within the United States (versus international travel-related) and the proportion transmitted by food. Finally, the CDC used an uncertainty model to generate a point estimate and 90 percent credible intervals for both hospitalizations and deaths (Figures 11.3 and 11.4).

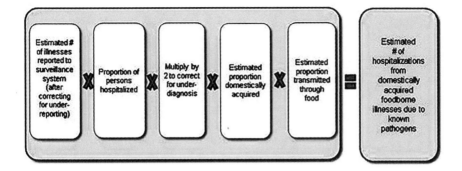

Figure 11.3. Estimating Hospitalizations from Foodborne Illnesses Due to Known Pathogens, 2011*
Probability distributions were used to model uncertainty in each of the data inputs. Point estimates were bounded by a 90 percent credible interval.

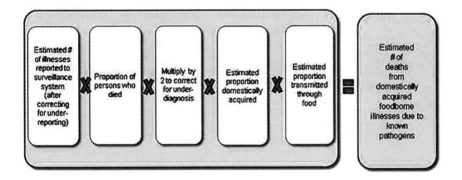

Figure 11.4. Estimating Deaths from Foodborne Illnesses Due to Known Pathogens, 2011*
Probability distributions were used to model uncertainty in each of the data inputs. Point estimates were bounded by a 90 percent credible interval.

Estimating Hospitalizations and Deaths from U.S. Foodborne Illnesses Due to Unspecified Agents

To estimate hospitalizations, the CDC applied the average hospitalization rate for all AGI, determined from survey data for 2000–2006, to 2006 U.S. population estimates and subtracted the estimated number of hospitalizations caused by the 24 known pathogens that cause AGI. For deaths, the CDC determined the death rate for acute gastroenteritis illnesses from U.S. death

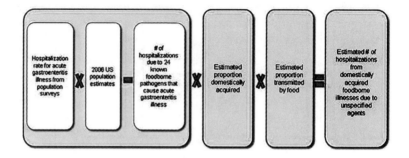

Figure 11.5. Estimating Hospitalizations from Foodborne
Illnesses Due to Unspecified Agents, 2011*
*Probability distributions were used to model uncertainty in
each of the data inputs. Point estimates were bounded by a 90
percent credible interval.*

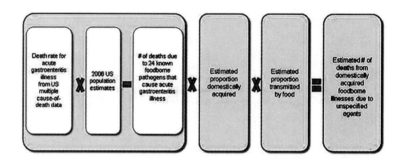

Figure 11.6. Estimating Deaths from Foodborne Illnesses Due to
Unspecified Agents, 2011*
*Probability distributions were used to model uncertainty in
each of the data inputs. Point estimates were bounded by a 90
percent credible interval.*

certificates (specifically, multiple-cause-of-death data) for 2000–2006 and
applied that rate to the 2006 U.S. population estimate. The CDC then
subtracted the estimated number of deaths from the 24 known gastroenteritis
pathogens. For both hospitalizations and deaths, the CDC multiplied the
overall number by the proportion of hospitalizations and deaths from the
24 known gastroenteritis pathogens that were domestically acquired and
foodborne. Finally, they used an uncertainty model to generate a point
estimate and 90 percent credible intervals (Figures 11.5 and 11.6).

Data Sources for Estimates

The CDC used five general types of data sources to create the 2011 estimates:

Active surveillance (public-health officials actively gather data from state and local health departments, laboratories, hospitals, etc.)

- Foodborne Diseases Active Surveillance Network (FoodNet)

Passive surveillance (public-health officials rely on state and local health departments, laboratories, hospitals, etc. to report data to surveillance systems)

- National Notifiable Diseases Surveillance System (NNDSS)
- National Tuberculosis Surveillance System (NTSS)
- Public Health Laboratory Information System (PHLIS)
- Cholera and other Vibrio Illness Surveillance System (COVIS)

Outbreak surveillance

- Foodborne Disease Outbreak Surveillance System

Surveys

- FoodNet Population Survey (FNPS)
- FoodNet Laboratory Survey
- National Ambulatory Medical Care Survey (NAMCS)
- National Hospital Ambulatory Medical Care Survey (NHAMCS)
- National Hospital Discharge Survey (NHDS)
- National Health and Nutrition Survey (NHANES)
- Nationwide Inpatient Sample (NIS)

Vital (government) statistics

- Multiple-cause-of-death data (from U.S. death certificates)
- U.S. Census

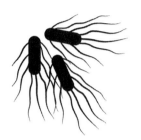

CHAPTER 12
Magnitude and Burden of Waterborne Disease in the United States

Much is known about the risk factors for waterborne illness, but the overall occurrence of waterborne illness in the United States is unknown. Regulatory and public-health agencies and academic researchers have published estimates of the number of illnesses associated with U.S. drinking water systems and marine water venues. These waterborne disease burden estimates provide a foundation for future work to quantify all U.S. waterborne illness, but these estimates do not include all types of waterborne disease nor waterborne disease from all possible types of water exposures and venues.

Pathogen-specific illness and cost estimates also provide important contributions to understanding the health impact of particular waterborne diseases. Many of these pathogens can also be spread in other ways in addition to water (for example, food, person-to-person). The total disease burden from each pathogen and the proportion due to waterborne transmission will both inform the comprehensive waterborne burden of disease estimate.

This chapter includes text excerpted from "Current Waterborne Disease Burden Data and Gaps," Centers for Disease Control and Prevention (CDC), August 9, 2017.

Pathogen-Specific Illness and Cost Estimates

Scope

- Deaths, emergency department (ED) visits, and hospitalizations associated with 13 diseases that can be transmitted by water.
- The 13 selected diseases have been implicated in waterborne disease outbreaks or are otherwise known to be transmitted by water:
- Acute otitis externa (AOE), campylobacteriosis, cryptosporidiosis, *Escherichia coli* (*E. coli*) infection, free-living ameba infection, giardiasis, hepatitis A virus (HAV) infection, Legionnaires' disease, nontuberculous mycobacterial (NTM) infection, *Pseudomonas*-related pneumonia or septicemia, salmonellosis, shigellosis, and vibriosis or cholera.
- Most of the diseases studied can also be transmitted through other routes, such as contaminated food or having contact with a sick person.

Estimates

- 6,939 annual total deaths were documented for 13 diseases caused by pathogens that can be transmitted by water.
- Of the 6,939 deaths, 91 percent were associated with three environmental pathogens that can grow in water system biofilms: *Legionella* (Legionnaires' disease) (250 deaths), NTM (1,216 deaths), and *Pseudomonas*-related pneumonia (1,618 deaths) or septicemia (3,217 deaths).
- Of the 6,939 deaths, 7 percent were associated with seven pathogens transmitted by the fecal–oral route: *Campylobacter, Cryptosporidium, E. coli, Giardia*, Hepatitis A, *Salmonella* nontyphoidal, and *Shigella*.
- 477,000 annual ED visits were documented for 13 diseases caused by pathogens that can be transmitted by water
- 101,000 (21%) of the ED visits resulted in immediate hospital admission; the remaining 376,000 annual treat-and-release ED visits resulted in $194 million in annual direct costs.
- Most treat-and-release ED visits (97%) and costs ($178 million/year) were associated with AOE (swimmer's ear); this condition had the lowest mean cost per visit ($487/visit).

- Overall, the annual hospitalization and treat-and-release ED visit costs associated with the selected diseases totaled to $3.8 billion.

What Is Not Included in the Scope of These 2017 Pathogen-Specific Illness and Cost Estimates?

- Estimates do not include all pathogens that could potentially be spread via water.
- Estimates do not include the percentage of each illness attributable to waterborne transmission.
- Estimates do not include less severe illness (i.e., illnesses that did not result in death or a visit to the emergency department)

Waterborne Disease Burden Estimates
Scope

- Cost of illness due to seafood consumption and contact with marine pathogens.
- Pathogen-specific cost estimates also included.

Estimates

- 5 million excess cases of gastrointestinal illness each year due to marine beach exposure, costing $300 million each year in healthcare expenses.
- In pathogen-specific analyses, researchers estimated that direct exposure to *Vibrio* species (*V. vulnificus*, *V. parahaemolyticus*, *V. alginolyticus*, and *K. brevis*) costs approximately $30 million each year in healthcare costs.

What Is Not Included in the Scope of the 2011 Marine Water Burden Estimates?

- Estimates do not include waterborne illness from nonmarine recreational water sources, including freshwater beaches and rivers, lakes, and streams.
- Estimates do not include recreational waterborne illness from chlorinated venues, including pools, splash parks, spas, and hot tubs.

Need for a Comprehensive Waterborne Disease Burden Estimate

Many stakeholders can benefit from a waterborne disease burden estimate. Surveillance and outbreak data suggest waterborne pathogens are still important causes of illness in the United States; however, the overall prevalence of waterborne illness in the United States is unknown. To determine how many people in the United States are affected by waterborne illnesses, which populations are most susceptible, and inform prevention-planning efforts, it is necessary to measure water-related illness across all water sectors, considering all water uses and exposures.

How a Waterborne Disease Burden Estimate Can Help Prevent Waterborne Illness in the United States

- Target resources and preventive measures
- Drive data collection that will refine the estimate over time
- Drive inclusion of items (such as chemicals)
- Drive partnerships
- Provide metrics to follow over time
- Address emerging issues

The Ideal Waterborne Disease Burden Estimate

The ideal waterborne disease burden estimate will provide a cohesive umbrella estimate that covers:

All water uses, including:
- Drinking and household uses
- Recreation and leisure
- Industry
- Agriculture and food production
- Medical and healthcare uses

All water venues, including:
- Drinking water systems (public, private)
- Natural swimming waters (beaches, freshwater)

- Chlorinated swimming venues (pools, hot tubs/spas, water parks, foot spas)
- Premise plumbing and building distribution systems
- Irrigation and food-processing water systems
- Reclaimed water, gray water

Premise Plumbing

Premise plumbing is the drinking water-system that is inside the housing, schools, and other buildings. It connects to the main drinking water distribution system, but the water utility does not monitor its safety. A large proportion of drinking water outbreaks are linked to pathogens that grow in premise plumbing and building water-system parts—such as hot-water tanks, cooling towers, decorative fountains, showerheads, and water taps—and are inhaled through steam or aerosol.

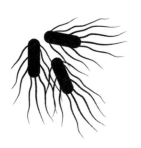

CHAPTER 13
Food Contamination and Food Poisoning

Chapter Contents

Section 13.1

How Food Gets Contaminated— the Food Production Chain

This section includes text excerpted from "How Food Gets Contaminated—the Food Production Chain," Centers for Disease Control and Prevention (CDC), September 5, 2017.

It takes several steps to get food from the farm or fishery to the dining table. These steps are called the "food production chain." Contamination can occur at any point along the chain—during production, processing, distribution, or preparation.

Production

"Production" means growing the plants we harvest or raising the animals we use for food. Most food comes from domesticated animals and plants, and their production occurs on farms or ranches. Some foods are caught or harvested from the wild, such as some fish, mushrooms, and game.

Examples of Contamination in Production

- If a hen's reproductive organs are infected, the yolk of an egg can be contaminated in the hen before it is even laid.
- If the fields are sprayed with contaminated water for irrigation, fruits and vegetables can be contaminated before harvest.
- Fish in some tropical reefs may acquire a toxin from the smaller sea creatures they eat.

Processing

"Processing" means changing plants or animals into what we recognize and buy as food. Processing involves different steps for different kinds of foods. For produce, processing can be as simple as washing and sorting,

227

or it can involve trimming, slicing, or shredding. Milk is usually processed by pasteurizing it; sometimes it is made into cheese. Nuts may be roasted, chopped, or ground (such as with peanut butter). For animals, the first step of processing is slaughter. Meat and poultry may then be cut into pieces or ground. They may also be smoked, cooked, or frozen and may be combined with other ingredients to make sausage or an entrée, such as a pot pie.

Examples of Contamination in Processing

- If contaminated water or ice is used to wash, pack, or chill fruits or vegetables, the contamination can spread to those items.
- During the slaughter process, germs on an animal's hide that came from the intestines can get into the final meat product.
- If germs contaminate surfaces used for food processing, such as a processing line or storage bins, these germs can spread to foods that touch those surfaces.

Distribution

"Distribution" means getting food from the farm or processing plant to the consumer or a food-service facility, such as a restaurant, cafeteria, or hospital kitchen. This step might involve transporting foods just once, such as trucking produce from a farm to the local farmers' market. Or it might involve many stages. For instance, frozen hamburger patties might be trucked from a meat-processing plant to a large supplier, stored for a few days in the supplier's warehouse, trucked again to a local distribution facility for a restaurant chain, and finally delivered to an individual restaurant.

Examples of Contamination in Distribution

- If refrigerated food is left on a loading dock for a long time in warm weather, it could reach temperatures that allow bacteria to grow.
- Fresh produce can be contaminated if it is loaded into a truck that was not cleaned after transporting animals or animal products.

Preparation

"Preparation" means getting the food ready to eat. This step may occur in the kitchen of a restaurant, home, or institution. It may involve following a complex recipe with many ingredients, simply heating and serving a food on a plate, or just opening a package and eating the food.

Examples of Contamination in Preparation

- If a food worker stays on the job while sick and does not wash his or her hands carefully after using the toilet, the food worker can spread germs by touching food.
- If a cook uses a cutting board or knife to cut raw chicken and then uses the same knife or cutting board without washing it to slice tomatoes for a salad, the tomatoes can be contaminated by germs from the chicken.
- Contamination can occur in a refrigerator if meat juices get on items that will be eaten raw.

Mishandling at Multiple Points

Sometimes, by the time a food causes illness, it has been mishandled in several ways along the food production chain. Once contamination occurs, further mishandling, such as undercooking the food or leaving it out on the counter at an unsafe temperature, can make a foodborne illness more likely. Many germs grow quickly in food held at room temperature; a tiny number can grow to a large number in just a few hours. Reheating or boiling food after it has been left at room temperature for a long time does not always make it safe because some germs produce toxins that are not destroyed by heat.

Section 13.2

Foodborne Contaminants: An Overview

This section includes text excerpted from "Food Borne
Contaminants," Centers for Disease Control and
Prevention (CDC), July 2, 2017.

What Are Foodborne Contaminants?

Most reported cases of foodborne illness are caused by ingestion of food
contaminated with pathogens or toxins of biological origin. While raw or
undercooked meat, poultry, shellfish, and eggs, and unpasteurized milk are
the foods most likely to be contaminated with pathogens, fresh fruits and
vegetables can also be contaminated. Foodborne toxins usually show up in
fish (fresh or cooked) and, to a lesser extent, mushrooms. Occasionally, food
contaminated with high concentrations of human-made, nonfood chemicals,
such as cleaners or pesticides, has sickened people. Adverse health outcomes
associated with chronic exposures to contaminants in the food supply chain
also contribute to the disease burden attributable to food contamination.

In some cases, such as mercury in fish, the data are compelling enough
to establish a link between chronic exposure to a foodborne contaminant
and a specific health outcome. In other cases, scientists are still investigating
possible connections. For example, long-term exposure to low levels of
pesticides and other endocrine disruptors found in food may contribute
to malformations and cancer, but the data are preliminary. (Endocrine
disruptors are chemicals that can disturb the body's endocrine system.)
These chemicals can produce negative developmental, reproductive,
neurological, and immune effects in humans. Monitoring food for the wide
range of possible chemical contaminants poses a formidable challenge,
especially as research suggests that even small doses of some chemicals may
cause adverse health effects over the long term.

Numerous programs are in place to detect the better-known chemical
contaminants, such as pesticides, mercury, and dioxins, and foods may be
removed from the food supply if they exceed certain health limits for those
contaminants. Many other foodborne chemical contaminants, however,

are not monitored. This section briefly reviews the status of foodborne contaminants in the United States, with particular attention to what is known about the types of contaminants and foods involved.

What Are the Health Effects of Foodborne Contaminants?

The bacterial and viral infections responsible for most reported cases of foodborne illness produce symptoms of gastroenteritis (inflammation of the stomach and intestines), including vomiting, diarrhea, and sometimes fever. Cases range from mild and short-lived to deadly. The very young, the elderly, and people with compromised immune systems generally have the most severe symptoms. People with mild symptoms are often cared for at home; more serious cases usually need treatment by a physician. However, the specific source of illness (e.g., food, contact with infected persons or animals) is rarely determined in individual cases.

Illnesses caused by foodborne toxins rather than pathogens often manifest as gastroenteritis, but can include additional symptoms. Most foodborne infections cause diarrheal illness, ranging from mild to severe. People in susceptible populations and some healthy people can develop severe complications, such as hemorrhagic colitis, bloodstream infection, meningitis, joint infection, kidney failure, paralysis, miscarriage, and other problems.

Skin flushing, palpitations, wheezing, itching, or dropping blood pressure can follow ingestion of fish-borne toxins. Several mushroom toxins cause life-threatening organ failure days to weeks after ingestion. Botulism is a rare, but serious paralytic illness caused by a nerve toxin that is produced by the bacterium *Clostridium botulinum* and sometimes by strains of *Clostridium butyricum* and *Clostridium baratii*. Foodborne botulism is caused by eating foods that contain the botulinum toxin. Infant botulism is caused by consuming the spores of the botulinum bacteria, which then grow in the intestines and release toxin. Adult intestinal toxemia (adult intestinal colonization) botulism is a very rare kind of botulism that occurs among adults via the same route as infant botulism. Finally, iatrogenic botulism can occur from accidental overdose of botulinum toxin. All forms of botulism can be fatal and are considered medical emergencies. Foodborne botulism is a public-health emergency because many people can be poisoned by eating a botulism-contaminated food.

Some foodborne illnesses can have severe sequelae (a condition that is a consequence of a previous disease or injury) in addition to the common signs of gastroenteritis. Examples of these include cases of Guillain-Barré syndrome (paralysis) associated with *Campylobacter* infection, hemolytic uremic syndrome (acute kidney failure) associated with Shiga toxin-producing *E. Coli* infection, and miscarriage and stillbirths associated with *Listeria monocytogenes* infection. Brain and nervous-system damage are linked with ingestion of foodborne mercury at high concentrations, but even low doses of mercury can interfere with fetal development. Other foodborne exposures, especially chronic exposure to foodborne endocrine disruptors (pesticides, phthalates, etc.) are believed to be linked with adverse health effects, but more data are needed to demonstrate an association.

How Are We Tracking Foodborne Contaminants?

At the federal level, monitoring the nation's food supply for pathogens and chemical contaminants is mainly the responsibility of the U.S. Food and Drug Administration (FDA) and the U.S. Department of Agriculture (USDA), although many other groups also play a role. The FDA oversees the safety of all food—domestic and imported—except meat, poultry, and processed egg products, which fall under the regulatory authority of the USDA.

The Food Safety and Inspection Service (FSIS) of the USDA inspects raw meat, poultry, and egg products sold in interstate and foreign commerce, including imported goods. Some states have their own inspection programs for meats sold only within the state, but these programs must be at least as stringent as that of the FSIS. If meat, poultry, or egg products are contaminated, the FSIS may issue a recall. Current and archived recall alerts are listed online. The FDA assists state and local agencies that assume primary responsibility for keeping the rest of the food supply safe. Foodborne contaminants detected by either a food facility's own monitoring or during inspections of the facility are generally handled at the facility or the local level unless "there is reasonable probability that an article of food will cause serious adverse health consequences." In those special cases, the facility must report the problem to the FDA's Reportable Food Registry.

Most recalls and reported food problems involve pathogens, such as *E. coli* O157: H7 or *Salmonella*, but both the USDA and FDA also have programs to monitor the food supply for a range of chemical contaminants. The USDA has been operating the Pesticide Data Program (PDP) since 1991. Each year, about 20 commodities (fresh fruits and vegetables, meat, dairy, grain, etc.) and drinking water are sampled from more than 500 food distribution sites across eleven states, and the raw samples are analyzed for a host of pesticides. The results are published in annual reports, which the U.S. Environmental Protection Agency (EPA) uses to set limits for pesticide residues in food.

The FDA's pesticide-residue monitoring program is a focused sampling program intended to detect pesticide-residue levels (in food) that exceed the EPA-established limits. Both domestic and imported foods, especially commodities that are not usually sampled during regulatory monitoring or that are suspected of having pesticide residues, are sampled and analyzed. The FDA has published annual reports since 1987 summarizing the results of the pesticide-residue monitoring program.

An ongoing complement to the FDA's pesticide-residue monitoring program is the Total Diet Study. A "market basket" of about 280 different foods that represent the average U.S. consumer's diet is collected four times per year, once from each of four different regions of the United States. The foods are prepared for consumption (peeled, cooked, etc.) and are then analyzed for a variety of industrial chemicals and toxic elements, such as pesticides, PCBs, and heavy metals. The analytical results are reported online.

Another program, directed jointly by representatives from the FDA, USDA, EPA, and numerous other agencies, has been monitoring dioxin levels in various foods, particularly meat, poultry, eggs, fish, and dairy products. This program is called the "Interagency Working Group on Dioxin" (Dioxin IWG). Some foods are tested for dioxins in the Total Diet Study, but the interagency group has collected and analyzed samples from other foods as well. The goal of the monitoring program is to find abnormally high levels of dioxin and to remove contaminated foods from the food supply.

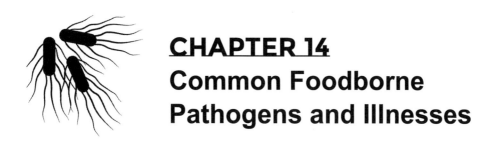

CHAPTER 14
Common Foodborne Pathogens and Illnesses

Causes of Food Poisoning

Many different disease-causing germs can contaminate foods, so there are many different foodborne infections.

- Researchers have identified more than 250 foodborne diseases.
- Most of them are infections, caused by a variety of bacteria, viruses, and parasites.
- Harmful toxins and chemicals also can contaminate foods and cause foodborne illness.

The Centers for Disease Control and Prevention (CDC) estimates that each year 48 million people get sick from a foodborne illness, 128,000 are hospitalized, and 3,000 die.

Do You Have Food Poisoning?

Common symptoms of foodborne diseases are nausea, vomiting, stomach cramps, and diarrhea. However, symptoms may differ among the different types of foodborne diseases. Symptoms can sometimes be severe and some foodborne illnesses can even be life-threatening. Although anyone can get a

This chapter includes text excerpted from "Foodborne Germs and Illnesses," Centers for Disease Control and Prevention (CDC), October 23, 2019.

foodborne illness, some people are more likely to develop one. Those groups include:

- Pregnant women
- Young children
- Older adults
- People with immune systems weakened from medical conditions, such as diabetes, liver disease, kidney disease, organ transplants, human immunodeficiency virus (HIV)/acquired immunodeficiency syndrome (AIDS), or from receiving chemotherapy or radiation treatment.

Most people with foodborne illness get better without medical treatment, but people with severe symptoms should see their doctor.

Some Common Foodborne Germs

The top five germs that cause illnesses from food eaten in the United States are:

- Norovirus
- *Salmonella*
- *Clostridium-perfringens*
- *Campylobacter*
- *Staphylococcus aureus* (Staph)

Some other germs do not cause as many illnesses, but when they do, the illnesses are more likely to lead to hospitalization. Those germs include:

- *Clostridium botulinum* (botulism)
- *Listeria*
- *Escherichia coli* (*E. coli*)
- *Vibrio*

Norovirus

Norovirus is a very contagious virus that causes vomiting and diarrhea. Anyone can get infected and sick with norovirus. You can get norovirus from:

- Having direct contact with an infected person

- Consuming contaminated food or water
- Touching contaminated surfaces and then putting your unwashed hands into your mouth

Salmonella

The CDC estimates *Salmonella* bacteria cause about 1.35 million infections, 26,500 hospitalizations, and 420 deaths in the United States every year. Food is the source for most of these illnesses.

- Most people who get ill from *Salmonella* have diarrhea, fever, and stomach cramps.
- Symptoms usually begin 6 hours to 6 days after infection and last 4 to 7 days.
- Most people recover without specific treatment and should not take antibiotics. Antibiotics are typically used only to treat people who have severe illness or who are at risk for it.
- Some people's illness may be so severe that they need to be hospitalized.

Clostridium Perfringens
What Is *Clostridium Perfringens?*

Clostridium perfringens (*C. perfringens*) is a spore-forming gram-positive bacterium that is found in many environmental sources as well as in the intestines of humans and animals. *C. perfringens* is commonly found on raw meat and poultry. It prefers to grow in conditions with very little or no oxygen, and under ideal conditions can multiply very rapidly. Some strains of *C. perfringens* produce a toxin in the intestine that causes illness.

What Are Common Food Sources of *Clostridium perfringens?*

Beef, poultry, gravies, and dried or precooked foods are common sources of *C. perfringens* infections. *C. perfringens* infection often occurs when foods are prepared in large quantities and kept warm for a long time before serving. Outbreaks often happen in institutions, such as hospitals, school cafeterias, prisons, and nursing homes, or at events with catered food.

Campylobacter

Campylobacter causes an estimated 1.5 million illnesses each year in the United States.

People can get *Campylobacter* infection by eating raw or undercooked poultry or eating something that touched it. They can also get it from eating other foods, including seafood, meat, and produce, by contact with animals, and by drinking untreated water.

Although people with *Campylobacter* infection usually recover on their own, some need antibiotic treatment.

Staphylococcus aureus (Staph)

Staph food poisoning is a gastrointestinal illness caused by eating foods contaminated with toxins produced by the bacterium *Staphylococcus aureus* (Staph) bacteria.

About 25 percent of people and animals have Staph on their skin and in their nose. It usually does not cause illness in healthy people, but Staph has the ability to make toxins that can cause food poisoning.

Clostridium botulinum (Botulism)

Botulism is a rare, but serious illness caused by a toxin that attacks the body's nerves.

Symptoms of botulism usually start with weakness of the muscles that control the eyes, face, mouth, and throat. This weakness may spread to the neck, arms, torso, and legs. Botulism also can weaken the muscles involved in breathing, which can lead to difficulty breathing and even death.

If you or someone you know has symptoms of botulism, see your doctor or go to the emergency room immediately.

Listeria

Listeriosis is a serious infection usually caused by eating food contaminated with the bacterium *Listeria monocytogenes*. An estimated 1,600 people get listeriosis each year, and about 260 die. The infection is most likely to sicken pregnant women and their newborns, adults aged 65 or older, and people with weakened immune systems.

Escherichia coli (E. coli)

Escherichia coli are bacteria found in the environment, foods, and intestines of people and animals. *E. coli* are a large and diverse group of bacteria. Although most strains of *E. coli* are harmless, others can make you sick. Some kinds of *E. coli* can cause diarrhea, while others cause urinary-tract infections, respiratory illness and pneumonia, and other illnesses.

Vibrio

Vibriosis causes an estimated 80,000 illnesses and 100 deaths in the United States every year. People with vibriosis become infected by consuming raw or undercooked seafood or exposing a wound to seawater. Most infections occur from May through October when water temperatures are warmer.

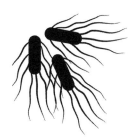

CHAPTER 15
Foodborne Illness: Especially Dangerous for the Vulnerable

The food supply in the United States is among the safest in the world. However, when certain disease-causing bacteria or pathogens contaminate food, they can cause foodborne illness, often called "food poisoning." The federal government estimates that there are about 48 million cases of foodborne illness annually—the equivalent of sickening 1 in 6 Americans each year. And each year, these illnesses result in an estimated 128,000 hospitalizations and 3,000 deaths. Although everyone is susceptible, some people are at greater risk of developing a foodborne illness.

Who Is At Risk?

If you—or someone you care for—are in one of these high-risk groups, it is especially important to practice safe food handling. Vulnerable people are not only at increased risk of contracting a foodborne illness, but are also more likely to have a lengthier illness, undergo hospitalization, or even die.

Pregnant Women

Changes during pregnancy alter the mother's immune systems, making pregnant women more susceptible to foodborne illness. Harmful bacteria can also cross the placenta and infect an unborn baby whose immune

This chapter includes text excerpted from "Food Safety: Importance for At-Risk Groups," U.S. Food and Drug Administration (FDA), February 28, 2019.

system is underdeveloped and not able to fight infection. Foodborne illness during pregnancy is serious and can lead to miscarriage, premature delivery, stillbirth, sickness, or the death of a newborn baby.

Young Children

Young children are more at risk for foodborne illness because their immune systems are still developing.

Older Adults

As people age, their immune systems and other organs become sluggish in recognizing and ridding the body of harmful bacteria and other pathogens that cause infections, such as foodborne illness. Many older adults have also been diagnosed with one or more chronic conditions, such as diabetes, arthritis, cancer, or cardiovascular disease, and are taking at least one medication. The chronic disease process and/or the side effects of some medications may also weaken the immune system. In addition, stomach acid decreases as people get older, and stomach acid plays an important role in reducing the number of bacteria in the intestinal tract—and the risk of illness.

People with Immune Systems Weakened by Disease or Medical Treatment

The immune system is the body's natural reaction or response to "foreign invasion." In healthy people, a properly functioning immune system readily fights off harmful bacteria and other pathogens that cause infection. However, the immune systems of transplant patients and people with certain illnesses, such as HIV/AIDS, cancer, and diabetes, are often weakened from the disease process and/or the side effects of some treatments, making them susceptible to many types of infections—such as those that can be brought on by harmful bacteria that cause foodborne illness. In addition, diabetes may lead to a slowing of the rate at which food passes through the stomach and intestines, allowing harmful foodborne pathogens an opportunity to multiply.

Foods to Avoid

If you are at greater risk of foodborne illness, you are advised not to eat:

- Raw or undercooked meat or poultry

- Raw fish, partially cooked seafood (such as shrimp and crab), and refrigerated smoked seafood
- Raw shellfish (including oysters, clams, mussels, and scallops) and their juices
- Unpasteurized (raw) milk and products made with raw milk, such as yogurt and cheese
- Soft cheeses made from unpasteurized milk, such as feta, Brie, Camembert, blue-veined, and Mexican-style cheeses (such as queso fresco, panela, asadero, and queso blanco)
- Raw or undercooked eggs or foods containing raw or undercooked eggs, including certain homemade salad dressings (such as Caesar salad dressing), homemade cookie dough and cake batters, and homemade eggnog

NOTE: Most premade foods from grocery stores, such as Caesar dressing, premade cookie dough, or packaged eggnog are made with pasteurized eggs.

- Unwashed fresh vegetables, including lettuce/salads
- Unpasteurized fruit or vegetable juices (these juices will carry a warning label)
- Hot dogs, luncheon meats (cold cuts), fermented and dry sausage, and other deli-style meats, poultry products, and smoked fish—unless they are reheated until steaming hot
- Salads (without added preservatives) prepared on-site in a deli-type establishment, such as ham salad, chicken salad, or seafood salad.
- Unpasteurized, refrigerated pâté or meat spreads
- Raw sprouts (alfalfa, bean, or any other sprout)

Foodborne Illness: Know the Symptoms

Symptoms of a foodborne illness usually appear 12 to 72 hours after eating contaminated food, but may occur between 30 minutes and 4 weeks later. Symptoms include:

- Nausea, vomiting, diarrhea (may be bloody), and abdominal pain
- Flu-like symptoms, such as fever, headache, and body ache

If you suspect that you could have a foodborne illness, contact your physician or healthcare provider right away!

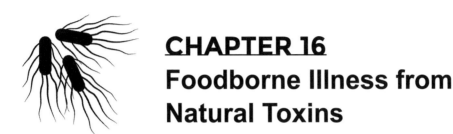

CHAPTER 16
Foodborne Illness from Natural Toxins

Natural Toxins

Food can be contaminated with naturally occurring chemicals that cause disease. Toxins such as mycotoxins and marine toxins are naturally produced under certain conditions. Given that these toxins generally occur in raw materials, especially crops and seafood, manufacturers should require suppliers to certify that the products they purchase are free from natural toxins.

Infestation of Mycotoxins
Infestation of Mycotoxins Due to Drought

Toxigenic fungi, or mycotoxins, are found primarily in foods of plant origin, although they can also pass through the food chain in milk and meat.

This chapter contains text excerpted from the following sources: Text beginning with the heading "Natural Toxins" is excerpted from "Good Manufacturing Practices for the 21st Century for Food Processing, Section 2: Literature Review of Common Food Safety Problems and Applicable Controls," U.S. Food and Drug Administration (FDA), September 14, 2018; Text under the heading "Food Poisoning from Marine Toxins" is excerpted from "Food Poisoning from Marine Toxins," Centers for Disease Control and Prevention (CDC), June 24, 2019; Text beginning with the heading "Ciguatoxin," is excerpted from "Bad Bug Book," U.S. Food and Drug Administration (FDA), November 8, 2019; Text beginning with the heading "Mushroom Toxins" is excerpted from "Bad Bug Book—Handbook of Foodborne Pathogenic Microorganisms and Natural Toxins," U.S. Food and Drug Administration (FDA), 2012. Reviewed March 2020.

Drought can encourage the growth of mycotoxins in certain crops. For example, drought stress can cause aflatoxin, a type of mycotoxin, to grow in corn and tree nuts. Drought can be minimized through adequate irrigation schedules. Thermal and chemical treatments are also available for use on the crop that is already affected by mycotoxins. Thermal inactivation, however, is not effective on certain types of mycotoxins, such as aflatoxin. Chemical treatments, such as ammoniation and activated carbons and clays, are other possible controls.

Infestation of Mycotoxins Due to Damage

Insect damage is associated with high levels of mycotoxin infection, as is mechanical damage from harvesters. Diseases, such as ear rot in corn, also cause damage that leaves the crop susceptible to mycotoxin infestation. Delayed harvesting can also make crops more susceptible to disease due to higher moisture levels. Damage to the product, whether through insect feeding or mechanical harvesters, provides a potential entry point for the mold that produces the mycotoxin. Controls available include pest management to prevent insect damage, breeding cultivars that are resistant to pest damage, timely harvesting, handpicking or electronic sorting to remove damaged crops, and thermal or chemical treatment as noted above. Possible biological control of insects and diseases in the field is also being investigated.

Infestation of Mycotoxins Due to Moisture/Heat during Storage

Post-harvest storage that protects the product from heat and moisture is essential to prevent mycotoxin infestation. Grains should be dried as soon as feasible, and storage under modified atmospheric conditions is desirable. Products should be dried rapidly to less than 10 percent moisture. Products can also be sampled for mycotoxins during storage. Methods include visual inspection with black light, enzyme-linked immunosorbent assay (ELISA) tests, and complex laboratory analysis using high-pressure liquid chromatography. While prevention with proper storage conditions is the best way to control mycotoxin infestation, thermal and chemical inactivation, as described earlier, can control any mycotoxins that do form under storage.

Food Poisoning from Marine Toxins
Ciguatera Fish Poisoning

Ciguatera fish poisoning occurs after eating reef fish contaminated with toxins such as ciguatoxin or maitotoxin. These potent toxins originate from *Gambierdiscus toxicus*, a small marine organism (dinoflagellate) that grows on and around coral reefs. Dinoflagellates are ingested by herbivorous fish. The toxins produced by *G. toxicus* are then modified and concentrated as they pass up the marine food chain to carnivorous fish and finally to humans. Ciguatoxins are concentrated in fish liver, intestines, roe, and heads.

G. toxicus may proliferate on dead coral reefs more effectively than other dinoflagellates. The risk of ciguatera poisoning is likely to increase as coral reefs deteriorate because of climate change, ocean acidification, offshore construction, and nutrient runoff.

Scombroid

Scombroid occurs worldwide in both temperate and tropical waters. One of the most common fish poisonings, it occurs after eating improperly refrigerated or preserved fish containing high levels of histamine and often resembles a moderate to severe allergic reaction.

Fish typically associated with scombroid have naturally high levels of histidine in the flesh and include tuna, mackerel, mahi mahi (dolphin fish), sardine, anchovy, herring, bluefish, amberjack, and marlin. Histidine is converted to histamine by bacterial overgrowth in fish improperly stored after capture. Histamine and other scombrotoxins are resistant to cooking, smoking, canning, or freezing.

Shellfish Poisoning

Several forms of poisoning may occur after ingesting toxin-containing shellfish, including filter-feeding bivalve mollusks (mussels, oysters, clams, scallops, and cockles), gastropod mollusks (abalone, whelks, and moon snails), or crustaceans (Dungeness crab, shrimp, and lobster). Toxins originate in small marine organisms (dinoflagellates or diatoms) that are ingested and are concentrated by the shellfish.

Paralytic Shellfish Poisoning

Paralytic shellfish poisoning (PSP) is the most common and most severe form of shellfish poisoning. PSP is caused by eating shellfish contaminated with saxitoxins. These potent neurotoxins are produced by various dinoflagellates. A wide range of shellfish may cause PSP, but most cases occur after eating mussels or clams.

PSP occurs worldwide but is most common in temperate waters, especially off the Pacific and Atlantic coasts of North America, including Alaska, the Philippines, China, Chile, Scotland, Ireland, New Zealand, and Australia, which have all reported cases.

Symptoms usually appear 30 to 60 minutes after eating toxic shellfish and include numbness and tingling of the face, lips, tongue, arms, and legs. There may be headache, nausea, vomiting, and diarrhea. Severe cases are associated with the ingestion of large doses of toxin and clinical features such as ataxia, dysphagia, mental-status changes, flaccid paralysis, and respiratory failure. The case–fatality ratio is dependent on the availability of modern medical care, including mechanical ventilation. The death rate may be particularly high in children.

Neurotoxic Shellfish Poisoning

Neurotoxic shellfish poisoning (NSP) is caused by eating shellfish contaminated with brevetoxins produced by the dinoflagellate Karinia brevis (K. brevis). Although predominately an illness of the Western Hemisphere (the southeastern coast of the United States, the Gulf of Mexico, and the Caribbean), there are also reports of the disease from New Zealand.

Neurotoxic shellfish poisoning (NSP) usually presents as gastroenteritis accompanied by neurologic symptoms resembling mild ciguatera or paralytic shellfish poisoning, 30 minutes to 3 hours after a shellfish meal. A syndrome known as "aerosolized red tide respiratory irritation" (ARTRI) occurs when aerosolized brevetoxins are inhaled in sea spray. This has been reported in association with a red tide (K. brevis HAB) in Florida. It can induce bronchoconstriction and may cause acute, temporary respiratory discomfort in healthy people. People with asthma may experience more severe and prolonged respiratory effects.

Diarrheic Shellfish Poisoning

Diarrheic shellfish poisoning (DSP) is caused by eating shellfish contaminated with toxins such as okadaic acid. It occurs worldwide, with outbreaks reported from China, Japan, Scandinavia, France, Belgium, Spain, Chile, Uruguay, Ireland, the United States, and Canada.

Most cases result from eating toxic bivalve mollusks such as mussels and scallops. Symptoms usually occur within 2 hours of eating contaminated shellfish and include chills, diarrhea, nausea, vomiting, and abdominal pain. Symptoms usually resolve within 2 to 3 days. No deaths have been reported.

Amnesic Shellfish Poisoning

Amnesic shellfish poisoning (ASP) is a rare form of shellfish poisoning caused by eating shellfish contaminated with domoic acid, produced by the diatom *Pseudonitzchia* spp. Outbreaks of ASP have been reported in Canada, Scotland, Ireland, France, Belgium, Spain, Portugal, New Zealand, Australia, and Chile. Implicated shellfish include mussels, scallops, razor clams, and other crustaceans.

In most cases, gastrointestinal symptoms such as diarrhea, vomiting, and abdominal pain develop within 24 hours of eating toxic shellfish, followed by headache, memory loss, and cognitive impairment. In severe cases, there may be hypotension, arrhythmias, ophthalmoplegia, coma, and death. Survivors may have severe anterograde, short-term memory deficits.

Mushroom Toxins

Some wild mushrooms contain poisons that can cause illness, with symptoms ranging from mild to deadly. The poisons are not likely to be destroyed by washing, cooking, freezing, or canning. Many poisonous wild mushrooms are almost impossible to tell apart from those that are not poisonous, and many cases of poisoning have happened in people who were using field guides and had a lot of experience and were "sure" they had picked the right kind of mushroom. Likewise, folklore is not a reliable way to avoid poisonous mushrooms.

Some of the deadliest wild mushrooms do not cause obvious symptoms for hours or even days or weeks after they are eaten, and, by the time symptoms appear, it is likely that liver or kidney damage has already occurred. These kinds of cases often begin with symptoms that go away after a few hours and seem to be gone for 3 to 5 days, making the person think that she or he is better—but then much worse symptoms appear, often leading to death.

The best way to keep from getting sick from wild mushrooms is not to eat them. Some can make you sick even from eating a sauce that contains them, even if you do not eat the mushrooms themselves. It is much safer to get mushrooms from grocery stores that sell the products grown on professional mushroom farms.

Aflatoxins

Aflatoxins are toxic substances produced by some kinds of fungus that can grow on food. People who eat food that contains high levels of aflatoxins can become sick. To date, there has never been a human illness outbreak caused by aflatoxins in the United States, where foods are carefully regulated and inspected to prevent such an occurrence, but some developing countries have had outbreaks. One of the aflatoxins is among the strongest known carcinogens (substances that cause cancer).

Scientists have pinpointed a site where this aflatoxin appears to cause a mutation in human deoxyribonucleic acid (DNA). Aflatoxins can lead to liver and immune-system problems. The combination of hepatitis B infection and eating foods contaminated with aflatoxin appears to make the risk of liver cancer especially high. Foods in which aflatoxins commonly are found (unless regulations and inspections prevent it, as in the United States) include corn, sorghum, rice, cottonseed, peanuts, tree nuts, dried coconut meat, cocoa beans, figs, ginger, and nutmeg.

Aflatoxins can cause illness in animals, and contaminated pet foods caused outbreaks and deaths among United States dogs and cats in 1998 and 2005. Cows are able to metabolize process aflatoxin. The substance (metabolite) that results after the cow processes the aflatoxin then may appear in the cow's milk, but is less toxic than the aflatoxin itself. Milk is routinely tested for this substance. In some developing countries, this metabolite also is found in the breast milk of human mothers who eat aflatoxin-contaminated foods.

Shellfish Toxins

Algae are plantlike life-forms that float or move on their own in the water. They vary in size from very small (microscopic) to very large (for example, seaweed, such as kelp). Some marine and freshwater algae make toxins (poisons). Many of the toxins that build up in shellfish—seafood, such as oysters, clams, and mussels, to name a few—are made by a small type of algae called "dinoflagellates," which swim and have characteristics of both plants and animals. When shellfish eat these algae, the poisons can build up in the shellfish and sicken people who eat them. The kind of illness depends on the poison. Some can be deadly, such as paralytic shellfish poisoning (PSP). Others, such as diarrhetic shellfish poisoning and azaspiracid shellfish poisoning, mostly cause symptoms such as nausea, vomiting, diarrhea, and stomach pain. Besides these kinds of symptoms, some shellfish poisonings, such as neurotoxic shellfish poisoning, also cause neurologic effects such as tingling or numbness of lips and throat, dizziness, and muscle aches. In extreme cases, amnesic shellfish poisoning has resulted in severe neurologic disorders, such as loss of short-term memory, in some people. These poisons are not destroyed by cooking, freezing, or other food preparation.

These realities highlight the importance of the U.S. Food and Drug Administration (FDA)'s seafood-safety programs, guidance to industry, and close working relationships with state regulators. For example, the levels of saxitoxins (which cause PSP) often become high in shellfish in New England waters at certain times of the year when the toxin-producing algae are present. When the level becomes too high for safety, state health agencies follow FDA guidance and ban shellfish harvesting, and PSP outbreaks from commercial products are very rare in the United States.

Scombrotoxin

Scombrotoxin is a combination of substances that form when certain fish are not properly refrigerated before being processed or cooked. One of the substances is histamine, which causes, for example, blood vessels to dilate and intestinal muscles to contract. Examples of fish that can form the toxin if they start to spoil include tuna, mahi mahi (dolphin fish), bluefish, sardines, mackerel, amberjack, and anchovies. The fish might not look or smell bad, but can cause illness.

In the United States, scombrotoxin is one of the most common illnesses caused by seafood. The symptoms, which should be treated with antihistamines by a health professional, usually are mild and start within minutes or hours after eating. They may include tingling or burning of the mouth or throat, rash or hives, low blood pressure, itching, headache, dizziness, nausea, vomiting, diarrhea, a fluttery heartbeat, and trouble breathing. The symptoms usually go away in a few hours, but may go on for days in severe cases. People who are on some medications, including tuberculosis drugs, or who have other medical conditions, are more likely to have severe reactions. Those are rare, but may include serious heart and lung problems. Be sure to tell your doctor if you ate fish, and when, to help with diagnosis.

Cooking, freezing, and canning does not "get rid of" this toxin after it has formed. The best prevention is to try to keep it from forming in the first place by keeping fish refrigerated at 40°F or lower.

Tetrodotoxin

In some parts of the world, especially Japan, pufferfish (also called "fugu" or "blowfish") are thought of as a delicacy—even though they contain a poison that is deadly to humans if the fish are not prepared by a highly trained expert. In some types of pufferfish, some organs, such as the liver and skin, contain the poison, which is called "tetrodotoxin." If the chef or trained cutter does not cut the fish in exactly the right way, the poison may get into the meat of the fish, and the person who eats it may become ill or even die without immediate medical treatment.

In mild cases of pufferfish poisoning, the person who eats it may get numbness and tingling in the lips, arms, and legs, and may feel lightheaded. In severe cases, death is from suffocation—often while awake until the end—because of paralyzed breathing muscles. There are many types (species) of pufferfish, and in most of them, only the organs, not the meat, naturally contain the poison. Other types do not contain any of the poison at all, such as the puffer from the Mid-Atlantic waters of the United States, called "northern puffer." This type of pufferfish used to be sold as "sea squab," but restaurants sell it under other names, such as "sugar toad." On the other hand, a few types of pufferfish naturally have large amounts of the poison in their meat (not just the organs), and it is never safe to eat them, no matter who prepares them. After a fish has been cleaned and processed (for example, turned into fillets or fish cakes), it can be hard to tell what kind it is. Because of this, the FDA allows only one type of puffer (*Takifugu rubripes*, also called "torafugu" or "tiger puffer") to be imported from Japan.

Only certain parts are allowed, and it has to be prepared by trained fish cutters before it is imported. It is sold only to restaurants belonging to a specific association. Because of these strict safety limitations, the availability of this pufferfish often is limited, and it is often expensive. Several times, the FDA has stopped illegally imported shipments of pufferfish. In some cases, unsafe importers have tried to get puffers into the country by labeling them as a different fish. Puffer—the dangerous kind—falsely labeled as monkfish was imported from China in 2007 and sickened people who had eaten bok go jim (blowfish casserole) or bok jiri (blowfish stew) in restaurants. ("Bok" is a Korean word for "puffer.") In Illinois, homemade puffer soup made from bok, from a local ethnic market, caused illness. The message to take away from all this is that if you choose to eat pufferfish, eat only those from sources known to be safe.

Ciguatoxin

The large majority of fish are safe to eat and provide good nutrition. But, if you plan to go fishing in tropical areas and plan to eat what you catch, be aware that some kinds of fish in those areas may contain a poison called "ciguatoxin." There is no way to tell if a fish contains ciguatoxin from the way it looks, tastes, or smells; the only way to tell is by testing it in a professional laboratory. Cooking and freezing do not get rid of the poison. The illness usually starts within six hours after the fish is eaten.

Symptoms and signs may include numbness and tingling around the mouth, nausea, vomiting, diarrhea, joint and muscle aches, headache, dizziness, muscle weakness, slow or fast heartbeat, low blood pressure, and being extremely sensitive to temperature. The symptoms usually go away in a few days, but in some cases, the neurologic symptoms (i.e., symptoms such as pain, numbness, tingling, etc.) may last much longer. These symptoms may go away and come back after many months, and it is thought that this return of symptoms may be somehow linked, in part, to eating or drinking alcohol, caffeine, nuts, and fish (even fish that do not contain poison).

There is no proven treatment for the poison itself, but treatment may be needed for some of the symptoms. If you will be fishing in tropical areas and plan to eat what you catch, it would be a good idea to ask local health authorities about which fish in the area are safe to eat. The list of the fish that are most likely to contain the poison includes, for example, barracuda, amberjack, other large jacks, and large groupers and snappers. This is not a complete list, however, since it tells only which fish are most likely to contain the poison based on experience.

It is possible that other fish in warm-water (tropical) areas also could contain the poison. Waters near the United States where fish containing this poison have been found include those of South Florida, the Bahamas, the United States, the British Virgin Islands, Puerto Rico, and Hawaii.

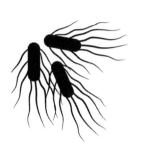

CHAPTER 17
Water Contamination and Its Effects

Chapter Contents

Major Sources of Water Contamination

This section contains text excerpted from the following sources: Text in this section begins with excerpts from "Water-Related Diseases and Contaminants in Public Water Systems," Centers for Disease Control and Prevention (CDC), April 7, 2014. Reviewed March 2020; Text under the heading "Water Contamination" is excerpted from "Water Contamination," Centers for Disease Control and Prevention (CDC), October 11, 2016. Reviewed March 2020.

The United States has one of the safest public drinking-water supplies in the world. Over 286 million Americans get their tap water from a community water system. The U.S. Environmental Protection Agency (EPA) regulates drinking-water quality in public water systems and sets maximum concentration levels for water chemicals and pollutants.

Sources of drinking water are subject to contamination and require appropriate treatment to remove disease-causing contaminants. Contamination of drinking-water supplies can occur in the source water as well as in the distribution system after water treatment has already occurred. There are many sources of water contamination, including naturally occurring chemicals and minerals (for example, arsenic, radon, and uranium), local land-use practices (fertilizers, pesticides, and concentrated feeding operations), manufacturing processes, and sewer overflows or wastewater releases.

The presence of contaminants in water can lead to adverse health effects, including gastrointestinal illness, reproductive problems, and neurological disorders. Infants, young children, pregnant women, the elderly, and people whose immune systems are compromised because of acquired immunodeficiency syndrome (AIDS), chemotherapy, or transplant medications, may be especially susceptible to illness from some contaminants.

Water Contamination

Over the past few decades, the increase in population and advances made in farming technology have increased the demand for crops and livestock from the agricultural industry. This growth in agricultural production has resulted in an increase in contaminants polluting soil and waterways. The increase in contaminants has prompted efforts to reduce the amount of pollutants in waterways in order to improve overall water quality.

Sources

Agriculture in many parts of the world is highly efficient in producing and delivering high-quality products to consumers. However, when agricultural activities are not well-monitored and managed, certain practices can negatively affect water quality.

Agricultural Runoff

According to the EPA, nonpoint source (NPS) pollution is pollution that comes from many diffuse sources, unlike pollution from point sources such as industrial and sewage-treatment plants. Finally depositing them into watersheds via lakes, rivers, wetlands, coastal waters, and even our underground sources of drinking water."

In 2002, in the National Water Quality Inventory report to United States Congress, the states reported that agricultural NPS pollution is the leading cause of river and stream impairment and the second leading cause of impairment in lakes, ponds, and reservoirs.

Agricultural activities that cause nonpoint source pollution include:
- Poorly managed animal feeding operations
- Overgrazing
- Overworking the land (for example, plowing too often)
- Poorly managed and ineffective application of pesticides, irrigation water, and fertilizer

Effects

Agricultural water can become contaminated through a variety of ways and can potentially spread bacteria, viruses, and parasites to crops and animals.

Crop Production

Fresh fruits and vegetables come into contact with water during various stages of the production process. Contaminated water that is used during crop production, harvesting, and processing can lead to health issues.

Below is a list of the potential food-production points where contaminated water sources can affect crop production:

- **Chemical application.** Crops with contaminated water used for pesticide or herbicide application. Water used for mixing chemicals should be of appropriate quality.
- **Irrigation.** Irrigating crops with contaminated water. Water used for irrigation should be of appropriate quality.
- **Worker hygiene.** Lack of potable water for hand hygiene. There should be an established handwashing and hygiene policy for farmworkers.
- **Food processing.** Wash crops in the final wash process with quality water. Water should be of drinking-water quality and should not be recycled.

People who consume fruits or vegetables that were exposed to contaminated water are at risk of developing a foodborne illness. Some of the bacteria that are spread through water within the United States include *E. coli, Salmonella* spp., Shigella spp., *Cryptosporidium, Giardia, Toxoplasma,* norovirus, and hepatitis A virus. Irrigation of foods imported from international locations can spread these and other microbes (for example, *Cyclospora)* not usually found in developed countries. Small amounts of any of these organisms can cause foodborne illness. In order to keep microbes out of water sources, growers should use practices that are appropriate for their operation and make sure that they are using the best quality water. Water quality is also important in ensuring postharvest quality by decreasing decay.

Animal Health

It is important that livestock are provided with adequate amounts of quality water, free of contamination. Contaminated water can contain disease-causing organisms which can rapidly spread if animals are drinking from the same trough. If there is reason to question the quality of the water that is provided to livestock, it is important to test the water to ensure its safety. There are many chemicals and microorganisms that can be potentially dangerous to livestock. Some chemicals include nitrates, sulfates, and chemicals found in pesticides such as DDT, Chlordane, and Endrin. Certain microorganisms such as blue-green algae, *Cryptosporidium*, or *Staphylococcus*, can be toxic to animals and cause symptoms such as diarrhea, lack of coordination, labored breathing, or death. Ill animals can then release millions of infectious microbes into the soil that can further contaminate other water sources.

Section 17.2
Top Waterborne Pathogens of Concern

This section includes text excerpted from "Water-Related Diseases and Contaminants in Public Water Systems," Centers for Disease Control and Prevention (CDC), April 7, 2014. Reviewed March 2020.

Bacteria
Legionella

Legionnaires' disease is a serious type of pneumonia (lung infection) caused by *Legionella* bacteria. People can get sick when they breathe in mist or accidently swallow water containing *Legionella* into the lungs.

Shigella

Shigellosis is an infectious disease caused by a group of bacteria called *Shigella*. Most people who are infected with *Shigella* develop diarrhea, fever, and stomach cramps starting a day or two after they are exposed to the bacteria. Shigellosis usually resolves in 5 to 7 days. Some people who are infected may have no symptoms at all, but may still pass the *Shigella* bacteria to others. The spread of *Shigella* can be stopped by frequent and careful handwashing with soap and taking other hygiene measures.

Campylobacter

Campylobacter causes an estimated 1.5 million illnesses each year in the United States.

People can get Campylobacteriosis by eating raw or undercooked poultry, or eating something that touched it. They can also get it from eating other foods, including seafood, meat, and produce, by contact with animals, and by drinking untreated water.

Although people with Campylobacteriosis usually recover on their own, some need antibiotic treatment.

Salmonella

The Centers for Disease Control and Prevention (CDC) estimates *Salmonella* bacteria cause about 1.35 million infections, 26,500 hospitalizations, and 420 deaths in the United States every year. Food is the source for most of these illnesses.

Most people who get ill from *Salmonella* have diarrhea, fever, and stomach cramps.

- Symptoms usually begin 6 hours to 6 days after infection and last 4 to 7 days.
- Most people recover without specific treatment and should not take antibiotics.
- Antibiotics are typically used only to treat people who have severe illness or who are at risk for it.

Some people's illness may be so severe that they need to be hospitalized.

Escherichia Coli

Escherichia coli (abbreviated as *E. coli*) are bacteria found in the environment, foods, and intestines of people and animals. *E. coli* are a large and diverse group of bacteria. Although most strains of *E. coli* are harmless, others can make you sick. Some kinds of *E. coli* can cause diarrhea, while others cause urinary-tract infections, respiratory illness and pneumonia, and other illnesses.

Virus
Norovirus

Norovirus is a very contagious virus that causes vomiting and diarrhea. Anyone can get infected and sick with norovirus. You can get norovirus from:

- Having direct contact with an infected person
- Consuming contaminated food or water
- Touching contaminated surfaces then putting your unwashed hands in your mouth

Hepatitis A

Hepatitis A is a vaccine-preventable, communicable disease of the liver caused by the hepatitis A virus (HAV). It is usually transmitted person to person through the fecal-oral route or consumption of contaminated food or water. Hepatitis A is a self-limited disease that does not result in chronic infection. Most adults with hepatitis A have symptoms, including fatigue, low appetite, stomach pain, nausea, and jaundice, that usually resolve within two months of infection; most children less than six years of age do not have symptoms or have an unrecognized infection. Antibodies produced in response to hepatitis A infection last for life and protect against reinfection. The best way to prevent hepatitis A infection is to get vaccinated.

Protozoa and Others
Giardia

Giardia is a microscopic parasite that causes the diarrheal illness known as "giardiasis." *Giardia* (also known as *Giardia intestinalis*, *Giardia lamblia*, or *Giardia duodenalis*) is found on surfaces or in soil, food, or water that has been contaminated with feces (poop) from infected humans or animals.

Giardia is protected by an outer shell that allows it to survive outside the body for long periods of time and makes it tolerant to chlorine disinfection. While the parasite can be spread in different ways, water (drinking water and recreational water) is the most common mode of transmission.

Cryptosporidium

Cryptosporidium is a microscopic parasite that causes the diarrheal disease cryptosporidiosis. Both the parasite and the disease are commonly known as "Crypto."

There are many species of *Cryptosporidium* that infect animals, some of which also infect humans. The parasite is protected by an outer shell that allows it to survive outside the body for long periods of time and makes it very tolerant to chlorine disinfection.

While this parasite can be spread in several different ways, water (drinking water and recreational water) is the most common way to spread the parasite. *Cryptosporidium* is a leading cause of waterborne disease among humans in the United States.

Section 17.3

Impact of Water Contamination on Children

This section includes text excerpted from "Drinking Water Contaminants," U.S. Environmental Protection Agency (EPA), October 30, 2015. Reviewed March 2020.

Variety of Contaminants

Drinking-water sources may contain a variety of contaminants that, at elevated levels, have been associated with increased risk of a range of diseases in children, including acute diseases such as gastrointestinal illness, developmental effects such as learning disorders, endocrine disruption, and cancer. Because children tend to take in more water relative to their body weight than adults do, children are likely to have higher exposure to drinking-water contaminants. Drinking-water sources include surface water, such as rivers, lakes, and reservoirs; and groundwater aquifers, which are subsurface layers of porous soil and rock that contain large collections of water. Groundwater and surface water are not isolated systems and are continually recharged by each other as well as by rain and other natural precipitation.

Several types of drinking-water contaminants may be of concern for children's health. Examples include microorganisms, (e.g., *E. coli, Giardia,* and noroviruses), inorganic chemicals (e.g., lead, arsenic, nitrates, and nitrites), organic chemicals (e.g., atrazine, glyphosate, trichloroethylene, and tetrachloroethylene), and disinfection byproducts (e.g., chloroform). The Environmental Protection Agency (EPA) and the U.S. Food and Drug Administration (FDA) are both responsible for the safety of drinking water. The FDA regulates bottled drinking water, while the EPA regulates drinking water provided by public water systems. The EPA sets enforceable drinking-water standards for public water systems, and unless otherwise specified, the term "drinking water" in this text refers to water provided by these systems. The drinking-water standards include maximum contaminant levels and treatment technique requirements for more than 90 chemical, radiological, and microbial contaminants, designed to protect people, including sensitive populations such as children, from adverse health effects. Microbial contaminants, lead, nitrates and nitrites, arsenic, disinfection byproducts, pesticides, and solvents are among the contaminants for which the EPA has set health-based standards.

Microbial Contaminants

Microbial contaminants include bacteria, viruses, and protozoa that may cause severe gastrointestinal illness. Children are particularly sensitive to microbial contaminants, such as *Giardia, Cryptosporidium, E. coli*, and noroviruses, because their immune systems are less developed than those of most adults.

Lead Exposure

Drinking water is a known source of lead exposure among children in the United States, particularly from corrosion of pipes and other elements of the drinking-water distribution systems. Exposure to lead via drinking water may be particularly high among very young children who consume baby formula prepared with drinking water that is contaminated by leaching lead pipes. The National Toxicology Program (NTP) has concluded that childhood lead exposure is associated with reduced cognitive function, reduced academic achievement, and increased attention-related behavioral problems.

Nitrates and Nitrites

Fertilizer, livestock manure, and human sewage can be significant contributors of nitrates and nitrites in groundwater sources of drinking water. High levels of nitrates and nitrites can cause the blood disorder methemoglobinemia (blue baby syndrome) and have been associated with thyroid dysfunction in children and pregnant women. Moderate deficits in maternal thyroid hormone levels during early pregnancy have been linked to reduced childhood IQ scores and other neurodevelopmental effects, as well as to unsuccessful or complicated pregnancies.

Arsenic

Arsenic enters drinking water sources from natural deposits in the earth, which vary widely from one region to another, or from agricultural and industrial sources where it is used as a wood preservative and a component of fertilizers, animal feed, and a variety of industrial products. Population studies of health effects associated with arsenic exposure have been conducted primarily in countries such as Bangladesh, Taiwan, and Chile, where arsenic levels in drinking water are generally much higher than in the United States due to high levels of naturally occurring arsenic in groundwater. Long-term consumption of arsenic-contaminated water has been associated with the development of skin conditions and circulatory-system problems, as well as increased risk of cancer of the bladder, lungs, skin, kidney, nasal passages, liver, and prostate.

In many cases, long-term exposure to arsenic begins during prenatal development or childhood, which increases the risk of mortality and morbidity among young adults exposed to arsenic long-term. A review of the literature concluded that epidemiological studies of associations between exposure to arsenic and some adverse health outcomes pertinent to children's health have mixed findings. These include studies of associations between high levels of exposure to arsenic and abnormal pregnancy outcomes, such as spontaneous abortion, stillbirths, reduced birth weight, and infant mortality, as well as associations between early-life exposure to arsenic and increased incidence of childhood cancer and reduced cognitive function.

Microorganisms

Water can contain microorganisms, such as parasites, viruses, and bacteria; the disinfection of drinking water to reduce waterborne infectious disease is one of the major public-health advances of the 20th century. The method by which infectious agents are removed or chemically inactivated depends on the type and quality of the drinking-water source and the volume of water to be treated. Surface water systems are more exposed than groundwater systems to weather and runoff; therefore, they may be more susceptible to contamination. Surface and groundwater systems use filtration and other treatment methods to physically remove particles. Disinfectants such as chlorine and chloramine, ultraviolet radiation, and ozone are added to drinking water provided by public-water systems to kill or neutralize microbial contaminants. However, this process can produce disinfection byproducts, which form when chemical disinfectants react with naturally occurring organic matter in water. The most common of these disinfection byproducts are chloroform and other trihalomethanes.

Consumption of drinking water from systems in the United States and other industrialized countries with relatively high levels of disinfection byproducts has been associated with bladder cancer and developmental effects in some studies. Some individual epidemiological studies have reported associations between the presence of disinfection byproducts in drinking water and increased risk of birth defects, especially neural-tube defects and oral clefts; however, articles reviewing the body of literature determined that the evidence is too limited to reach conclusions about a possible association between exposure to disinfection byproducts and birth defects.

Agricultural Pesticides

Some of the most widely used agricultural pesticides in the United States, such as atrazine and glyphosate, are also drinking-water contaminants. Pesticides can enter drinking-water sources as runoff from crop production in agricultural areas and enter groundwater through abandoned wells on farms. Some epidemiological studies have reported associations between prenatal exposure to atrazine and reduced fetal growth. The use of glyphosate, an herbicide used to kill weeds, has increased dramatically in recent years because of the growing popularity of crops genetically modified to survive glyphosate treatment. Previous safety assessments have concluded that glyphosate does not affect fertility or reproduction in laboratory animal studies. However, more studies in laboratory animals have found that male rats exposed to high levels of glyphosate, either during prenatal or pubertal development, may suffer from reproductive problems, such as delayed puberty, decreased sperm production, and decreased testosterone production. Very few epidemiological human studies have investigated effects of glyphosate exposure on reproductive endpoints. In contrast to the results of animal studies, one such epidemiological study of women living in regions with different levels of exposure to glyphosate found no associations between glyphosate exposure and delayed time to pregnancy.

Chemical Contaminants

A variety of other chemical contaminants can enter the water supply after use in industry. Examples include trichloroethylene and tetrachloroethylene (also known as "perchloroethylene"), which are solvents widely used in industry as degreasers, dry-cleaning agents, paint removers, chemical extractors, and components of adhesives and lubricants. Potential health concerns from exposure to trichloroethylene, based on limited epidemiological data and evidence from animal studies, include decreased fetal growth and birth defects, particularly cardiac birth defects. A study conducted in Massachusetts reported associations between birth defects and maternal exposure to drinking water contaminated with high levels of tetrachloroethylene around the time of conception.

An additional study reported that older mothers or mothers who had previously miscarried, and who were exposed to high levels of tetrachloroethylene in contaminated drinking water, had a higher risk of delivering a baby with reduced birth weight. However, other studies did not find associations between maternal exposure to tetrachloroethylene and pregnancy loss, gestational age, or birth weight. Studies in laboratory animals indicate that mothers exposed to high levels of tetrachloroethylene can have spontaneous abortion, and their fetuses can suffer from altered growth and birth defects. The EPA has not determined whether standards are necessary for some drinking-water contaminants, such as personal-care products. Personal-care products, such as cosmetics, sunscreens, and fragrances; and pharmaceuticals, including prescription, over-the-counter, and veterinary medications, can enter water systems after use by humans or domestic animals and have been measured at very low levels in drinking water sources.

Many concentrated animal feeding operations treat livestock with hormones and antibiotics, and can be one significant source of pharmaceuticals in water. Other major sources of pharmaceuticals in water are human waste, manufacturing plants and hospitals, and other human activities, such as showering and swimming. Any potential health implications of long term exposure to levels of pharmaceuticals and personal-care products found in drinking water are unclear.

Personal-Care Products

The EPA has not determined whether standards are necessary for some drinking water contaminants, such as personal-care products. Personal-care products, such as cosmetics, sunscreens, and fragrances; and pharmaceuticals, including prescription, over-the-counter, and veterinary medications, can enter water systems after use by humans or domestic animals and have been measured at very low levels in drinking water sources.

Manganese

Manganese is a naturally occurring mineral that can enter drinking water sources from rocks and soil or from human activities. While manganese is an essential nutrient at low doses, chronic exposure to high doses may be harmful, particularly to the nervous system. Many of the reports on adverse effects from manganese exposure are based on inhalation exposures in occupational settings. Fewer studies have examined health effects associated with oral exposure to manganese. However, some epidemiological studies have reported associations between long-term exposure to high levels of manganese in drinking water during prenatal development or childhood and intellectual impairment; decreased nonverbal memory, attention, and motor skills; hyperactivity; and other behavioral effects.

Most studies on the health effects of manganese have been conducted in countries where manganese exposure is generally higher than in the United States. However, two individual studies conducted in specific areas of relatively high manganese contamination in the United States reported associations between prenatal or childhood manganese exposure and problems with general intelligence, memory, and behavior. Although there is no health-based regulatory standard for manganese in drinking water, the EPA has set a voluntary standard for manganese as a guideline to assist public water systems in managing their drinking water for aesthetic considerations, such as taste, color, and odor.

Perchlorate

Perchlorate is a naturally occurring and human-made chemical that has been found in surface and groundwater in the United States. Perchlorate is used in the manufacture of fireworks, explosives, flares, and rocket fuel. Perchlorate was detected in just over 4 percent of public water systems in a nationally representative monitoring study conducted from 2001 to 2005. Some infant formulas have been found to contain perchlorate, and the perchlorate content of the formula is increased if it is prepared with perchlorate-contaminated water. Exposure to elevated levels of perchlorate can inhibit iodide uptake into the thyroid gland, possibly disrupting the function of the thyroid and potentially leading to a reduction in the production of thyroid hormone. As noted above, thyroid hormones are particularly important for growth and development of the central nervous system in fetuses and infants.

In January 2009, the EPA issued an interim health advisory level to help state and local officials manage local perchlorate contamination issues in a health-protective manner, in advance of the EPA regulatory determination. In February 2011, the EPA decided to develop a federal drinking water standard for perchlorate, based on the concern for effects on thyroid hormones and the development and growth of fetuses, infants, and children. The process for developing the standard will include receiving input from key stakeholders as well as submitting any formal rule to a public comment process.

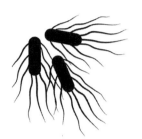

CHAPTER 18
Assessing the Impact of Climate Change on Water-Related Illnesses

Across most of the United States, climate change is expected to affect fresh and marine water resources in ways that will increase people's exposure to water-related contaminants that cause illness. Water-related illnesses include waterborne diseases caused by pathogens, such as bacteria, viruses, and protozoa. Water-related illnesses are also caused by toxins produced by certain harmful algae and cyanobacteria (also known as "blue-green algae") and by chemicals introduced into the environment by human activities. Exposure occurs through ingestion, inhalation, or direct contact with contaminated drinking or recreational water and through consumption of fish and shellfish.

Factors related to climate change—including temperature, precipitation and related runoff, hurricanes, and storm surge—affect the growth, survival, spread, and virulence or toxicity of agents (causes) of water-related illness. Heavy downpours are already on the rise and increases in the frequency and intensity of extreme precipitation events are projected for all United States regions. Projections of temperature, precipitation, extreme events such as flooding and drought, and other climate factors vary by region of the United States, and thus the extent of climate health impacts will also vary by region.

This chapter includes text excerpted from "Water-Related Illness," GlobalChange.gov, U.S. Global Change Research Program (USGCRP), May 15, 2000. Reviewed March 2020.

Waterborne pathogens are estimated to cause 8.5 percent to 12 percent of acute gastrointestinal illness cases in the United States, affecting between 12 million and 19 million people annually. Eight pathogens, which are all affected to some degree by climate, account for approximately 97 percent of all suspected waterborne illnesses in the United States: the enteric viruses norovirus, rotavirus, and adenovirus; the bacteria *Campylobacter jejuni*, *E. coli* O157:H7, and *Salmonella enterica*; and the protozoa *Cryptosporidium* and *Giardia*.

Health risks associated with changes in natural marine, coastal, and freshwater systems and water infrastructure for drinking water, wastewater, and stormwater are explained below, and include fish and shellfish illnesses associated with the waters in which they grow and are affected by the same climate factors that affect drinking and recreational waters. Sources of contamination, exposure pathways, and health outcomes are also included when available. Based on the available data and research, many of the examples are regionally focused and make evident that the impact of climate change on water-related illness is inherently regional.

Whether or not illness results from exposure to contaminated water, fish, or shellfish is dependent on a complex set of factors, including human behavior and social determinants of health that may affect a person's exposure, sensitivity, and adaptive capacity. Water-resource, public-health, and environmental agencies in the United States provide many public-health safeguards to reduce risk of exposure and illness even if water becomes contaminated. These include water-quality monitoring, drinking-water treatment standards and practices, beach closures, and issuing advisories for boiling drinking water and harvesting shellfish.

Many water-related illnesses are either undiagnosed or unreported, and therefore, the total incidence of waterborne disease is underestimated. On average, illnesses from pathogens associated with water are thought to be underestimated by as much as 43-fold, and may be underestimated by up to 143 times for certain *Vibrio* species.

Sources of Water-Related Contaminants

The primary sources of water contamination are human and animal waste and agricultural activities, including the use of fertilizers. Runoff and flooding resulting from expected increases in extreme precipitation, hurricane rainfall, and storm surge may increase risks of contamination. Contamination occurs when agents of water-related illness and nutrients, such as nitrogen and phosphorus, are carried from urban, residential, and agricultural areas into surface waters, groundwater, and coastal waters. The nutrient loading can promote growth of naturally occurring pathogens and algae. Human exposure occurs via contamination of drinking-water sources, recreational waters, and fish and shellfish.

Water contamination by human waste is tied to failure of local urban or rural water infrastructure, including municipal wastewater, septic, and stormwater conveyance systems. Failure can occur either when rainfall and subsequent runoff overwhelm the capacity of these systems—causing, for example, sewer overflows, basement backups, or localized flooding—or when extreme events, such as flooding and storm surges damage water conveyance or treatment infrastructure and result in reduction or loss of performance and functionality. Many older cities in the Northeast and around the Great Lakes region of the United States have combined sewer systems (with stormwater and sewage sharing the same pipes), which are prone to discharging raw sewage directly into surface waters after moderate to heavy rainfall. The amount of rain that causes combined sewer overflows is highly variable between cities because of differences in infrastructure capacity and design, and ranges from 5 mm (about 0.2 inches) to 2.5 cm (about 1 inch).

Overall, combined sewer overflows are expected to increase, but site-specific analysis is needed to predict the extent of these increases. Extreme precipitation events will exacerbate existing problems with inadequate, aging, or deteriorating wastewater infrastructure throughout the country. These problems include broken or leaking sewer pipes and failing septic systems that leach sewage into the ground. Runoff or contaminated groundwater discharge also carries pathogens and nutrients into surface water, including freshwater and marine coastal areas and beaches.

Water contamination from agricultural activities is related to the release of microbial pathogens or nutrients in livestock manure and inorganic fertilizers that can stimulate rapid and excessive growth, or blooms, of harmful algae. Agricultural land covers about 900 million acres across the United States, comprising over 2 million farms, with livestock sectors concentrated in certain regions of the United States. Depending on the type and number of animals, a large livestock operation can produce between 2,800 and 1,600,000 tons of manure each year. With the projected increases in heavy precipitation for all United States regions, agricultural sources of contamination can affect water quality across the nation. Runoff from lands where manure has been used as fertilizer or where flooding has caused wastewater lagoons to overflow can carry contamination agents directly from the land into bodies of water.

Management practices and technologies, such as better timing of manure application and improved animal feeds, help reduce or eliminate the risks of manure-borne contaminant transport to public water supplies and shellfish-harvesting waters and reduce nutrients that stimulate harmful algal blooms. Drinking-water treatment and monitoring practices also help to decrease or eliminate exposure to waterborne illness agents originating from agricultural environments.

Water contamination from wildlife (e.g., rodents, birds, deer, and wild pigs) occurs via the feces and urine of infected animals, which are reservoirs of enteric and other pathogens. Warmer winters and earlier springs are expected to increase animal activity and alter the ecology and habitat of animals that may carry pathogens. This may lengthen the exposure period for humans and expand the geographic ranges in which pathogens are transmitted.

Exposure Pathways and Health Risks

Humans are exposed to agents of water-related illness through several pathways, including drinking water (treated and untreated), recreational waters (freshwater, coastal, and marine), and fish and shellfish.

Drinking Water

Although the United States has one of the safest municipal drinking-water supplies in the world, water-related outbreaks (more than one illness case linked to the same source) still occur. Public drinking-water systems provide treated water to approximately 90 percent of Americans at their places of residence, work, or schools. However, about 15 percent of the population relies fully or in part on untreated private wells or other private sources for their drinking water. These private sources are not regulated under the Safe Drinking Water Act. The majority of drinking water outbreaks in the United States are associated with untreated or inadequately treated groundwater and distribution-system deficiencies.

Pathogen and Algal Toxin Contamination

Between 1948 and 1994, 68 percent of waterborne disease outbreaks in the United States were preceded by extreme precipitation events, and heavy rainfall and flooding continue to be cited as contributing factors in more recent outbreaks in multiple regions of the United States. Extreme precipitation events have been statistically linked to increased levels of pathogens in treated drinking-water supplies and to an increased incidence of gastrointestinal illness in children. This established relationship suggests that extreme precipitation is a key climate factor for waterborne disease. The Milwaukee *Cryptosporidium* outbreak of 1993—the largest documented waterborne disease outbreak in United States history, causing an estimated 403,000 illnesses and more than 50 deaths—was preceded by the heaviest rainfall event in 50 years in the adjacent watersheds. Various treatment-plant operational problems were also key contributing factors. Observations in England and Wales also show waterborne disease outbreaks were preceded by weeks of low cumulative rainfall and then heavy precipitation events, suggesting that drought or periods of low rainfall may also be important climate-related factors.

Small community or private groundwater wells or other drinking-water systems where water is untreated or minimally treated are especially susceptible to contamination following extreme precipitation events. For example, in May 2000, following heavy rains, livestock waste containing *E. coli* O157:H7 and *Campylobacter* was carried in runoff to a well that served as the primary drinking-water source for the town of Walkerton, Ontario, Canada, resulting in 2,300 illnesses and 7 deaths. High rainfall amounts were an important catalyst for the outbreak, although nonclimate factors, such as well infrastructure, operational and maintenance problems, and lack of communication between public-utilities staff and local health officials were also key factors.

Likewise, extreme precipitation events and subsequent increases in runoff are key climate factors that increase nutrient loading in drinking-water sources, which in turn increases the likelihood of harmful cyanobacterial blooms that produce algal toxins. The EPA has established health advisories for two algal toxins (microcystins and cylindrospermopsin) in drinking water. Lakes and reservoirs that serve as sources of drinking water for between 30 million and 48 million Americans may be periodically contaminated by algal toxins. Certain drinking-water treatment processes can remove cyanobacterial toxins; however, efficacy of the treatment processes may vary from 60 percent to 99.9 percent. Ineffective treatment could compromise water quality and may lead to severe treatment disruption or treatment-plant shutdown. Such an event occurred in Toledo, Ohio, in August 2014, when nearly 500,000 residents of the state's fourth-largest city lost access to their drinking water after tests revealed the presence of toxins from a cyanobacterial bloom in Lake Erie near the water plant's intake.

Water Supply

Climate-related hydrologic changes, such as those related to flooding, drought, runoff, snowpack and snowmelt, and saltwater intrusion (the movement of ocean water into fresh groundwater) have implications for freshwater management and supply. Adequate freshwater supply is essential to many aspects of public health, including provision of drinking water and proper sanitation and personal hygiene. For example, following floods or storms, short-term loss of access to potable water has been linked to increased incidence of illnesses, including gastroenteritis and respiratory-tract and skin infections. Changes in precipitation and runoff, combined with changes in consumption and withdrawal, have reduced surface and groundwater supplies in many areas, primarily in the western United States. These trends are expected to continue under future climate change, increasing the likelihood of water shortages for many uses.

Future climate-related water shortages may result in more municipalities and individuals relying on alternative sources for drinking water, including reclaimed water and roof-harvested rainwater. "Water reclamation" refers to the treatment of stormwater, industrial wastewater, and municipal wastewater for beneficial reuse. States such as California, Arizona, New Mexico, Texas, and Florida are already implementing wastewater reclamation and reuse practices as a means of conserving and adding to freshwater supplies. However, no federal regulations or criteria for public-health protection have been developed or proposed specifically for potable water reuse in the United States. Increasing household rainwater collection has also been seen in some areas of the country (primarily Arizona, Colorado, and Texas), although in some cases, exposure to untreated rainwater has been found to pose health risks from bacterial or protozoan pathogens, such as *Salmonella enterica* and *Giardia lamblia*.

Projected Changes

Runoff from more frequent and intense extreme precipitation events will contribute to contamination of drinking-water sources with pathogens and algal toxins and place additional stresses on the capacity of drinking-water treatment facilities and distribution systems. Contamination of drinking-water sources may be exacerbated or insufficiently addressed by treatment processes at the treatment plant or by breaches in the distribution system, such as during water-main breaks or low-pressure events. Untreated groundwater drawn from municipal and private wells is of particular concern.

Climate change is not expected to substantially increase the risk of contracting illness from drinking water for those people who are served by treated drinking-water systems, if appropriate treatment and distribution is maintained. However, projections of more frequent or severe extreme precipitation events, flooding, and storm surge suggest that drinking-water infrastructure may be at greater risk of disruption or failure due to damage or exceedance of system capacity. Aging drinking-water infrastructure is one long-standing limitation in controlling waterborne disease, and may be especially susceptible to failure. For example, there are more than 50,000 systems providing treated drinking water to communities in the United States, and most water-distribution pipes in these systems are already failing or will reach their expected lifespan and require replacement within 30 years. Breakdowns in drinking-water treatment and distribution systems, compounded by aging infrastructure, could lead to more serious and frequent health consequences than those we experience now.

Recreational Waters

Humans are exposed to agents of water-related illness through recreation (such as swimming, fishing, and boating) in freshwater and marine or coastal waters. Exposure may occur directly (ingestion and contact with water) or incidentally (inhalation of aerosolized water droplets).

Pathogen and Algal Toxin Contamination

Enteric viruses, especially noroviruses, from human waste are a primary cause of gastrointestinal illness from exposure to contaminated recreational fresh and marine water. Although there are comparatively few reported illnesses and outbreaks of gastrointestinal illness from recreating in marine waters compared to freshwater, marine contamination still presents a significant health risk. Illnesses from marine sources are less likely to be reported than those from freshwater beaches, in part because the geographical residences of beachgoers are more widely distributed (for example, tourists may travel to marine beaches for vacation) and illnesses are less often attributed to marine exposure as a common source.

Key climate factors associated with risks of exposure to enteric pathogens in both freshwater and marine recreational waters include extreme precipitation events, flooding, and temperature. For example, *Salmonella* and *Campylobacter* concentrations in freshwater streams in the southeastern United States increase significantly in the summer months and following heavy rainfall. In the Great Lakes—a freshwater system— changes in rainfall, higher lake temperatures, and low lake levels have been linked to increases in fecal bacteria levels. The zoonotic bacteria *Leptospira* are introduced into water from the urine of animals, and increased illness rates in humans are linked to warm temperatures and flooding events.

In marine waters, recreational exposure to naturally occurring bacterial pathogens (such as *Vibrio* species) may result in eye, ear, and wound infections, diarrheal illness, or death. Reported rates of illness for all *Vibrio* infections have tripled since 1996, with *V. alginolyticus* infections having increased 40-fold. *Vibrio* growth rates are highly responsive to rising sea-surface temperatures, particularly in coastal waters, which generally have high levels of the dissolved organic carbon required for *Vibrio* growth. The distribution of species changes with salinity patterns related to sea-level rise and to changes in delivery of freshwater to coastal waters, which is affected by flooding and drought. For instance, *V. parahaeomolyticus* and *V. alginolyticus* favor higher salinities while *V. vulnificus* favors more moderate salinities.

Harmful algal blooms caused by cyanobacteria were responsible for nearly half of all reported outbreaks in untreated recreational freshwater in 2009 and 2010, resulting in approximately 61 illnesses, primarily reported in children/young adults age 1 to 19. (Health effects included dermatologic, gastrointestinal, respiratory, and neurologic symptoms.) Cyanobacterial blooms are strongly influenced by rising temperatures, altered precipitation patterns, and changes in freshwater discharge or flushing rates of water bodies. Higher temperatures (77°F and greater) favor surface-bloom-forming cyanobacteria over less harmful types of algae. In marine water, the toxins associated with harmful "red tide" blooms of Karenia brevis can aerosolize in water droplets through wind and wave action and cause acute respiratory illness and eye irritation in recreational beachgoers. People with preexisting respiratory diseases, specifically asthma, are at increased risk of illness. Prevailing winds and storms are important climate factors influencing the accumulation of *K. brevis* cells in the water. For example, in 1996, Tropical Storm Josephine transported a Florida panhandle bloom as far west as Louisiana, the first documented occurrence of *K. brevis* in that state.

Projected Changes

Overall, climate change will contribute to contamination of recreational waters and increased exposure to agents of water-related illness. Increases in flooding, coastal inundation, and nuisance flooding (linked to sea-level rise and storm surge from changing patterns of coastal storms and hurricanes) will negatively affect coastal infrastructure and increase chances for pathogen contamination, especially in populated areas. In areas where increasing temperatures lengthen the seasons for recreational swimming and other water activities, exposure risks are expected to increase.

As average temperatures rise, the seasonal and geographic range of suitable habitat for cyanobacterial species is projected to expand. For example, tropical and subtropical species such as *Cylindrospermopsisraciborskii, Anabaena* spp. and *Aphanizomenon* spp. have already shown poleward expansion into midlatitudes of Europe, North America, and South America. Increasing variability in precipitation patterns and more frequent and intense extreme precipitation events (which will increase nutrient loading) will also affect cyanobacterial communities. If such events are followed by extended drought periods, the stagnant, low-flow conditions accompanying droughts will favor cyanobacterial dominance and bloom formation.

In recreational waters, projected increases in sea-surface temperatures are expected to lengthen the seasonal window of growth and expand geographic range of *Vibrio* species, although the certainty of regional projections is affected by underlying model structure. While the specific response of *Vibrio* and degree of growth may vary by species and locale, in general, longer seasons and expansion of *Vibrio* into areas where it had not previously been will increase the likelihood of exposure to *Vibrio* in recreational waters. Regional climate changes that affect coastal salinity (such as flooding, drought, and sea-level rise) can also affect the population dynamics of these agents, with implications for human exposure risk. Increases in hurricane intensity and rainfall are projected as the climate continues to warm. Such increases may redistribute toxic blooms of *K. brevis* ("red tide" blooms) into new geographic locations, which would change human exposure risk in newly affected areas.

Fish and Shellfish

Water-related contaminants as well as naturally occurring harmful bacteria and algae can be accumulated by fish or shellfish, providing a route of human exposure through consumption. Shellfish, including oysters, are often consumed raw or very lightly cooked, which increases the potential for ingestion of an infectious pathogen.

Pathogens Associated with Fish and Shellfish

Enteric viruses (for example, noroviruses and hepatitis A virus) found in sewage are the primary causes of gastrointestinal illness due to shellfish consumption. Rainfall increases the load of contaminants associated with sewage delivered to shellfish-harvesting waters and may also temporarily reduce salinity, which can increase persistence of many enteric bacteria and viruses. Many enteric viruses also exhibit seasonal patterns in infection rates and detection rates in the environment, which may be related to temperature.

Among naturally occurring water-related pathogens, *Vibrio vulnificus* and *V. parahaemolyticus* are the species most often implicated in foodborne illness in the United States, accounting for more than 50 percent of reported shellfish-related illnesses annually. Cases have increased significantly since 1996. Rising sea-surface temperatures have contributed to an expanded geographic and seasonal range in outbreaks associated with shellfish.

Precipitation is expected to be the primary climate driver affecting enteric pathogen loading to shellfish-harvesting areas, although temperature also affects bioaccumulation rates of enteric viruses in shellfish. There are currently no national projections for the associated risk of illness from shellfish consumption. Many local and state agencies have developed plans for closing shellfish beds in the event of threshold-exceeding rain events that lead to loading of these contaminants and deterioration of water quality.

Increases in sea-surface temperatures, changes in precipitation and freshwater delivery to coastal waters, and sea-level rise will continue to affect *Vibrio* growth and are expected to increase human exposure risk. Regional models project increased abundance and extended seasonal windows of growth of *Vibrio* pathogens. The magnitude of health impacts depends on the use of intervention strategies and on public and physician awareness.

Harmful Algal Toxins

Harmful algal blooms (HABs) that contaminate seafood with toxins are becoming increasingly frequent and persistent in coastal marine waters, and some have expanded into new geographic locations. Attribution of this trend has been complicated for some species, with evidence to suggest that human-induced changes (such as ballast water exchange, aquaculture, nutrient loading to coastal waters, and climate change) have contributed to this expansion.

Among HABs associated with seafood, ciguatera fish poisoning (CFP) is most strongly influenced by climate. CFP is caused by toxins produced by the benthic algae *Gambierdiscus* and is the most frequently reported fish poisoning in humans. There is a well-established link between warm sea-surface temperatures and increased occurrences of CFP and, in some cases, increases have also been linked to El Niño–Southern Oscillation events. The frequency of tropical cyclones in the United States has also been associated with CFP, but with an 18-month lag period associated with the time required for a new *Gambierdiscus* habitat to develop.

Paralytic shellfish poisoning (PSP) is the most globally widespread shellfish poisoning associated with algal toxins, and records of PSP toxins in shellfish tissues (an indicator of toxin-producing species of *Alexandrium*) provide the longest time series in the United States for evaluating climate impacts. Warm phases of the naturally occurring climate pattern known as the "Pacific Decadal Oscillation" co-occur with increased PSP toxins in Puget Sound shellfish on decadal timescales. Further, it is very likely that the 20th-century warming trend also contributed to the observed increase in shellfish toxicity since the 1950s. Warm spring temperatures also contributed to a bloom of *Alexandrium* in a coastal New York estuary in 2008. Decadal patterns in PSP toxins in Gulf of Maine shellfish show no clear relationships with long-term trends in climate but ocean–climate interactions and changing oceanographic conditions are important factors for understanding *Alexandrium* bloom dynamics in this region.

There is less agreement on the extent of climate impacts on other marine HAB-related diseases in the United States. Increased abundances of *Pseudo-nitzschia* species, which can cause amnesic shellfish poisoning, have been attributed to nutrient enrichment in the Gulf of Mexico. On the United States West Coast, increased abundances of at least some species of *Pseudo-nitzschia* occur during warm phases associated with El Niño events. For *Dinophysis* species that can cause diarrhetic shellfish poisoning, data records are too short to evaluate potential relationships with climate in the United States, but studies in Sweden have found relationships with natural climate oscillations.

The projected impacts of climate change on toxic marine harmful algae include geographic-range changes in both warm- and cold-water species, changes in abundance and toxicity, and changes in the timing of the seasonal window of growth. These impacts will likely result from climate change-related impacts on one or more of:

- Water temperatures
- Salinities
- Enhanced surface stratification
- Nutrient availability and supply to coastal waters (upwelling and freshwater runoff)
- Altered winds and ocean currents

Limited understanding of the interactions among climate and nonclimate stressors and, in some cases, limitations in the design of experiments for investigating decadal- or century-scale trends in phytoplankton communities, makes forecasting the direction and magnitude of change in toxic marine HABs challenging. Still, changes to the community composition of marine microalgae, including harmful species, will occur. Conditions for the growth of dinoflagellates—the algal group containing numerous toxic species—could potentially be increasingly favorable with climate change because these species possess certain physiological characteristics that allow them to take advantage of climatically driven changes in the structure of the ocean (for example, stronger vertical stratification and reduced turbulence).

Climate change, especially continued warming, will dramatically increase the burden of some marine HAB-related diseases in some parts of the United States, with strong implications for disease surveillance and public-health preparedness. For example, the projected 4.5°F to 6.3°F increase in sea surface temperature in the Caribbean over the coming century is expected to increase the incidence of ciguatera fish poisoning by 200 percent to 400 percent. In the Puget Sound, warming is projected to increase the seasonal window of growth for *Alexandrium* by approximately

30 days by 2040, allowing blooms to begin earlier in the year and persist for longer.

Populations of Concern

Climate-change impacts on the drinking-water exposure pathway will act as an additional stressor on top of existing exposure disparities in the United States. Lack of consistent access to potable drinking water and inequities in exposure to contaminated water disproportionately affect the following populations: Native tribes and Alaska Natives, especially those in remote reservations or villages; residents of low-income rural subdivisions known as "colonias" along the United States–Mexico border; migrant farm workers; the homeless; and low-income communities not served by public-water utilities—which can be urban, suburban, or rural, and some of which are predominately Hispanic or Latinx and Black or African American communities in certain regions of the country. In general, the heightened vulnerability of these populations primarily results from unequal access to adequate water and sewer infrastructure, and various environmental, political, economic, and social factors jointly create these disparities.

Children, older adults (primarily 65 years of age and older), pregnant women, and immunocompromised individuals have a higher risk of gastrointestinal illness and severe health outcomes from contact with contaminated water. Pregnant women who develop severe gastrointestinal illness are at high risk for adverse pregnancy outcomes (pregnancy loss and preterm birth). Because children swallow roughly twice as much water as adults while swimming, they have higher recreational-exposure risk for both pathogens and freshwater HABs. Recent cryptosporidiosis and giardiasis cases have frequently been reported in children one to nine years of age, with onset of illness peaking during the summer months. In addition, 40 percent of swimming-related eye and ear infections from *Vibrio alginolyticus* during the period 1997–2006 were reported in children (median age of 15).

Traditional tribal consumption of fish and shellfish in the Pacific Northwest and Alaska can be on average 3 to 10 times higher than that of average United States consumers, or even up to 20 times higher.

Climate change will contribute to increased seafood contamination by toxins and potentially by chemical contaminants with potential health risks and cultural implications for tribal communities. Those who continue to consume traditional diets may face increased health risks from contamination. Alternatively, replacing these traditional nutrition sources may involve consuming less nutritious processed foods and the loss of cultural practices tied to fish and shellfish harvest.

Emerging Issues

A key emerging issue is the impact of climate on new and reemerging pathogens. While cases of nearly-always-fatal primary amoebic meningoencephalitis due to the amoeba *Naegleria fowleri* and other related species remain relatively uncommon, a northward expansion of cases has been observed in the last five years. Evidence suggests that, in addition to detection in source water (ground and surface waters), these amoebae may be harbored in biofilms associated with water distribution systems, where increased temperatures decrease efficacy of chlorine disinfection and support survival and potentially growth.

Climate change may also alter the patterns or magnitude of chemical contamination of seafood, leading to altered effects on human health—most of which are chronic conditions. Rising temperatures and reduced ice cover are already linked to increasing burdens of mercury and organohalogens in arctic fish, a sign of increasing contamination of the arctic food chain. Changes in hydrology resulting from climate change are expected to alter releases of chemical contaminants into the nation's surface waters, with as-yet-unknown effects on seafood contamination.

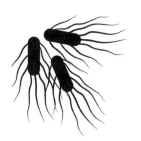

CHAPTER 19
Water Safety for Travelers

Risk for Travelers

Waterborne disease is a risk for international travelers who visit countries that have poor hygiene and inadequate sanitation, and for wilderness visitors who rely on surface water in any country, including the United States. The list of potential waterborne pathogens is extensive and includes bacteria, viruses, protozoa, and parasitic helminths. Most of the organisms that can cause travelers' diarrhea can be waterborne. Many types of bacteria and viruses can cause intestinal (enteric) infection through drinking water. Protozoa that are commonly waterborne include *Cryptosporidium*, *Giardia*, and *Entamoeba histolytica* (the cause of amebic dysentery). Parasitic worms are not commonly transmitted through drinking water, but it is a potential means of transmission for some.

Where treated tap water is available, aging or inadequate water treatment infrastructure may not effectively disinfect water or maintain water quality during distribution. Some larger hotels and resorts may provide additional onsite water treatment to provide potable water. Travelers can ask the facility manager about the safety of their water; however, if there is concern, it may be easiest for travelers to treat the water themselves. Where untreated surface or well water is used and there is no sanitation infrastructure, the risk of waterborne infection is high.

This chapter includes text excerpted from "Water Disinfection," Centers for Disease Control and Prevention (CDC), June 24, 2019.

Bottled water has become the convenient solution for most travelers, but in some places it may not be superior to tap water. Moreover, plastic bottles create an ecological problem, since most developing countries do not recycle plastic bottles. All international travelers, especially long-term travelers or expatriates, should become familiar with and use simple methods to ensure safe drinking water. Several methods are scalable and some can be improvised from local resources, allowing adaptation to disaster relief and refugee situations.

Field Techniques for Water Treatment
Heat

Common intestinal pathogens are readily inactivated by heat. Microorganisms are killed in a shorter time at higher temperatures, whereas temperatures as low as 140°F (60°C) are effective with a longer contact time. Pasteurization uses this principle to kill foodborne enteric pathogens and spoilage-causing organisms at temperatures between 140°F (60°C) and 158°F (70°C), well below the boiling point of water (212°F [100°C]).

Although boiling is not necessary to kill common intestinal pathogens, it is the only easily recognizable end point that does not require a thermometer. All organisms except bacterial spores, which are rarely waterborne enteric pathogens, are killed in seconds at boiling temperature. In addition, the time required to heat the water from 60°C to boiling works toward heat disinfection. Any water that is brought to a boil should be adequately disinfected; however, if fuel supplies are adequate, travelers should consider boiling for 1 minute to allow for a margin of safety. Although the boiling point decreases with altitude, at common terrestrial travel elevations it is still well above the temperature required to inactivate enteric pathogens (for example, at 16,000 ft [4,877 m] the boiling temperature of water is 182°F [84°C]). In hot climates with sunshine, a water container placed in a simple reflective solar oven can reach pasteurization temperature of 65°C. Travelers with access to electricity can bring a small electric heating coil or a lightweight beverage warmer to boil water.

Filtration and Clarification

Portable hand-pump or gravity-drip filters with various designs and types of filter media are commercially available to international travelers. Filter pore size is the primary determinant of a filter's effectiveness, unless the filter is designed to remove microbes by electrochemical attachment to filter media. Filter pore size will be described as being "absolute" or "nominal": absolute pore-size filters will remove all microbes of the identified pore size or larger, whereas nominal pore-size filters allow 20 percent to 30 percent of particles or microorganisms of the pore size to pass through. Progressively smaller pore-size filters require higher pressure to push water through the filter, often at a slower rate and higher cost. Filters that claim Environmental Protection Agency (EPA) designation of water "purifier" undergo company-sponsored testing to demonstrate removal of at least 106 bacteria (99.9999%), 104 viruses (99.99%), and 103 *Cryptosporidium oocysts* or *Giardia* cysts (99.9%). (The EPA does not independently test the validity of these claims.)

Filters with an absolute pore size of 1 µm or smaller should effectively remove protozoan parasites such as *Cryptosporidium* and *Giardia*. Microfilters with "absolute" pore sizes of 0.1–0.4 µm are usually effective at removing bacteria as well as cysts, but may not adequately remove enteric viruses, like norovirus. Water in remote alpine areas with little human and animal activity generally has little contamination with enteric pathogens, so microfilters with ceramic, synthetic fiber, compressed carbon, or large-pore hollow-fiber filter elements are sufficient to remove bacteria and protozoan cysts, the primary pathogens.

For areas with high levels of human and animal activity in the watershed or developing areas with poor sanitation, higher levels of filtration discussed below or other techniques to remove viruses are preferred. If using a microfilter, one option to remove viruses is pretreatment with chlorine. Progressively finer levels of filtration known as "ultrafiltration," "nanofiltration," and "reverse osmosis" can remove particles of 0.01, 0.001, and 0.0001 µm, respectively. All of these filters can remove viruses. Portable ultrafilters are the most commonly available "purifying" filters and may operate by gravity, hand-pump, or drink-through. Ultrafilter-based filters will have a rated pore size of 0.01 µm, and should be effective for removing viruses, bacteria, and parasites. All are effective, although drink-through is least practical because of the negative pressure required to draw water through the filter.

Nanofilters will have rated pore sizes of 0.001 μm and thus will remove chemicals and organic molecules. Reverse osmosis filters (having pore sizes of 0.0001 μm [0.1 nm] and smaller) will remove monovalent salts and dissolved metals, thus achieving desalination. The high price and slow output of small hand-pump reverse osmosis units prohibit use by land-based travelers; however, they are survival aids for ocean voyagers, and larger powered devices are used for military and refugee situations.

In resource-limited international settings, filters may be used in the communities and households that are made from ceramic clay or simple sand and gravel (slow sand or biosand). Gravel and sand filters can be improvised in remote or austere situations when no other means of disinfection is available.

Water can be clarified by using chemical products that coagulate and flocculate (clump together) suspended particles that cause a cloudy appearance and bad taste and do not settle by gravity. This process removes many, but not all, microorganisms, unless the product also contains a disinfectant. Alum, an aluminum salt that is widely used in food, cosmetic, and medical applications, is the principal agent for coagulation/flocculation, but many other natural substances are used throughout the world. When using alum, a 1/4 teaspoon of alum powder can be added to a quart of cloudy water and the water stirred frequently for a few minutes. The process can be repeated, if necessary, until clumps form. The clumped material is allowed to settle, and then the water is poured through a coffee filter or clean, fine cloth to remove the sediment. Most microbes are removed, but not all, so a second disinfection step is necessary. Tablets or packets of powder that combine flocculant and a chemical disinfectant are available commercially (for example, Chlor-floc and P and G Purifier of Water).

Granular-activated carbon (GAC) treats water by adsorbing organic and inorganic chemicals (including chlorine or iodine compounds) and most heavy metals, thereby improving odor, taste, and safety. GAC is a common component of household and field filters. It may trap microorganisms, but

GAC filters are generally not designed or rated for microbe removal and do not kill microorganisms.

Chemical Disinfection
Liquid and Tablet Products

Chemical disinfectants for drinking-water treatment, including chlorine compounds, iodine, and chlorine dioxide, are commonly available as commercial products. Sodium hypochlorite, the active ingredient in common household bleach, is the primary disinfectant promoted by the Centers for Disease Control and Prevention (CDC) and World Health Organization (WHO). Other chlorine-containing compounds such as calcium hypochlorite and sodium dichloroisocyanurate, available in granular or tablet formulation, are equally effective for water treatment. An advantage of chemical-water disinfection products is flexible dosing that allows use by individual travelers, small or large groups, or communities. In emergency situations, or when other commercial chemical-disinfection water-treatment products are not available, household bleach can be used for flexible dosing based on water volume and clarity.

Given adequate concentrations and length of exposure (contact time), chlorine and iodine have similar activity and are effective against bacteria and viruses. Giardia cysts are more resistant to chemical disinfection; however, field-level concentrations are effective with longer contact times. For this reason, dosing and concentrations of chemical-disinfection products are generally targeted to the cysts. Some common waterborne parasites, such as *Cryptosporidium* and possibly *Cyclospora*, are poorly inactivated by chlorine- and iodine-based disinfection at practical concentrations, even with extended contact times.

Chemical disinfection may be supplemented with filtration to remove resistant oocysts from drinking water. Cloudy water contains substances that will neutralize disinfectant, so it will require higher concentrations or contact times or, preferably, clarification through settling, coagulation/flocculation, or filtration before disinfectant is added.

Because iodine has physiologic activity, the WHO recommends limiting iodine water disinfection to a few weeks. Iodine use is not recommended for people with unstable thyroid disease or known iodine allergy. In addition, pregnant women should not use iodine to disinfect water over the long-term because of the potential effect on the fetal thyroid. Pregnant travelers who have other options should use an alternative means such as heat, chlorine, or filtration.

Some prefer the taste of iodine to chlorine, but neither is appealing in doses often recommended for field use. The taste of halogens in water can be improved by running water through a filter containing activated carbon or adding a 25-mg tablet of vitamin C, a tiny pinch of powdered ascorbic acid, or a small amount of hydrogen peroxide (5 to 10 drops of 3% peroxide per quart), then stir or shake. Repeat until the taste of chlorine or iodine is gone.

Chlorine Dioxide

Chlorine dioxide (ClO_2) can kill most waterborne pathogens, including *Cryptosporidium* oocysts, at practical doses and contact times. Tablets and liquid formulations are commercially available to generate chlorine dioxide in the field for personal use.

Salt (Sodium Chloride) Electrolysis

Electrolytic water purifiers generate a mixture of oxidants, including hypochlorite, by passing an electrical current through a simple brine salt solution. Purifier products sold for personal and group travel use produce an oxidant solution that can be added to water to kill microorganisms. This technique has been engineered into portable, battery-powered products that are commercially available.

Ultraviolet Light

Ultraviolet (UV) light kills bacteria, viruses, and *Cryptosporidium* oocysts in water. The effect depends on UV dose and exposure time. Portable battery-operated units that deliver a metered, timed dose of UV are an effective way to disinfect small quantities of clear water in the field. Larger units with higher output are available where a power source is available. These units have limited effectiveness in water with high levels of suspended solids and turbidity, because suspended particles can shield microorganisms from UV light.

Solar Irradiation and Heating

UV irradiation of water using sunlight (solar disinfection or SODIS) can improve the microbiologic quality of water and may be used in austere emergency situations. Solar disinfection is not effective on turbid water. If the headlines in a newspaper cannot be read through the bottle of water, then the water must be clarified before solar irradiation is used. Under cloudy weather conditions, water must be placed in the sun for 2 consecutive days.

Silver and Other Products

Silver ion has bactericidal effects in low doses, and some attractive features include lack of color, taste, and odor, and the ability of a thin coating on the container to maintain a steady, low concentration in water. Silver is widely used by European travelers as a primary drinking-water disinfectant. In the United States, silver is approved only for maintaining the microbiologic quality of stored water because its concentration can be strongly affected by adsorption onto the surface of the container, and there has been limited testing on viruses and cysts. Silver is available alone or in combination with chlorine in tablet formulation.

Several other common products, including hydrogen peroxide, citrus juice, and potassium permanganate, have antibacterial effects in water and are marketed in commercial products for travelers. None have sufficient data to recommend them for primary water disinfection at low doses in the field.

Photocatalytic Disinfection

Advanced oxidation processes use UV light or natural sunlight to catalyze the production of potent disinfectants for microorganisms and can break down complex organic contaminants and even most heavy metals into nontoxic forms. Titanium dioxide (TiO_2) is the most effective substance, but other metal oxides, chitins, and nanoparticles also have oxidative potential. A TiO_2-impregnated membrane incorporated into a portable bag is available commercially.

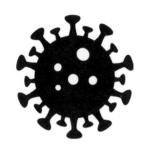

PART 4 · DISEASES AND OUTBREAKS TRANSMITTED TO HUMANS FROM ANIMALS, INSECTS, AND CONTAMINATED FOOD AND WATER

CHAPTER 20
Zoonoses and Outbreaks

Chapter Contents

Section 20.1

Prioritizing and Preventing Deadly Zoonotic Diseases

This section includes text excerpted from "Prioritizing and Preventing Deadly Zoonotic Diseases," Centers for Disease Control and Prevention (CDC), April 30, 2019.

Public-Health Threat

Diseases shared between animals and humans pose one of the greatest threats to our health, safety, and security.

Stopping the spread of zoonotic diseases requires a One Health approach that brings human, animal, and environmental health sectors together.

Response

The Centers for Disease Control and Prevention (CDC) led the development of the One Health Zoonotic Disease Prioritization tool to help countries with limited resources focus their most urgent global-health security efforts. The Division of Global Health Protection (DGHP) has supported 17 multisectoral One Health Zoonotic Disease Prioritization Workshops across the globe, using the tool to help countries identify which zoonotic diseases are of greatest national concern.

Workshop participants include a wide range of people who protect health — of people, animals, or the environment. Together, they select the country's top five diseases to target for One Health collaborations. Commonly prioritized zoonotic diseases include rabies, influenza viruses, viral hemorrhagic fevers, such as Ebola virus and Rift Valley fever, brucellosis, and anthrax.

One Health teams then develop strategies to tackle newly prioritized diseases. For example, having a rabies vaccination campaign for dogs can lead to fewer rabies deaths in people in a country.

Impact

The CDC is working with disease experts in countries, using the prioritization tool to guide improvements in laboratory capacity, surveillance, outbreak response, and prevention activities for prioritized diseases. By building One Health capacities and strengthening partnerships, countries will more effectively address priority threats and respond to new and emerging zoonotic diseases.

Facts about Zoonotic Diseases

- Six out of every ten infectious diseases in humans are spread from animals.
- Three out of four new or emerging infectious diseases come from animals.
- Zoonotic diseases are responsible for an estimated 2.5 billion cases of illness and 2.7 million deaths worldwide each year.

Section 20.2

The Novel Coronavirus (COVID-19) Pandemic

This section includes text excerpted from "Coronavirus Disease 2019 (COVID-19) Situation Summary," Centers for Disease Control and Prevention (CDC), March 3, 2020.

The Centers for Disease Control and Prevention (CDC) is responding to an outbreak of respiratory disease caused by a novel (new) coronavirus that was first detected in China and which has now been detected in over 100 locations internationally, including in the United States. The virus has been named "SARS-CoV-2" and the disease it causes has been named "coronavirus disease 2019" (abbreviated "COVID-19").

On January 30, 2020, the International Health Regulations Emergency Committee of the World Health Organization (WHO) declared the outbreak a "public health emergency of international concern" (PHEIC). On January 31, 2020, U.S. Department of Health and Human Services (HHS) Secretary Alex M. Azar II declared a public-health emergency (PHE) for the United States to aid the nation's healthcare community in responding to COVID-19.

Source and Spread of the Virus

Coronaviruses are a large family of viruses that are common in people and many different species of animals, including camels, cattle, cats, and bats. Rarely, animal coronaviruses can infect people and then spread between people, such as with Middle East respiratory syndrome coronavirus (MERS-CoV), severe acute respiratory syndrome coronavirus (SARS-CoV), and now with this new virus (named SARS-CoV-2).

The SARS-CoV-2 virus is a betacoronavirus, like MERS-CoV and SARS-CoV. All three of these viruses have their origins in bats. The sequences from U.S. patients are similar to the one that China initially posted, suggesting a likely single, recent emergence of this virus from an animal reservoir.

Early on, many of the patients at the epicenter of the outbreak in Wuhan, Hubei Province, China had some link to a large seafood and live-animal market, suggesting animal-to-person spread. Later, a growing number of patients reportedly did not have exposure to animal markets, indicating person-to-person spread. Person-to-person spread was subsequently reported outside Hubei and in countries outside China, including in the United States. Some international destinations now have apparent community spread with the virus that causes COVID-19, including in some parts of the United States. "Community spread" means some people have been infected and it is not known how or where they became exposed.

Situation in United States

- Imported cases of COVID-19 in travelers have been detected in the United States.

- Person-to-person spread of COVID-19 was first reported among close contacts of returned travelers from Wuhan.
- During the week of February 23, the CDC reported community spread of the virus that causes COVID-19 in California (in two locations), Oregon, and Washington state. Community spread in Washington state resulted in the first death in the United States from COVID-19, as well as the first reported case of COVID-19 in a U.S. healthcare worker, and the first potential outbreak in a long-term care facility.

Illness Severity

Both MERS-CoV and SARS-CoV have been known to cause severe illness in people. The complete clinical picture with regard to COVID-19 is not fully understood. Reported illnesses have ranged from mild to severe, including illness resulting in death. While information so far suggests that most COVID-19 illness is mild, a report out of China suggests serious illness occurs in 16 percent of cases. Older people and people with certain underlying health conditions like heart disease, lung disease and diabetes, for example, seem to be at greater risk of serious illness.

Risk Assessment

Outbreaks of novel virus infections among people are always of public-health concern. The risk from these outbreaks depends on characteristics of the virus, including how well it spreads between people, the severity of resulting illness, and the medical or other measures available to control the impact of the virus (for example, vaccine or treatment medications). The fact that this disease has caused illness, including illness resulting in death, and sustained person-to-person spread is concerning. These factors meet two of the criteria of a pandemic. As community spread is detected in more and more countries, the world moves closer toward meeting the third criteria, worldwide spread of the new virus.

Reported community spread of COVID-19 in parts of the United States raises the level of concern about the immediate threat for COVID-19 for those communities. The potential public-health threat posed by COVID-19 is very high, to the United States and globally.

At this time, however, most people in the United States will have little immediate risk of exposure to this virus. This virus is NOT currently spreading widely in the United States. However, it is important to note that current global circumstances suggest it is likely that this virus will cause a pandemic. This is a rapidly evolving situation and the risk assessment will be updated as needed.

Current risk assessment:

- For most of the American public, who are unlikely to be exposed to this virus at this time, the immediate health risk from COVID-19 is considered low.
- People in communities where ongoing community spread with the virus that causes COVID-19 has been reported are at elevated, though still relatively low, risk of exposure.
- Healthcare workers caring for patients with COVID-19 are at elevated risk of exposure.
- Close contacts of people with COVID-19 also are at elevated risk of exposure.
- Travelers returning from affected international locations where community spread is occurring also are at elevated risk of exposure.

What May Happen

More cases of COVID-19 are likely to be identified in the coming days, including more cases in the United States. It's also likely that person-to-person spread will continue to occur, including in communities in the United States. It's likely that at some point, widespread transmission of COVID-19 in the United States will occur.

Widespread transmission of COVID-19 would translate into large numbers of people needing medical care at the same time. Schools, childcare centers, workplaces, and other places for mass gatherings may experience more absenteeism. Public-health and healthcare systems may become overloaded, with elevated rates of hospitalizations and deaths. Other critical infrastructure, such as law enforcement, emergency medical services, and the transportation industry may also be affected. Healthcare providers and hospitals may be overwhelmed. At this time, there is no vaccine to protect against COVID-19 and no medications approved to treat it. Nonpharmaceutical interventions would be the most important response strategy.

The CDC's Response

Global efforts at this time are focused concurrently on containing the spread and mitigating the impact of this virus. The federal government is working closely with state, local, tribal, and territorial partners, as well as public-health partners, to respond to this public-health threat. The public-health response is multi-layered, with the goal of detecting and minimizing introductions of this virus in the United States. The CDC is operationalizing all of its pandemic preparedness and response plans, and working on multiple fronts to meet these goals, including specific measures to prepare communities to respond to local transmission of the virus that causes COVID-19. There is an abundance of pandemic guidance developed in anticipation of an influenza pandemic that is being repurposed and adapted for a COVID-19 pandemic.

Highlights of the CDC's Response

- The CDC established a COVID-19 Incident Management System on January 7, 2020. On January 21, the CDC activated its Emergency Operations Center to better provide ongoing support to the COVID-19 response.
- The U.S. government has taken unprecedented steps with respect to travel in response to the growing public-health threat posed by this new coronavirus:
  - Effective February 2, at 5 p.m., the U.S. government suspended entry of foreign nationals who have been in China within the past 14 days.
    - U.S. citizens, residents, and their immediate family members who have been in Hubei province and other parts of mainland China are allowed to enter the United States, but they are subject to health monitoring and possible quarantine for up to 14 days.
  - On February 29, the U.S. government announced it was suspending entry of foreign nationals who have been in Iran within the past 14 days.

- The CDC has issued the following travel guidance related to COVID-19:
  - China—Level 3, Avoid Nonessential Travel—updated February 22;
  - Hong Kong—Level 1, Practice Usual Precautions—issued February 19;
  - Iran—Level 3, Avoid Nonessential Travel—updated February 28;
  - Italy—Level 3, Avoid Nonessential Travel—updated February 28;
  - Japan—Level 2, Practice Enhanced Precautions—updated February 22;
  - South Korea—Level 3, Avoid Nonessential Travel—updated February 24.
  - The CDC also recommends that all travelers reconsider cruise ship voyages into or within Asia at this time.
- The CDC is issuing clinical guidance, including:
  - On January 30, the CDC published guidance for healthcare professionals on the clinical care of COVID-19 patients.
  - On February 3, the CDC posted guidance for assessing the potential risk for various exposures to COVID-19 and managing those people appropriately.
  - On February 27, the CDC updated its criteria to guide evaluation of persons under investigation for COVID-19.
  - On February 28, the CDC issued a Health Alert Network (HAN): Update and Interim Guidance on Outbreak of COVID-19.
- The CDC has deployed multidisciplinary teams to support state health departments in case identification, contact tracing, clinical management, and communications.
- The CDC has worked with the U.S. Department of State, supporting the safe return of Americans who have been stranded as a result of the ongoing outbreaks of COVID-19 and related travel restrictions. The CDC has worked to assess the health of passengers as they return to the United States and provided continued daily monitoring of people who are quarantined.
- An important part of the CDC's role during a public-health emergency is to develop a test for the pathogen and equip state and local public-health labs with testing capacity.

- After distribution of a CDC rRT-PCR test to diagnose COVID-19 to state and local public-health labs started, performance issues were identified related to a problem in the manufacturing of one of the reagents. Laboratories were not able to verify the test performance.
- The CDC worked on two potential resolutions to this problem.
  - The CDC developed a new protocol that uses two of the three components of the original CDC test kit to detect the virus that causes COVID-19 after establishing that the third component, which was the problem with the original test, can be excluded from testing without affecting accuracy. The CDC is working with the U.S. Food and Drug Administration (FDA) to amend the existing Emergency Use Authorization (EUA) for the test, but in the meantime, the FDA granted discretionary authority for the use of the original test kits.
    - Public-health laboratories can use the original CDC test kit to test for the virus that causes COVID-19 using the new protocol.
  - Further, newly manufactured kits have been provided to the International Reagent Resource icon for distribution.
- Combined with other reagents that the CDC has procured, there are enough testing kits to test more than 75,000 people.
- In addition, the CDC has two laboratories conducting testing for the virus that causes COVID-19. The CDC can test approximately 350 specimens per day.
- Commercial labs are working to develop their own tests that hopefully will be available soon. This will allow a greater number of tests to happen close to where potential cases are.
- The CDC has grown the COVID-19 virus in cell culture, which is necessary for further studies, including for additional genetic characterization. The cell-grown virus was sent to the National Institutes of Health (NIH)'s BEI Resources Repository for use by the broad scientific community.

The CDC Recommends

- Everyone can do their part to help CDC respond to this emerging public-health threat:

- It's currently flu and respiratory disease season and the CDC recommends getting a flu vaccine, taking everyday preventive actions to help stop the spread of germs, and taking flu antivirals if prescribed.
- If you are a healthcare provider, be on the lookout for:
  - People who recently traveled from China or another affected area and who have symptoms associated with COVID-19, and
  - People who have been in close contact with someone with COVID-19 or pneumonia of unknown cause. (Consult the most recent definition for patients under investigation [PUIs].)
- If you are a healthcare provider or a public-health responder caring for a COVID-19 patient, please take care of yourself and follow recommended infection-control procedures.
- If you are a close contact of someone with COVID-19 and develop symptoms of COVID-19, call your healthcare provider and tell them about your symptoms and your exposure.
- If you are a resident in a community where person-to-person spread of COVID-19 has been detected and you develop COVID-19 symptoms, call your healthcare provider and tell them about your symptoms.
- For people who are ill with COVID-19, but are not sick enough to be hospitalized, please follow CDC guidance on how to reduce the risk of spreading your illness to others. People who are mildly ill with COVID-19 are able to isolate at home during their illness.
- If you have been in China or another affected area or have been exposed to someone sick with COVID-19 in the last 14 days, you will face some

limitations on your movement and activity for up to 14 days. Please follow instructions during this time. Your cooperation is integral to the ongoing public-health response to try to slow spread of this virus.

Section 20.3

Zoonoses Preparedness and Response Plan

This section includes text excerpted from "Emerging Animal Disease Preparedness and Response Plan," U.S. Department of Agriculture (USDA), July 2017.

Identifying and Characterizing Global and Domestic Threats to Animal Health
Global and Domestic Awareness and Assessment

The U.S. Department of Agriculture (USDA) risk identification (RI) team is responsible for monitoring the distribution of animal diseases domestically and globally to identify potential threats to U.S. agriculture. The team works collaboratively with personnel across veterinary services (VS) and others in the community responsible for animal and public health (federal, state, territory, tribal, industry, and private sector) to identify and describe global emerging animal-disease risks. The RI team identifies and characterizes animal-disease risks using information from relationships established directly or through VS points of contacts (POCs) from other U.S. Department of Agriculture (USDA) units and other United States and international sources, including the following:

- U.S. Department of Homeland Security (DHS)
- U.S. Department of the Interior (DOI)
- U.S. Department of Commerce (DOC)
- U.S. Department of Defense (DOD)

- U.S. Department of Justice (DOJ)
- Centers for Disease Control and Prevention (CDC)
- Inter-American Institute for Cooperation on Agriculture (IICA)
- International Regional Organization for Plant and Animal Health (OIRSA)
- Pan-American Foot and Mouth Disease Centre (PANAFTOSA)
- World Organization for Animal Health (OIE)
- Food and Agriculture Organization (FAO) of the United Nations
- World Health Organization (WHO)

The team reviews open-source information available from international agencies and organizations, various media outlets, and peer-reviewed scientific literature daily to maintain a baseline situational awareness of global animal-health issues and disease events.

Domestically, the team uses information from a variety of resources, including:

- National Veterinary Services Laboratories (NVSL)
- National Animal Health Laboratory Network (NAHLN), voluntary National Animal Health Reporting System (NAHRS)
- National Animal Health Monitoring System surveys
- Mandatory reporting, such as that required by the "Reporting, Herd Monitoring and Management of Novel Swine Enteric Coronavirus Diseases Federal Order"
- Data provided by VS certification and surveillance programs

In addition, the team utilizes existing relationships with animal industry groups; state and tribal animal-health, public-health, and wildlife health officials, laboratories, accredited veterinarians, producers, livestock-market operators, universities, and other agencies to access, share, and evaluate a broad scope of information.

VS personnel also serve as agency liaisons to industry organizations, such as the Swine Health Information Center (SHIC) and Equine Disease Communication Center (EDCC), that have implemented systems to gather animal-disease information in order to facilitate effective communication and collaboration.

Roles and Responsibilities

Successful emerging-disease response requires a collaborative effort between the Animal and Plant Health Inspection Service (APHIS), state and tribal animal-health officials, and animal industries. While the VS leads this effort, the input and cooperation of states and animal industries are essential.

Veterinary Services Business Units

The general responsibilities of VS business units are as follows:

Science, Technology and Analysis Services

The RI team, as part of the Center for Epidemiology and Animal Health's (CEAH) risk identification and risk assessment (RIRA) unit, is the primary unit responsible for monitoring domestic and international information sources, conducting preliminary evaluations of information pertaining to risks to U.S. animal health, and leading further analyses and data-gathering when possible emerging diseases are identified. The team maintains a database of diseases that are actively monitored and a time interval for updating information used to assign a risk level to each.

In addition to RIRA, CEAH, and Science, Technology and Analysis Services (STAS), other units participate in emerging-disease assessment and response. In CEAH, these include the information management and analytic support unit, the monitoring and modeling unit, and the surveillance, design, and analysis unit. Within STAS, they include the Center for Veterinary Biologics (CVB), the NVSL, and the Office of STAS Interagency Coordination. Directors in STAS designate the emerging-diseases POCs responsible for assisting RI team analysts with the collection of information and initial risk-category assignment. In addition, STAS designates directors to serve as liaisons to the RIRA director and review information prepared by the RI team and their POCs.

Surveillance, Preparedness and Response Services

As the VS business unit responsible for implementation of surveillance, preparedness, and response activities, the Surveillance, Preparedness and

Response Services (SPRS) routinely receive information about potentially emerging animal-health issues. SPRS staff designate emerging-diseases POCs for each animal commodity, the National Preparedness and Incident Coordination Center (NPICC), and the One Health Coordination Office (OHCO).

In addition, directors of the Avian, Swine, and Aquatic Animal Health Center; Cattle Health Center; Sheep, Goat, Cervid, and Equine Health Center; OHCO; and NPICC serve as liaisons to the RIRA director and review information prepared by the RI team and their POCs.

National Import and Export Services
The National Import and Export Services (NIES) designates emerging-diseases POCs and assists RI team analysts with the collection of information and initial risk-category assignments. NIES also designates the unit directors to serve as liaisons who review information prepared by the RI team and their POCs.

Emerging-diseases POCs are responsible for the following activities:
- Communicating information regarding potential emerging diseases to RI team analysts for situational awareness
- Providing subject-matter expertise to the RI team to determine a risk-level category assignment for each agent
- Assisting with the review of laboratory-testing results
- Estimating trade issues
- Communicating issues up their respective supervisory chains

For each international agent designated a risk category 2, domestic agent designated a risk category 1 or greater, or each agent for which additional information is required before a risk category can be assigned, the appropriate VS liaisons will determine if additional information, analyses, or field response is required and will assign appropriate subject-matter experts within their units to participate with the cross-unit emerging-disease team to evaluate these needs and make recommendations.

States. States' responsibilities include reporting under the NAHRS. However, states are encouraged to contact the appropriate SPRS assistant director concerning any unusual disease event in their state to discuss the results of diagnostic testing and available epidemiological information. State animal-health officials may also participate with cross-unit emerging-disease teams, by assisting the VS with the evaluation and analysis of information and data gathering when possible emerging diseases are identified. In addition to providing input into the discussion and development of possible response options, further state responsibilities include the issuance of holds or quarantines and participation in any monitoring, control, or eradication activity, as appropriate.

Industry. The VS uses previously established communication links with industry organizations to communicate information, evaluate and discuss data related to potential disease risks and concerns, and develop response options. Industry organizations also may establish POCs for regular information exchange and provide subject-matter experts to participate in cross-unit emerging-disease team tasks. For those industries, such as the SHIC and EDCC, that have implemented systems to gather animal-disease information, VS personnel serve as agency liaisons who facilitate rapid communication and collaboration.

Agency and nonagency partners. Other federal partners in the USDA, DHS, CDC, DOI, DOJ, etc., as well as NAHLN laboratories, universities, tribes and accredited veterinarians, provide information, review data, and provide subject-matter expertise as needed. Depending on the situation, these partners may provide subject-matter experts to help analyze preliminary information and determine the level of risk to U.S. animal or public health and assist cross-unit emerging-disease teams in the evaluation and characterization of the disease incident, communications, and other related emerging-disease response activities.

Initial Assessment of Information

Based on information from global and domestic sources provided by federal, state, academic, and industry partners, the RI team will work with emerging-diseases POCs to conduct a preliminary assessment and assign the disease to one of the following risk-level categories:

- Level 1: Nominal risk to U.S. animal or public health
- Level 2: Potential risk to U.S. animal or public health

- Level 3: Impending risk to U.S. animal or public health
- Level 4: Current risk to U.S. animal or public health

The RI team will maintain a tracking system documenting each agent being actively monitored and its assigned risk-level category. For each international emerging-disease risks designated at risk level 2 or greater, domestic diseases designated at any level, or diseases for which additional information is needed before a risk level can be assigned, the RI team summarizes the information used to make the risk-category assignment in a short briefing document. The RI team will share the briefing documents with appropriate VS Liaisons for review.

If, based on the results of the review, the severity and complexity of a disease incident warrants additional communication, evaluation, characterization, or response, VS liaisons will identify appropriate subject-matter experts to form a cross-unit emerging-disease team. The team will determine the additional information, communications, analyses, or field response needed to thoroughly evaluate, characterize, or mitigate the disease incident, including the possible creation of partnerships with other entities.

Evaluation of Disease Incidents and Recommendations for Response

When the RIRA director and VS liaisons' initial review determines an emerging-disease incident requires communication, evaluation, characterization, or response, VS liaisons, in collaboration with RI analysts and emerging-diseases POCs, will identify appropriate subject-matter experts to form the cross-unit and, if needed, interagency or agency-stakeholder emerging-disease team to conduct these activities. For public-health concerns associated with emerging zoonotic-disease issues, the team closely collaborates with the CDC through the OHCO and the APHIS liaison position co-located at the CDC.

The RI team lead will initially organize and lead the team to review information, determine gaps in data or preparedness, and outline additional communications, analyses, research, field epidemiological investigations, or mitigations needed to fully characterize, communicate, and respond to the emerging-disease incident. The emerging-disease team will document and provide results of all evaluations, including any communication materials and recommendations for response, to VS liaisons for presentation and decision-making by the VS executive team (VSET), as appropriate. Recommendations will outline any regulatory issues or financial needs associated with each action.

The VSET will approve and authorize resources for the appropriate response measures. Depending on the scale, scope, and urgency of the situation, the VSET may need to designate responsibility to the appropriate VS business unit for each recommendation. For instance, further field investigations would be the responsibility of and coordinated through SPRS, pathway analyses would be the responsibility of and coordinated through RIRA or NIES, and questions about existing surveillance data would be coordinated by STAS.

Response Coordination

If the evaluation of an emerging-disease incident includes response-option recommendations, the cross-unit emerging-disease team will take the lead in coordinating the response option(s) selected by the VSET. The actions necessary to develop and implement specific responses are outside the scope of this document. However, VS will follow standard program, regulatory, and budgetary business practices, including the use of VS Guidance 12001.2 Potential Foreign Animal Disease Incidents (FAD/EDI) and response evaluation tools such as the "Technique for the Assessment of Intervention Options" (TAIO) and Decision Lens, as needed.

If the emerging disease impacts a single species, the appropriate SPRS Commodity Center director (or designee) will become the leader of the cross-unit emerging-disease team and will be responsible for developing and implementing response options, and coordinating as needed with affected commodity groups and state animal-health officials. If a disease impacts more than one commodity or a commodity not represented in an existing VS health center, then it will be the responsibility of the SPRS associate deputy administrator to designate a leader for the team. The team leader may request further analyses to clarify response options. The analyses should consider impacts to international trade, animal health, public health, food security, agricultural production, and the environment; geographic distribution of disease; political pressures; resource intensity; available subject matter expertise; diagnostic capabilities; regulatory authorities; and the potential for bioterrorism.

Possible response options are listed by risk-level category below and will depend on the specific situation. Response options outlined for each risk level also include all options listed for lower risk-level categories. Additionally, there may be responses not identified that might be relevant to a certain emerging-disease incident.

Possible Responses to Emerging International Threats
Risk Level 1 (Nominal Risk to U.S. Animal or Public Health)
- Provide continual monitoring of emerging-disease incidents and situational awareness updates, as needed.

Risk Level 2 (Potential Risk to U.S. Animal or Public Health)
- Continue to monitor emerging-disease incidents and provide situational awareness updates, as needed.
- Assess preparedness status for introduction (e.g., lab capacity, presence of valid diagnostic tests, and vaccines).
- Identify existing disease mitigations.

Risk Level 3 (Impending Risk to U.S. Animal or Public Health) or Insufficient Information Available to Assign a Risk Level
- All options in levels 1 and 2
- Work with APHIS International Services personnel in relevant countries to obtain additional information on disease incidents.
- Determine need for further evaluation and characterization of incidents by an emerging-disease team.
- Conduct pathways, import risk assessments, and determine data gaps and needs for additional information to inform high-risk entry points.
- Increase laboratory diagnostic capacity and evaluation or development of effective vaccines. Implement import restrictions or increased surveillance, as needed.

- Develop and distribute communication materials to relevant partners and stakeholders.

Possible Responses to Emerging Domestic Threats
Risk Level 1 (Nominal Risk to U.S. Animal or Public Health)

- Contact diagnostician(s), state, territory, tribal, and federal partners, and relevant diagnostic laboratories to obtain additional information and confirmation of disease incidents.
- Identify and conduct additional needed research (e.g., animal inoculation studies, additional molecular characterization of pathogen).
- Determine reservoirs, transmission pathways, and potential impacts on U.S. animal or public health.
- Implement increased surveillance, as needed.
- Develop a case definition based on known epidemiological or agent-specific characteristics. Conduct an investigation on farms meeting case definition, as needed, to characterize the incident. Develop and distribute communication materials to relevant agency and nonagency partners and stakeholders.
- Increase diagnostic capacity, as needed.

Risk Level 2 (Potential Risk to U.S. Animal or Public Health)

- All options in level 1
- Increase laboratory diagnostic capacity and evaluation or development of effective vaccines. Develop a case definition for reporting based on laboratory criteria.
- Define laboratory data formats and data flows.
- Provide guidance to states, territories, tribes, industry, and other stakeholders for prevention, detection, and response to emerging disease.

Risk Level 3 (Impending Risk to U.S. Animal or Public Health)

- All options in levels 1 and 2
- Determine need for and establish regulations and/or new policies.

Risk Level 4 (Risk to U.S. Animal or Public Health)

- All options in levels 1 to 3
- Develop a surveillance plan and conduct active surveillance (situation dependent).
- Conduct analytical epidemiologic investigations.
- Determine need for and establish regulations for a new program (certification, control, or eradication) or new policies.

Section 20.4

Epidemiologic and Economic Modeling

This section includes text excerpted from
"Epidemiologic and Economic Modeling," U.S.
Department of Agriculture (USDA), February 3, 2017.

About Epidemiologic and Economic Modeling

The modeling team leads the evaluation, acquisition, and enhancement of applied animal-disease models based on supportable epidemiologic and economic principles to effectively communicate modeling results through training and outreach, and supports federal and state emergency management in animal-disease outbreak response and preparedness. Specifically, the models address animal diseases that are highly contagious and may cause disruption to the food supply.

Monitoring and Modeling (M&M) uses several software applications to accomplish its objectives. InterSpread Plus® (ISP) and the North American Animal Disease Spread Model/Animal Disease Spread Model (NAADSM/ADSM) are the most commonly used applications to simulate animal-disease spread and control. Both applications are stochastic state-transition models and provide a flexible SIR (susceptible/infected/removed) framework for users to simulate disease progression and spread by contact or air. Outbreak-control measures such as vaccination and depopulation can be implemented while accounting for resource limitations in personnel or supplies.

The economic impacts of an animal-disease outbreak are broad. Response costs associated with control of the outbreak include human resources needed for an emergency response, indemnity for animals which are depopulated to control disease, and the costs of eliminating the pathogen from the farm. There are also costs, such as trade restrictions and changes in consumer demand, which often have further-reaching consequences on the U.S. economy than the response costs.

Parameter Documentation

The applications used by the modeling team create a framework for the development of epidemiologic models that can simulate the spread and control of a variety of infectious diseases. User-defined input parameters broadly represent animal populations, disease dynamics within herds/flocks, disease transmission between herds/flocks, disease detection and surveillance, and disease control. Parameter values are derived from multiple sources, often including a review of the literature, available data, data generated from separate modeling tools, and subject-matter elicitation.

Section 20.5

Laboratory Information and Services

This section includes text excerpted from "Laboratory Information and Services," U.S. Department of Agriculture (USDA), May 24, 2019.

National Veterinary Services Laboratories

Animal and Plant Health Inspection Service (APHIS) laboratory services are provided by the National Veterinary Services Laboratories (NVSL) in Ames, Iowa, and Orient Point (Plum Island), New York. The NVSL provides a wide variety of information and services centered around diagnosis of domestic and foreign animal diseases, support of disease-control and eradication programs, reagents for diagnostic testing, training, and laboratory certification.

Diagnostic Testing

Authorized individuals may submit specimens to the NVSL facilities for diagnostic testing. The NVSL website describes the types of tests performed at the NVSL and provides instructions for submitting samples. The site also includes statements regarding ownership of specimens.

Reagents and Proficiency Tests

Diagnostic reagents are produced by the NVSL as needed when a commercial source of reagent is not available or when commercial sources are not fulfilling diagnostic needs. A list of available reagents, including proficiency tests, and instructions for ordering, and more can be found at https://www.aphis.usda.gov/aphis/ourfocus/animalhealth/lab-info-services/sa_reagents/ct_reagents.

Approved Laboratories

Some diagnostic testing may be conducted by APHIS-approved state, federal, or private laboratories. The United States Department of Agriculture (USDA) NVSL site describes the t https://www.aphis.usda.gov/aphis/ourfocus/animalhealth/lab-info-services/sa_diagnostic_tests/ct_diagnostic_tests

Diagnostic Training

The NVSL provides a variety of courses on diagnostic testing, specimen collection, and disease recognition. Descriptions of courses, instructions to register for a course, and more can be found at https://www.aphis.usda.gov/aphis/ourfocus/animalhealth/lab-info-services/sa_nvsl_training/ct_training.

National Animal Health Laboratory Network

The National Animal Health Laboratory Network (NAHLN) is part of a nationwide strategy to coordinate the work of all organizations providing veterinary surveillance and testing services.

Section 20.6

One Health

This section includes text excerpted from "One Health,"
U.S. Department of Agriculture (USDA),
February 14, 2019.

One Health (OH) is a collaborative, multisectoral, and transdisciplinary approach—working at the local, regional, national, and global levels—with the goal of achieving optimal health outcomes recognizing the interconnection between people, animals, plants, and their shared environment.

A One Health approach embraces the idea that complex problems that affect the health of humans, animals, and the environment are best solved through improved communication, cooperation, and collaboration across disciplines and sectors. Complex problems require a "whole system" approach to identify the elements, see relationships and patterns, identify potential root causes, and determine the course of action.

Throughout its history, the U.S. Department of Agriculture (USDA) has played a central role in protecting the health of American animal agriculture. The organization has offered essential services related to the import and export of animals, animal products, and biologics; emergency preparedness and response; animal disease diagnostics; animal vaccine development; and disease surveillance, control, and eradication.

It is part of the USDA's Animal and Plant Health Inspection Service (APHIS)'s vision that Veterinary Services (VS) division will be nationally engaged in response, research, and service by continuing to build an organization that encourages innovative thinking, action, and productive collaborations. The One Health realm is an area where VS contributes its extensive animal-health expertise and experience to address the animal component of One Health issues.

The VS coordinates and helps implement the One Health aspects of the USDA's mission, as outlined in *Veterinary Services: A New Perspective*. Since 2012, VS has strengthened multisector responses to zoonotic diseases and other complex issues that intersect with the Alternate Healthy Eating Index (AHEI) and promote a One Health approach to these issues.

VS works with internal and external partners to strengthen interagency coordination and address One Health issues. VS helps promote collaboration across sectors by identifying and developing policies, procedures, and tools that help define when and how different sectors can work together.

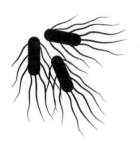

CHAPTER 21
Vector-Borne Disease Identification and Outbreaks

Chapter Contents

Section 21.1

Combatting Vector-Borne Illnesses: An Overview

This section includes text excerpted from "Illnesses on the Rise," Centers for Disease Control and Prevention (CDC), May 1, 2018.

Almost everyone has been bitten by a mosquito, tick, or flea. These can be vectors for spreading pathogens (germs). A person who gets bitten by a vector and gets sick has a vector-borne disease, such as dengue, Zika, Lyme, or plague. More than 640,000 cases of these diseases were reported, and 9 new germs spread by bites from infected mosquitoes and ticks were discovered or introduced in the United States from 2004 to 2016. State and local health departments and vector-control organizations are the nation's main defense against this increasing threat. Yet, 84 percent of local vector-control organizations lack at least 1 of 5 core vector-control competencies. Better control of mosquitoes and ticks is needed to protect people from these costly and deadly diseases.

State and Local Public-Health Agencies Can

- Build and sustain public-health programs that test and track germs and the mosquitoes and ticks that spread them.
- Train vector-control staff on 5 core competencies for conducting prevention and control activities.
- Educate the public about how to prevent bites and control germs spread by mosquitoes, ticks, and fleas in their communities.

Increasing Threat, Limited Capacity to Respond

More Cases in the United States (2004–2016)

- The number of reported cases of disease from mosquito, tick, and flea bites has more than tripled.
- More than 640,000 cases of these diseases were reported from 2004 to 2016.
- Disease cases from ticks have doubled.
- Mosquito-borne disease epidemics happen more frequently.

More Germs (2004–2016)

- Chikungunya and Zika viruses caused outbreaks in the United States for the first time.
- Seven new tick-borne germs can infect people in the United States.

More People at Risk

- Commerce moves mosquitoes, ticks, and fleas around the world.
- Infected travelers can introduce and spread germs across the world.
- Mosquitoes and ticks move germs into new areas of the United States, causing more people to be at risk.

The United States Is Not Fully Prepared

- Local and state health departments and vector-control organizations face increasing demands to respond to these threats.
- More than 80 percent of vector-control organizations report needing improvement in 1 or more of 5 core competencies, such as testing for pesticide resistance.
- More proven and publicly accepted mosquito and tick-control methods are needed to prevent and control these diseases.

Controlling Diseases from Mosquitoes and Ticks Requires 5 Core Competencies

Local health departments and vector-control organizations must be able to:
1. Monitor and track mosquitoes and ticks locally.

2. Use data to drive local decisions about vector control.
3. Have an action plan to kill mosquitoes and ticks at every life stage.
4. Control vectors using multiple types of methods.
6. Conduct pesticide-resistance testing.

What Can Be Done
The Federal Government Is

- Funding states, territories, industry, university, and international groups to detect and respond to infections from mosquitoes, ticks, and fleas and to report the cases to the Centers for Disease Control and Prevention (CDC).
- Convening a Tick-Borne Disease Working Group established by the 21st Century Cures Act to improve federal coordination of tick-borne disease efforts.
- Supporting 5 regional centers of excellence to address emerging diseases from mosquitoes and ticks.
- Conducting and developing diagnostic tests, vaccines, and treatments for these diseases.
- Educating the public about protecting themselves from diseases resulting from an infective mosquito, tick, or flea bite.

State and Local Government Agencies Can

- Build and sustain public-health programs that test and track germs and the mosquitoes and ticks that spread them.
- Train vector-control staff on 5 core competencies for conducting prevention and control activities.
- Educate the public about how to prevent bites and control germs spread by mosquitoes, ticks, and fleas in their communities.

Universities and Companies Can

- Study mosquitoes and ticks to better understand how to control them.
- Develop new or better methods and products to kill mosquitoes and ticks at each stage of life.

- Discover or improve tests for diagnosing new and known diseases from infective mosquito and tick bites.
- Create and sustain information-sharing networks.
- Train the next generation of entomologists and vector-control professionals.

Everyone Can

- Use a U.S. Environmental Protection Agency (EPA)-registered insect repellent.
- Wear long-sleeved shirts and long pants.
- Treat items, such as boots, pants, socks, and tents, with permethrin or buy permethrin-treated clothing and gear.
- Take steps to control ticks and fleas on pets.
- Find and remove ticks daily from family and pets.
- Take steps to control mosquitoes, ticks, and fleas inside and outside your home.

Section 21.2

Vital Signs: Trends in Vector-Borne Diseases

This section includes text excerpted from "Vital Signs: Trends in Reported Vector-Borne Disease Cases— United States and Territories, 2004–2016," Centers for Disease Control and Prevention (CDC), May 3, 2018.

Vectors are blood-feeding insects and ticks capable of transmitting pathogens between hosts. Wide varieties of pathogens have evolved to exploit vector transmission, including some viruses, bacteria, rickettsia, protozoa, and helminths. Dengue viruses are estimated to infect nearly 400 million persons worldwide each year, and malaria is a major cause of pediatric mortality in equatorial Africa. Plague and rickettsioses cause deadly epidemics abroad.

In the United States, 16 vector-borne diseases are reportable to state and territorial health departments, which are encouraged to report them to the National Notifiable Disease Surveillance System (NNDSS). Among the diseases on the list that are caused by indigenous pathogens are Lyme disease (*Borrelia burgdorferi*); West Nile, dengue and Zika virus diseases; plague (*Yersinia pestis*); and spotted fever rickettsioses (e.g., *Rickettsia rickettsii*). Malaria and yellow fever are no longer transmitted in the United States but have the potential to be reintroduced. As a group, vector-borne diseases in the United States are notable for their wide distribution and resistance to control. A U.S. Food and Drug Administration (FDA)-approved vaccine is available to prevent only one of the notifiable diseases, yellow fever.

Despite the dissimilarities among vector-borne pathogens and the many vector species that can transmit them, commonalities exist. Vector-borne disease epidemiology is complex because of environmental influences on the biology and behavior of the vectors. The longevity, distribution, biting habits, and propagation of vectors, which ultimately affect the intensity of transmission, depend on environmental factors such as rainfall, temperature, and shelter. Most vector-borne pathogens are zoonoses, often with wild-animal reservoirs, such as rodents or birds, making them difficult or impossible to eliminate. Arthropod vectors can bridge the gap between animals and humans that would not ordinarily intersect, as happens in Lyme disease, plague, and West Nile virus (WNV), facilitating the introduction of emerging animal pathogens to humans.

Trends of Reported Vector-Borne Disease Cases in the United States

The pace of emergence of new or obscure vector-borne pathogens through introduction or belated recognition appears to be increasing. Since 2004, these have included two previously unknown, life-threatening tick-borne

RNA viruses, Heartland and Bourbon, both reported from the U.S. Midwest. A tick-borne relapsing fever agent, *Borrelia miyamotoi*, first described in Japan, has been found widely distributed in the United States and another bacterial spirochete, *Borrelia mayonii*, was discovered in the upper U.S. Midwest. Two tick-borne spotted fevers, *Rickettsiae*, *R. parkeri* and *Rickettsia species 364D*, and a tick-borne *Ehrlichia* (*E. muris eauclairensis*) were discovered to be pathogenic to humans.

The mosquito-borne viruses chikungunya and Zika were introduced to Puerto Rico in 2014 and 2015, respectively. Zika virus is emblematic of the dangers of emergence. Zika was one of a number of obscure, mosquito-borne viruses known to be pathogenic to humans that are rarely encountered or studied. In the 60 years following its discovery in a monkey in Uganda, it was seldom reported as a human pathogen. In 2016, more than 36,000 cases were reported in Puerto Rico; limited autochthonous, or local, transmission in Florida and Texas; and nearly 5,000 cases among travelers to the United States. The teratogenic consequences of the 2015–2017 epidemic in the region of the Americas were unexpected.

Vector-Borne Disease Key Findings

- A total of 642,602 cases of 16 diseases caused by bacteria, viruses, or parasites transmitted through the bites of mosquitoes, ticks, or fleas were reported to CDC during 2004–2016. Indications are that cases were substantially underreported.

- Tick-borne diseases more than doubled in 13 years and were 77 percent of all vector-borne disease reports. Lyme disease accounted for 82 percent of all tick-borne cases, but spotted fever rickettsioses, babesiosis, and anaplasmosis/ehrlichiosis cases also increased.

- Tick-borne disease cases predominated in the eastern continental United States and areas along the Pacific coast. Mosquito-borne dengue, chikungunya, and Zika viruses were almost exclusively transmitted in Puerto Rico, American Samoa, and the U.S. Virgin Islands, where they were periodically epidemic. West Nile virus, also occasionally epidemic, was widely distributed in the continental United States, where it is the major mosquito-borne disease.

- During 2004–2016, nine vector-borne human diseases were reported for the first time from the United States and U.S. territories. The discovery or introduction of novel vector-borne agents will be a continuing threat.
- Vector-borne diseases have been difficult to prevent and control. An FDA- approved vaccine is available only for the yellow fever virus. Many of the vector-borne diseases, including Lyme disease and West Nile virus, have animal reservoirs. Insecticide resistance is widespread and increasing.
- Preventing and responding to vector-borne disease outbreaks are high priorities for the CDC and will require additional capacity at state and local levels for tracking, diagnosing, and reporting cases; controlling vectors; and preventing transmission.

Section 21.3
Impact of Climate on Vector-Borne Diseases

This section includes text excerpted from "Vector-Borne Diseases," Centers for Disease Control and Prevention (CDC), 2016. Reviewed March 2020.

The seasonality, distribution, and prevalence of vector-borne diseases are influenced significantly by climate factors, primarily high and low-temperature extremes and precipitation patterns. Climate change can result in modified weather patterns and an increase in extreme events that can affect disease outbreaks by altering biological variables such as vector population size and density, vector survival rates, the relative abundance of disease-carrying animals (zoonotic reservoir hosts), and pathogen reproduction rates. Collectively, these changes may contribute to an increase in the risk of the pathogen being carried to humans.

Climate change is likely to have both short- and long-term effects on vector-borne disease transmission and infection patterns, affecting both seasonal risk and broad geographic changes in disease occurrence over decades. However, models for predicting the effects of climate change on vector-borne diseases are subject to a high degree of uncertainty, largely due to two factors: (1) vector-borne diseases are maintained in nature in complex transmission cycles that involve vectors, other intermediate zoonotic hosts, and humans; and (2) there are a number of other significant social and environmental drivers of vector-borne disease transmission in addition to climate change. For example, while climate variability and climate change both alter the transmission of vector-borne diseases, they will likely interact with many other factors, including how pathogens adapt and change, the availability of hosts, changing ecosystems and land use, demographics, human behavior, and adaptive capacity. These complex interactions make it difficult to predict the effects of climate change on vector-borne diseases.

The risk of introducing exotic pathogens and vectors not currently present in the United States, while likely to occur, is similarly difficult to project quantitatively. In recent years, several important vector-borne pathogens have been introduced or reintroduced into the United States. These include the West Nile virus, dengue virus, and chikungunya virus. In the case of the 2009 dengue outbreak in southern Florida, climate change was not responsible for the reintroduction of the virus in this area, which arrived via infected travelers from disease-endemic regions of the Caribbean. In fact, vector populations capable of transmitting dengue have been present for many years throughout much of the southern United States, including Florida. Climate change has the potential to increase human exposure risk or disease transmission following shifts in extended spring and summer seasons as dengue becomes more established in the United States. Climate change effects, however, are difficult to quantify due to the adaptive capacity of a population that may reduce exposure to vector-borne pathogens through such means as air conditioning, screens on windows, vector control, and public-health practices.

Section 21.4

Detection, Prevention, and Response to Pathogens Spread by Vectors

This section includes text excerpted from "About
the Division of Vector-Borne Diseases," Centers for
Disease Control and Prevention (CDC),
January 24, 2019.

Division of Vector-Borne Diseases

The Division of Vector-Borne Diseases (DVDB) is part of the Centers for
Disease Control and Prevention (CDC)'s National Center for Emerging
and Zoonotic Infectious Diseases (NCEZID). DVBD has four branches:

- **Arboviral Diseases Branch.** It focuses on viruses spread by
  mosquitoes and ticks. This branch is responsible for viruses like
  chikungunya, West Nile, yellow fever, and Zika. This branch also
  serves as the World Health Organization (WHO) Collaborating
  Centre for Arthropod-Borne Viruses Reference and Research.

- **Bacterial Diseases Branch.** Focuses on bacteria spread by ticks
  and fleas. This branch is responsible for bacteria such as Lyme
  disease, plague, and tularemia. This branch also serves as the WHO
  Collaborating Centre for Bacterial Vector-Borne Diseases.

- **Dengue Branch.** Focuses on the four dengue viruses spread by
  mosquitoes.

- **Rickettsial Zoonoses Branch.** Focuses on a special category of
  bacteria primarily spread by ticks, lice, and fleas. This branch is
  responsible for bacteria such as Q fever, Rocky Mountain spotted
  fever, and typhus fevers.

DVBD's Vision, Mission, and Goals

- **Vision.** To create a future where vector-borne diseases no longer threaten
  public health

- **Mission.** Reduce illness and death from vector-borne diseases
- **Goals:**
  - Identify and detect vector-borne pathogens that cause diseases in people.
  - Understand when, where, how often, and how people are exposed to vector-borne pathogens.
  - Prevent exposure to vector-borne pathogens and mitigate the consequences of infection.
  - Implement vector-borne disease diagnostics, surveillance, control, and prevention programs.

Addressing Vector-Borne Diseases Threats
A Coordinated Strategy for Vector-Borne Threats

In 2016, Congress provided the CDC with $350 million in supplemental funding to perform the critical work needed to prevent, detect, and respond to the public-health emergency posed by Zika virus. The funding is vital to protect areas at the highest risk of impact from Zika.

Building on that investment, a strong, sustained, national infrastructure for the vector-borne disease is needed. This infrastructure must advance innovation and discovery, and build comprehensive vector programs.

Steps Being Taken to Prepare the Nation

Currently, DVBD is working on several fronts to prepare the nation. As part of the CDC's strategy for securing global health and America's preparedness, Dr. Redfield, CDC Director, has made vector-borne threats a priority. The DVBD funds state, local, and territorial health departments, five centers for excellence in vector-borne diseases, and innovative research.

Advance Innovation and Discovery

As a nation, we need:
- Cutting-edge diagnostic tools for fast and accurate detection of vector-borne infections.

- Identification of new and emerging vector-borne diseases and increased understanding of the magnitude of existing vector-borne threats.
- Research and development by government, universities, and industry to develop ways to foster new vector-control technologies and monitor and prevent insecticide resistance.

Build Comprehensive Vector-Control Programs

To build local vector-control programs, we need:

- A skilled vector workforce that can respond to the full variety of pathogens and the vectors that transmit them.
- Robust state and local vector programs with expertise in laboratory, case and outbreak investigation, and vector control that can identify and mobilize for action against existing and emerging threats.

Responding to Threats

The DVBD responds to disease threats by providing technical assistance and by preparing public-health agencies for potential bioterrorism events.

Provide Technical Support

The DVBD provides technical assistance and disease investigation services to local, state, territorial, and international agencies making the request. Short-term assistance to United States and international agencies can improve understanding of an emerging disease and help prevent further spread of a vector-borne disease. For example, when a Zika virus outbreak hit the Pacific island of Yap, DVBD disease detectives studied the outbreak. This work provided valuable information needed when Zika came to the Western Hemisphere.

Prepare for Bioterrorism and Exotic Pathogens

Some bacteria and viruses can be used to deliberately cause harm or fear. Laboratory personnel play an important role in prevention and response to biological emergencies. Some pathogens of concern include anthrax, botulism, Ebola, plague, smallpox, *Coxiella burnetii* (Q fever), and tularemia. The DVBD experts research plague, Q fever, and tularemia to help protect Americans.

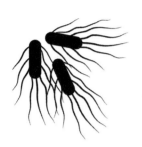

CHAPTER 22
Foodborne Disease and Outbreaks

Chapter Contents

Size and Extent of Foodborne Outbreaks

This section includes text excerpted from "Size and Extent of Foodborne Outbreaks," Centers for Disease Control and Prevention (CDC), March 24, 2015. Reviewed March 2020.

When two or more people get the same illness from the same contaminated food or drink, the event is called a "foodborne outbreak." Illnesses that are not part of outbreaks are called "sporadic." Public-health officials investigate outbreaks to control them, so more people do not get sick in the outbreak, and to learn how to prevent similar outbreaks from happening in the future.

The size and scope of a foodborne outbreak can vary based on which pathogen or toxin is involved, how much food is contaminated, where in the food production chain contamination occurs, where the food is served, and how many people eat it. For example:

- **Small, local outbreak** — A contaminated casserole served at a church supper may cause a small outbreak among church members who know each other.
- **Statewide or regional outbreak** — A contaminated batch of ground beef sold at several locations of a grocery-store chain may lead to illnesses in several counties or even in neighboring states.
- **Multistate outbreak** — Contaminated produce from one farm may be shipped to grocery stores nationwide and make hundreds of people sick in many states.

Section 22.2

Identifying Commercial Entities during Outbreak Investigations

This section includes text excerpted from "Identifying Commercial Entities during Outbreak Investigations," Centers for Disease Control and Prevention (CDC), March 24, 2015. Reviewed March 2020.

When investigating outbreaks of infectious disease, public-health investigators sometimes find that the way people get sick involves a commercial entity (e.g., a store or restaurant they patronized), an institution or company (e.g., a hotel or hospital they stayed at), or a particular product they bought.

The Centers for Disease Control and Prevention (CDC) has a long-standing practice of regularly disclosing names of commercial entities implicated in infectious-disease outbreaks in order to protect public health. These disclosures have helped the public reduce their health risks and have helped commercial entities improve the safety of their practices and products. As each situation is unique, it is important that the CDC programs evaluate whether to identify an implicated entity on a case-by-case basis, working in partnership with affected states and other partners.

Timing matters. Early in an ongoing investigation, releasing the name of a "suspected" source may interfere with the investigative process. Once a specific source is implicated in an infectious disease outbreak, the CDC routinely provides information during an ongoing investigation if there are actions that individuals can take to protect their health. When an outbreak is over and the investigation has been completed, the CDC usually provides specific information when there is conclusive evidence regarding the root cause of contamination.

Generally, the decision to disclose names of commercial entities should be made with the involved state or states. Long after the outbreak is controlled, in publications that add to the body of knowledge on public-health topics, the CDC typically refers to implicated entities anonymously (e.g., "Restaurant A" or "Supplier B") rather than by name, as the specific implications have little relevance for public health in the longer term. In some situations, federal law will dictate whether the CDC may disclose or must protect the identity of commercial entities, for example a requirement to protect commercial confidential information.

Section 22.3

Key Players in Foodborne Outbreak Response

This section includes text excerpted from "Key Players in Foodborne Outbreak Response," Centers for Disease Control and Prevention (CDC), August 5, 2019.

Local, State, and Federal Agencies

Public-health agencies that identify and investigate foodborne illnesses operate on several levels. Which agency or agencies participate in an investigation depends on the size and scope of the outbreak. Sometimes one agency starts an investigation and then calls on other agencies as more illnesses are reported across county or state lines.

- **Local agencies** — Most foodborne outbreaks are local events. Public-health officials in just one city or county health department investigate these outbreaks.
- **State agencies** — Typically, the state health department investigates outbreaks that spread across several cities or counties. This department often works with the state department of agriculture and with federal food safety agencies.

- **Federal agencies** — For outbreaks that involve large numbers of people or severe or unusual illness, a state may ask for help from the Centers for Disease Control and Prevention (CDC). The CDC usually leads investigations of widespread outbreaks — those that affect many states at once. States communicate regularly with one another and with the CDC about outbreaks and ongoing investigations. The CDC routinely collaborates with federal food-safety agencies, such as the U.S. Food and Drug Administration (FDA) or Food Safety and Inspection Service (FSIS), part of the U.S. Department of Agriculture (USDA), throughout all phases of an outbreak investigation. The FDA and FSIS, by law, oversee U.S. food safety and regulate the food industry with inspection and enforcement. In the case of an outbreak of foodborne illness, they work to find out why it occurred, take steps to control it, and look for ways to prevent future outbreaks. They may trace foods to their origins, test foods, assess food safety measures in restaurants and food-processing facilities, lead farm investigations, and announce food recalls.

Outbreak Investigation Teams

Outbreak investigative teams are usually made up of a variety of professionals, including:

- **Epidemiologists** — disease detectives
- **Microbiologists** — laboratory scientists who study germs
- **Environmental health specialists** (sometimes called "sanitarians") — inspectors who help restaurants serve safe food
- **Regulatory compliance officers and inspectors** — officials who make sure food safety laws are followed
- **Health communication specialists**

A team may add other professionals as the investigation proceeds.

Food Industry's Role

The food industry itself plays an important role in preventing and responding to outbreaks of foodborne illness.

Safety Standards and Inspections

Larger companies that produce, process, and package foods often have food safety managers on staff to identify and prevent problems. Some companies require their suppliers to meet specific food-safety standards. They may also inspect their suppliers or hire outside auditors to inspect them.

Outbreak Control Measures

Based on findings of an outbreak investigation, the food company involved often takes steps to help stop the outbreak and avoid a similar one in the future. Such measures include stopping processing, cleaning and disinfecting facilities and equipment, training or retraining employees, recalling food, and changing industry-wide practices.

Section 22.4

Investigating Outbreaks

This section includes text excerpted from "Steps in a Foodborne Outbreak Investigation," Centers for Disease Control and Prevention (CDC), June 21, 2018.

A foodborne outbreak investigation goes through several steps. They are described here in order, but in reality investigations are dynamic and several steps may happen at the same time.

Step 1: Detect a Possible Outbreak

Detecting an outbreak is the first step in investigating a multistate foodborne outbreak.

- An outbreak with multiple sick people can be missed if they are spread out over a wide area.

- Outbreaks are detected by using public-health surveillance methods, including PulseNet, formal reports of illnesses, and informal reports of illnesses.

Step 2: Define and Find Cases

Finding sick people is important to help public-health officials understand the size, timing, severity, and possible sources of an outbreak.

- A case definition is developed to define who will be included as part of an outbreak.
- Investigators use the case definition to search for illnesses related to the outbreak.
- Illnesses are plotted on an epidemic curve (epi curve) so that public-health officials can track when illnesses occur over time.

Step 3: Generate Hypotheses about Likely Sources

Hypothesis generation is an ongoing process.

- Possible explanations of an outbreak are continually changed or disproved as more information is gathered.
- Interviews, questionnaires, and home visits are helpful in narrowing down how and where people in the outbreak got sick.

Step 4: Test Hypotheses

A hypothesis is tested to determine if the outbreak source has been correctly identified.

- Investigators use many methods to test their hypotheses.
- Two main methods are analytic epidemiologic studies and food testing.

Step 5: Solve Point of Contamination and Source of the Food

Health officials use three types of data to link illnesses to contaminated foods and solve outbreaks: epidemiologic, traceback, and food and environmental testing.

- Health officials assess all of these types of data together to try to find the likely source of the outbreak.
- A contamination can happen anywhere along the chain of food production, processing, transportation, handling, and preparation.

Step 6: Control an Outbreak

Once the food source of an outbreak is determined, control measures must be taken.

- If contaminated food stays on store shelves, in restaurant kitchens, or in home pantries, more people may get sick.
- There are several different outbreak control measures that can be taken.
- Public-health officials choose measures based on the information available to them.
- Measures can change as the investigation goes on.

Step 7: Decide an Outbreak Is Over

An outbreak is over when the number of new illnesses drops back to what investigators normally expect.

- With continued public-health surveillance, if the number of illnesses rises again, the investigation continues or restarts.

Section 22.5

Public Communication during Foodborne Outbreaks

This section includes text excerpted from "Public Communication during Foodborne Outbreaks," Centers for Disease Control and Prevention (CDC), December 4, 2017.

Warning consumers quickly about contaminated food can save lives. Public health and regulatory officials work quickly to find the source of foodborne disease outbreaks so they can take action to prevent more people from getting sick.

During a foodborne outbreak investigation, officials collect three types of data: epidemiologic, traceback, and food and environmental test results. Health officials assess all of these data to try to find the likely source of the outbreak. They take action when there is clear and convincing information linking illness to contaminated food. One of the most important actions public-health officials can take to prevent illness is warning consumers quickly about contaminated food.

Deciding to Communicate

Multistate contaminated-food outbreak investigations are complex and involve many partners at local, state, and federal health and regulatory agencies. The Centers for Disease Control and Prevention (CDC) makes the decision to communicate about a multistate outbreak with input from all of these partners.

The CDC follows a consistent process for evaluating the need to warn consumers about ongoing multistate foodborne outbreaks. The process includes considering why communication might or might not be needed. Rather than designing a rigid set of communication rules or policies, the CDC and investigation partners developed a flexible and comprehensive guide on when, what, and how to communicate during an outbreak.

The CDC is most likely to warn consumers when the investigation identifies a specific food linked to illness, and there is a continuing risk to public health because the food is still in stores or homes. In this scenario, there are specific, clear, and actionable steps for consumers to take to protect themselves from contaminated food. The company also may have recalled the food in this scenario.

Some factors the CDC considers when deciding to warn consumers:

- Illnesses continue to be reported (an outbreak is ongoing)
- The data have identified a specific brand or type of food linked to illness
- The number of new illnesses is increasing rapidly
- Illnesses are unusually severe
- A specific group of people is at higher risk for illness

Informing the Public

If the decision is made to notify the public of an outbreak, the CDC posts a Web announcement. This announcement tells people what they can do to protect their health.

Web announcements typically include:

- How many people are sick in each state
- What contaminated food is linked to the outbreak
- Signs and symptoms of the illness
- Advice to consumers and retailers about foods to avoid eating or selling
- Other investigation details, including food-testing results, if available

The CDC posts Web updates during outbreak investigations to ensure the website reflects the most accurate and current information. Updates are posted on an as-needed basis, and the timing differs depending on the outbreak.

The CDC posts a final Web update once an investigation ends. The final Web update indicates to the public that the immediate risk of illness is over.

Outbreak Reports and Publications

Public-health officials do not solve every outbreak. Sometimes the outbreak ends before enough information is gathered to identify the likely source and warn the public. The source also may be identified after the outbreak ends and the risk to the public is over.

Even if an urgent warning is no longer needed, the CDC often writes outbreak reports after an investigation ends. These reports provide valuable information for people interested in food safety topics, such as the media, food-safety educators, and consumer advocacy groups, as well as for food industries and regulatory officials as they work to make our food safer.

Section 22.6

Surveillance and Reporting

This section includes text excerpted from "Surveillance and Reporting," Centers for Disease Control and Prevention (CDC), October 14, 2016. Reviewed March 2020.

The Centers for Disease Control and Prevention (CDC) has a long history of summarizing outbreak reports from local and state health departments.

State and local public-health authorities investigate all foodborne disease outbreaks. The CDC coordinates those that involve multiple states, since such outbreaks usually result from contaminated food that is widely distributed to many states. Data reported to the CDC for each outbreak include the number of illnesses, hospitalizations, and deaths; the pathogens, toxins, and chemical agents that caused illnesses; the implicated food; the settings of food preparation and consumption; and factors contributing to food contamination.

Foodborne disease-outbreak surveillance and reporting provides valuable insights into the agents and foods that cause illness and the settings where contamination occurs.

Knowing more about the foods, germs, and settings where outbreaks occur increases our understanding of its impact on human health and is the first step toward prevention.

Section 22.7

Partnerships That Help Early in Foodborne Outbreak Investigations

This section includes text excerpted from "Partnerships That Help Early in Foodborne Outbreak Investigations," Centers for Disease Control and Prevention (CDC), March 24, 2015. Reviewed March 2020.

Consultation with Food-Industry Representatives during Multistate Foodborne Outbreaks

Food-industry experts are important for many reasons, including their knowledge of food production practices, distribution patterns, consumer purchasing information, and other relevant information, such as product testing and supply-chain information.

Consultation with industry experts early in an outbreak investigation can provide important clues to help focus the investigation on the foods or food ingredients that may be making people sick. Insights from industry can increase the speed and ensure greater accuracy of the investigation.

Knowing How Food Is Produced and Distributed Can Help Solve Foodborne Outbreaks

The U.S. food marketplace has millions of different foods and food products. When exposure to contaminated food is suspected as the source of an outbreak, public-health investigators must consider the large number of foods that may be making people sick.

Even when the list of foods is narrowed to only those that ill people ate, or remember eating, before they got sick, it still may not point the investigators to the specific food making people sick.

Information about how food is produced and distributed can help investigators narrow the list of suspected contaminated foods and food ingredients.

Why Partnering Helps

Consultation with the food industry early in the investigation of a foodborne-disease outbreak can help reduce the amount of time needed to form an accurate picture of what is causing the outbreak and implement control measures, such as a food recall.

Goal of Partnership

This consultation process is aimed at using current industry information to speed up the investigation and make it more effective, all with a goal of keeping people from getting sick.

Who Participates

Participants include:

- Federal government public-health and regulatory officials
- Food industry subject-matter experts
- Other experts, such as people from industry associations or academia, who may provide information needed

How the Process Works

Not every investigation requires the use of this process. If a decision is made to use the process, one or more telephone calls with consultants would be held over the course of an investigation. Typically, the process happens early in an outbreak investigation, when the list of possible contaminated foods has been narrowed to two or three.

How the Process Was Created

This process was created from a series of meetings through the Collaborative Food Safety Forum (CFSF) hosted by the Pew Charitable Trusts and the Robert Wood Johnson Foundation (RWJF), and involving the Centers for Disease Control and Prevention (CDC), U.S. Food and Drug Administration (FDA), U.S. Department of Agriculture's (USDA) Food Safety and Inspection Service (FSIS), and industry and consumer groups.

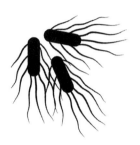

CHAPTER 23
Detecting and Tracking Waterborne Disease and Outbreaks

Chapter Contents

Section 23.1

Importance of Waterborne Disease Outbreak Surveillance

This section includes text excerpted from "Importance of Outbreak Investigations," Centers for Disease Control and Prevention (CDC), April 25, 2019.

Importance of Outbreak Investigations

Outbreak investigations help learn more about the causes of outbreaks. Officials can learn what germs are causing waterborne illness, what types of water are involved, and what groups of people become ill. This knowledge can be used to control an outbreak and prevent additional illnesses. The lessons learned from these investigations are routinely used to develop recommendations on how to prevent similar outbreaks from happening in the future.

Determining the type of water causing an illness may seem straightforward, but it is more complicated than you might think. People rarely know whether contaminated water made them ill, and it can be difficult or impossible to figure out. Many of the germs that are spread by water can also be spread in other ways, including by eating contaminated food or by contact with an ill person or animal. People come in contact with water often each day, making it even harder to know which exposure might have made a person sick. Finally, it can take several days or even weeks to become ill after being exposed to a germ, making it difficult to pinpoint the place and time of exposure. Without an outbreak investigation, it can be difficult or impossible to link illnesses to water.

When a group of people become ill at the same time, an investigation that collects information on timing and location of exposures and illnesses (known as an "epidemiologic investigation") can help determine where and when the outbreak started and what caused it. An outbreak investigation can sometimes identify a direct link between the illnesses and contaminated water and might identify the type of water, systems, or settings involved. This information is difficult to gather outside of an outbreak (such as with individual infections).

Learning from Outbreaks

When a group of people becomes ill at the same time, local or state health departments may:

- Investigate to understand what caused the outbreak
- Take steps to control the outbreak and prevent additional illnesses
- Learn how to prevent similar outbreaks from happening in the future

Following an investigation, health departments report outbreak summary data to the Centers for Disease Control and Prevention (CDC). The information includes the number of outbreak-associated illnesses, hospitalizations, and deaths; agents; and implicated types of water, water systems, and water settings.

CDC disease detectives (epidemiologists) review the reported outbreak data and follow up with health departments to verify it and to gather more information as needed. CDC researchers analyze the reported outbreak data periodically and summarize outbreak characteristics and trends in waterborne disease-outbreak surveillance reports.

Public-health agencies, policy makers, and the public can access waterborne disease-outbreak surveillance reports and use the findings to guide health communication, policy, and prevention efforts to reduce the future spread and occurrence of waterborne disease.

Section 23.2

Outbreak Investigation: Role of Public-Health Departments

This section includes text excerpted from "Waterborne Disease and Outbreak Surveillance," Centers for Disease Control and Prevention (CDC), April 25, 2019.

Investigating and Reporting

Investigating Outbreaks

Public-health officials investigate outbreaks to control them and prevent additional illnesses and to learn how to prevent similar outbreaks from happening in the future. Anyone who suspects an outbreak occurrence should contact their local or state health department.

The public-health community works to detect, investigate, control, and prevent future waterborne disease outbreaks. The 8 steps in an outbreak investigation are:

- DETECT a possible outbreak
- DEFINE and FIND cases
- GENERATE hypotheses
- TEST hypotheses using epidemiology, clinical data, and environmental investigation
- IDENTIFY source of outbreak
- CONTROL outbreak through remediation and outreach
- DECIDE outbreak is over
- PREVENT future outbreaks through summarizing, interpreting, and reporting findings

Several steps may happen at the same time in an outbreak investigation. Once a waterborne disease outbreak investigation ends, public-health departments report outbreaks to the CDC's Waterborne Disease and Outbreak Surveillance System (WBDOSS) using a standard reporting form.

Reporting Outbreaks

Waterborne disease outbreaks became nationally notifiable in the United States in 2009. Public-health agencies in all 50 states, the District of Columbia, U.S. territories, and Freely Associated States have primary responsibility for identifying and investigating waterborne outbreaks and reporting outbreaks voluntarily to CDC. From 1971 to 2008, outbreaks were reported using a paper form. Since 2009, outbreaks have been reported electronically through the CDC's National Outbreak Reporting System (NORS). WBDOSS collects data reported to NORS on waterborne disease and outbreaks associated with recreational water, drinking water, and other nonrecreational water exposures.

Detecting and Investigating Waterborne Diseases and Outbreaks

By collecting data on the types of water, water systems, settings, and agents (what spreads the disease) that are linked to waterborne illness, the CDC's Waterborne Disease and Outbreak Surveillance System (WBDOSS) improves the understanding of waterborne illnesses to better guide future prevention efforts.

Although we generally enjoy safe and healthy drinking and recreational water in the United States, waterborne diseases still pose a threat to our health and productivity. We interact with water in many ways during our day-to-day activities. Drinking and household, recreation and leisure, industry, agricultural, and medical uses are just a few examples of our daily interactions with water.

Water contaminated with germs, chemicals, or toxins can lead to waterborne illness if you drink it, breathe it in, or it touches your skin, eyes, ears, or other mucous membranes. A waterborne disease outbreak occurs when two or more people get the same illness from the same contaminated water. Public-health officials have been tracking waterborne disease in the United States for more than 100 years, and the CDC has been overseeing waterborne disease and outbreak tracking since 1971.

Tracking Disease

Surveillance is the term for tracking illness and injury. Surveillance data help guide efforts to reduce and prevent future outbreaks. Waterborne disease surveillance data have supported national efforts to develop drinking water regulations and have provided guidance for recreational water activities, such as the CDC's Healthy Swimming program.

The national Waterborne Disease and Outbreak Surveillance System (WBDOSS) collects data on waterborne disease and outbreaks associated with recreational water, drinking water, and environmental and undetermined exposures to water. The system collects data on the number of outbreak-associated illnesses, hospitalizations, and deaths; agents; implicated types of water; water systems; and water settings. WBDOSS also collects information on single cases of waterborne illness caused by certain types of chemicals or germs.

Role of Public-Health Departments

The Centers for Disease Control and Prevention (CDC) has a long history of working with state, local, territorial, and tribal public-health departments to investigate waterborne disease cases and outbreaks. The size and scope of the outbreak and the capacity of the health department to complete the investigation determines which public-health departments participate in an investigation. Sometimes one department starts an investigation and then calls on others for assistance as more illnesses are reported across county or state lines.

Public-health departments collect information on potential outbreaks to protect people from becoming ill.

- **Local health department role.** Most waterborne outbreaks are local events, rarely occurring on a national scale. Public-health officials in just one city or county health department investigate most waterborne outbreaks.
- **State health department role.** Typically, a state health department investigates outbreaks that spread across several cities or counties.

The state health department may also assist the local health department in conducting an investigation.

- **The Centers for Disease Control and Prevention (CDC)'s role.** A state might ask for help from the CDC to investigate outbreaks that involve a large number of people, have novel or unknown transmission routes, or involve unusual illness. The CDC helps investigate only after the state health department invites it to participate. States communicate regularly with one another and with the CDC about outbreaks and ongoing investigations.

Section 23.3

Waterborne Disease and Outbreak Surveillance System

This section includes text excerpted from "Interpreting Waterborne Disease Outbreak Data," Centers for Disease Control and Prevention (CDC), April 25, 2019.

Detecting waterborne disease outbreaks is challenging because many waterborne pathogens can also be spread in other ways (such as through food, person-to-person, or animal-to-person). Linking illness to drinking water is difficult during investigations because most people drink water every day. Recreational water (such as lakes and swimming pools) is often not considered as the source of infection, particularly when illness occurs days after the exposure or the exposure occurs while traveling.

Environmental investigations provide information on factors and deficiencies that contribute to outbreaks and strengthen evidence implicating drinking or recreational water as a common source of infection. However, these investigations might not be conducted if the evidence does not implicate water.

Outbreak-Investigation Capacity and Reporting Activities Vary across States and Localities

For state and local public-health agencies to recognize, investigate, and report outbreaks, public-health agencies must have the necessary financial and personnel resources. They must recognize and link cases of illness to a common contaminated water source, which requires appropriate epidemiologic, environmental, and laboratory capacity to conduct investigations. This surveillance, investigation, and reporting capacity varies across states and localities. Therefore, it is challenging to interpret reported geographic differences in the occurrence and types of waterborne disease outbreaks.

Public-Health Practices Have Changed Over Time

Practices related to outbreak investigation and reporting have changed over time, and these changes make certain germs more or less likely to be detected during outbreak investigations.

For example, new diagnostic tests can increase clinicians' awareness of certain diseases, leading to increased reporting and outbreak detection for these diseases.

Improved laboratory methods for detecting germs and microbial indicators of contamination may also mean that certain diseases are detected more often.

Generally, outbreak reporting may increase when more is known about how waterborne diseases are spread and as the ability to track and test increases. On the other hand, as local jurisdictions develop the capacity to identify illness clusters by molecular subtyping, they might investigate fewer clusters with unknown causes (for example, cases of illness without a laboratory-confirmed germ diagnosis), which could lead to a decrease in waterborne disease-outbreak reporting because most cases of illness are not laboratory confirmed.

Changes in public-health practice do not affect the validity of the data in surveillance reports but might limit the ability to interpret trends in the number of outbreaks and types of problems with water systems across reporting periods.

Information from Laboratory Investigations Is Often Unavailable, Incomplete, or Inconsistent

Analyses of water or environmental samples for specific germs and indicators of water quality depend on the availability of certified or approved laboratories. Although many laboratories are certified to conduct standard environmental-sample analyses for fecal indicators and chemicals, few laboratories have the capability to identify waterborne germs in environmental samples. In addition, the tests needed to do these analyses can be expensive. Waterborne contaminants are usually very dilute, so collecting water samples to identify germs often requires sampling large quantities of water or filtering large volumes of water through special membranes. Environmental samples also traditionally contain many other contaminants that decrease the ability to detect germs compared to common diagnostic samples, such as blood, stool, and urine.

Water samples are often collected late in an investigation or not collected at all, which limits the ability to link clinical and environmental data. Molecular epidemiologic or other laboratory testing that identifies a direct match or link between the germs in patient specimens and those in environmental water samples can establish a water-related exposure. Even with improved water sampling and pathogen testing, water samples collected during an outbreak investigation might not contain the germs that were present when people were exposed. Negative water sample tests do not rule out water as the source of the outbreak.

PART 5 · HOW TO PROTECT YOURSELF AND YOUR FAMILY FROM DISEASES AND ILLNESSES TRANSMITTED TO HUMANS BY ANIMALS, INSECTS, AND CONTAMINATED WATER

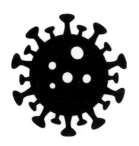

CHAPTER 24
Protect Yourself and Your Family from Zoonotic Diseases

Chapter Contents

How to Stay Healthy around Pets

This section contains text excerpted from the following sources: Text beginning with the heading "Tips to Stay Healthy around Pets" is excerpted from "Pets and Other Animals—Cats," Centers for Disease Control and Prevention (CDC), April 1, 2019; Text beginning with the heading "Safely Clean Up after Your Dog" is excerpted from "Pets and Other Animals—Dogs," Centers for Disease Control and Prevention (CDC), February 21, 2020; Text under the heading "Prevent Ferret Scratches and Bites" is excerpted from "Pets and Other Animals—Ferrets," Centers for Disease Control and Prevention (CDC), April 8, 2019.

Tips to Stay Healthy around Pets

Before buying or adopting a pet, make sure your pet is the right type of pet for your family. Pets can sometimes carry germs that can make people sick, even when they appear clean and healthy. Visit your veterinarian for routine care to keep your pet healthy and to prevent infectious diseases.

Wash Your Hands

- Wash your hands with soap and running water:
  - After handling pets, their food and water dishes, or their supplies
  - After contact with your pet's saliva or poop
  - After cleaning a litter box
  - After gardening, especially if outdoor cats or dogs live in the area
  - Before you eat or drink
- Adults should supervise handwashing for children under 5 years of age.
- Use hand sanitizer if soap and water are not readily available.
- Wear gloves while gardening, particularly if you know that outdoor cats live in the area.

Safely Clean Up after Your Cat

In the case of pet cats:

- To stay healthy, take precautions when cleaning your cat's litter boxes.
- Change litter boxes daily.
- Always wash your hands after cleaning the litter box, even if you use a scoop to remove the poop.
- People with weakened immune systems and pregnant women should not clean litter boxes if possible, as they are more at risk for complications from germs spread by cats. If no one else can perform the task, wear disposable gloves and wash your hands afterward.
- Keep your cat's litter box away from other animals, children, and food-preparation areas.

Prevent Cat Scratches and Bites

Cat bites and scratches can spread germs, even if the wound does not seem deep or serious. For example, cat-scratch disease can happen if a scratch only breaks the surface of the skin. Data on exactly how many people are bitten or scratched by cats each year is unknown because incidents often are not reported. However, it is known that about 20 to 80 percent of reported cat bites and scratches become infected.

How to Prevent Cat Bites and Scratches

- Be cautious with unfamiliar animals. Approach cats with care, even if they seem friendly.
- Avoid rough play with cats and kittens. Rough play causes cats to be defensive toward people.
- Avoid rough play when animals are young. This will lead to fewer scratches and bites as animals become older. Studies have shown cats generally bite when provoked.
- Trim your cat's nails regularly. If you need help, ask your veterinarian.
- Parents should tell children to let them know if they are ever bitten or scratched by any animal, including cats.

What to Do If You Are Bitten or Scratched by a Cat

If you are bitten or scratched by a cat, you should:

- Wash wounds with warm soapy water immediately.
- Seek medical attention if:
  - You do not know if the cat has been vaccinated against rabies
  - The cat appears sick
  - The wound is serious
  - The wound becomes red, painful, warm, or swollen
  - It has been more than five years since your last tetanus shot
- Report the bite to animal control or your local health department if the bite is unprovoked and
  - The cat is a stray, or
  - You are unsure if the cat has been vaccinated against rabies
- Because of the risk of rabies, ensure that the cat is seen by a veterinarian and contact your local health department if it becomes sick or dies shortly after the bite.

Safety Clean Up after Your Dog

Cleaning up after your dog helps to keep the environment clean and reduces the risk of diseases spreading to people and other animals.

- Always pick up dog poop and dispose of it properly.
- Dog poop should be picked up, even in your own yard, and especially in areas where children may play.

Prevent Dog Scratches and Bites

Dog bites can cause pain and injury, but they can also spread germs that cause infection. Nearly 1 in 5 people bitten by a dog requires medical attention. Any dog can bite, especially when scared, nervous, eating, or when playing or protecting toys or puppies. Dogs may also bite when they are not feeling well and want to be left alone. Any dog can bite, but most dog bites are preventable, and there are many things you can do at home and within your community to help prevent them. Practicing the safe handling tips below can help you avoid dog bites.

Know the Risks

Children are more likely than adults to be bitten by a dog, and when they are, the injuries can be more severe. Most dog bites affecting young children occur during everyday activities and while interacting with familiar dogs. Having a dog in the household is linked to a higher likelihood of being bitten than not having a dog. As the number of dogs in the home increases, so does the likelihood of being bitten. Adults with two or more dogs in the household are five times more likely to be bitten than those living without dogs at home. Among adults, men are more likely than women to be bitten by a dog.

How to Prevent Dog Bites and Scratches

- Always ask if it is ok to pet someone else's dog before reaching out to pet it even if the dog appears friendly.
- Let the new dog approach you first.
- When a new dog approaches you, remain still to allow the dog to feel comfortable.
- Always make sure a dog has seen you and sniffed you before you reach out to pet it.
- Do not approach an unfamiliar dog, even if it seems friendly or healthy. Call animal control if you see a dog in trouble or a dog running loose.
- Do not let young children play with dogs without supervision, even if the child has met the dog before or if the dog is your family pet.
- Responsible pet ownership, including socializing your dog and using a leash in public, which can help prevent dog bites.
- Do not disturb a dog while it is eating, sleeping, or caring for puppies.
- Do not pet a dog if it appears to be hiding or needing time alone.
- Do not continue petting a dog if it seems scared, sick, or angry.
- If a dog knocks you over, curl into a ball with your head tucked and your hands over your ears and neck. You can also put a purse, bag, or jacket between you and the dog.
- Do not encourage your dog to play aggressively or roughhouse.
- Do not panic or make loud noises, and never run from a dog.
- Do not try to break up dog fights.

If an unfamiliar dog approaches you, stay still and be calm, and avoid direct eye contact with the dog. Say "no" or "go home" in a firm, deep voice and stand with the side of your body facing the dog. Slowly raise your hands to your neck with your elbows in and wait for the dog to pass or slowly back away.

What to Do If You Are Bitten or Scratched by a Dog

Germs can be spread from dog bites and scratches, even if the wound does not seem deep or serious.
- For minor wounds:
  - Wash the wound thoroughly with soap and water.
  - Apply an antibiotic cream.
  - Cover the wound with a clean bandage.
- For deep wounds:
  - Apply pressure with a clean, dry cloth to stop the bleeding. Then seek medical attention.
  - If you cannot stop the bleeding or you feel faint or weak, call 911 or your local emergency medical services immediately.

See a healthcare provider if:
- The wound is serious or deep (uncontrolled bleeding, extreme pain, loss of function)
- The wound becomes red, painful, or swollen, or if you develop a fever
- If you do not know if the dog has been vaccinated against rabies
- If it has been more than 5 years since your last tetanus shot and the bite is deep
- Let the healthcare provider know that you were bitten by a dog. The healthcare provider may consult with your state or local health department to help you decide if you need rabies postexposure prophylaxis (PEP) treatment.

Report the Bite

Because anyone who is bitten by a dog is at risk of getting rabies, consider contacting your local animal-control agency or police department to report the incident, especially:

- If you do not know if the dog has been vaccinated against rabies
- If the dog appears sick or is acting strangely
- If possible, contact the owner and ensure the animal has a current rabies vaccination. You will need the rabies vaccine license number, the name of the veterinarian who administered the vaccine, and the owner's name, address, and phone number.

Prevent Ferret Scratches and Bites

Germs can spread from ferret bites and scratches, even if the wound does not seem deep or serious. Ferret bites can become seriously infected or spread rabies, especially if the ferret is unvaccinated and has had contact with a rabid animal. Young children are especially at risk for bites from ferrets.

How to Prevent Ferret Bites and Scratches

- Avoid bites and scratches from ferrets. Ferret bites can become seriously infected or spread rabies, especially if the ferret is unvaccinated.
- Be cautious with unfamiliar animals. Approach ferrets with care, even if they seem friendly.
- Do not play roughly with ferrets, especially when they are young. This will lead to fewer scratches and bites as animals become older.
- Always supervise children around ferrets.

What to Do If You Are Bitten or Scratched by a Ferret

Many types of germs can be spread from animal bites and scratches, even if the wound does not look very bad. Unvaccinated ferrets are at risk for rabies and can spread rabies to you if they become infected.

If you are bitten or scratched by a ferret, you should:

- Wash the wound with warm, soapy water immediately.

- Seek medical attention if:
  - You are unsure if the ferret has been vaccinated against rabies
  - The ferret appears sick or is acting unusual
  - The wound or injury is serious (uncontrolled bleeding, unable to move, extreme pain, muscle or bone is showing, or the bite is over a joint)
  - The wound or site of injury becomes red, painful, warm, or swollen (especially if the person bitten is 5 years of age or younger, elderly, pregnant, or has a weak immune system)
  - It has been more than 5 years since your last tetanus shot
- If you were bitten by a ferret you do not know, report the bite to animal control or your local health department.
- If possible, contact the owner and ensure the animal has a current rabies vaccination. You will need the rabies license number, name of the veterinarian who administered the vaccine, and the owner's name, address, and phone number.
- Make sure a veterinarian sees the ferret and contact your local health department if the ferret becomes sick or dies shortly after you were bitten.

Section 24.2

How to Stay Healthy around Farm Animals

This section includes text excerpted from "Farm Animals," Centers for Disease Control and Prevention (CDC), February 19, 2020.

Health Tips to Follow When around Farm Animals

Before interacting with farm animals, be aware that they can sometimes carry germs that can make people sick.

Wash Your Hands

- Wash your hands with soap and running water:
  - After contact with farm animals
  - After contact with animal saliva, birthing tissue or fluid, or other body fluids
  - After contact with animal products (for example, milk and eggs)
  - After cleaning up animal stalls or feces (poop)
  - After handling animal food, supplies, bowls, or equipment
  - After touching items such as fences, buckets, or other equipment used on the farm
- Adults should supervise handwashing for children under 5 years of age.
- Washing hands with soap and water is the best way to get rid of germs in most situations. If soap and water are not readily available, you can use an alcohol-based hand sanitizer that contains at least 60 percent alcohol.

Protect Yourself While Caring for Farm Animals

Be aware that animals can still spread germs even if they look healthy and clean.

- If you keep or work with farm animals:
  - Always wear protective equipment such as masks, gloves, and boots when cleaning animal stalls, assisting an animal in giving birth, or doing any activities that would involve touching bodily fluids from animals.
  - Have dedicated shoes and gloves that you only use when working with your animals. Keep and store these items outside of your home.
- If you visit another farm, be sure to scrub your shoes and change your clothes before interacting with their animals and before coming back to your animals.
- Cover open wounds or cuts when visiting or working around farm animals.

Prevent Bites and Kicks

Germs can spread from bites and scratches, even if the wound does not seem deep or serious.

- Be cautious when around farm animals. Always be aware of your surroundings and know where animals and escape routes are at all times.
- Do not stand directly behind a farm animal or approach a farm animal from the rear, even when the animal stands in stocks or is restrained.
- Supervise children around farm animals so the child does not get injured.
- Teach children about safety around farm animals, including keeping fingers away from the mouth and not approaching an animal from behind.

What to Do If You Are Bitten, or Scratched by a Farm Animal

Bites and scratches can become infected, even if the wound does not seem deep or serious. Being kicked by an animal can result in serious injury. If kicked by an animal, move away from the animal as quickly as possible and seek medical attention, especially if you were kicked in the head.

To prevent infection from bites and scratches:

- Wash wounds with soap and warm water immediately.
- Seek medical attention if:
  - The animal appears sick or is acting unusual
  - The wound or injury is serious (uncontrolled bleeding, unable to move, extreme pain, muscle or bone is showing, or the bite is over a joint)
  - The wound or site of injury becomes red, painful, warm, or swollen
  - It has been more than 5 years since your last tetanus shot

Stay Healthy at Petting Zoos and Animal Exhibits

- Wash your hands thoroughly with soap and water immediately after touching farm animals or anything in the area where they live and roam.
  - Avoid touching your mouth before washing your hands.
  - Adults should supervise handwashing for young children.
  - Use hand sanitizer if soap and water are not readily available.
  - Wash hands after removing clothes and shoes.
- Supervise children when they are around farm animals:
  - Prevent hand-to-mouth activities, such as nail-biting, finger sucking, and eating dirt.
  - Help children wash hands well with soap after interaction with any farm animal.
  - Do not let children stand behind animals, grab their tails, or put their fingers near an animal's mouth. This can lead to serious injury if the animal bites, scratches, or kicks.
- Do not let children five years of age or younger handle or touch chicks, ducklings, or live poultry.
- Do not bring baby or children's items (for example, toys, pacifiers, spill-proof cups, baby bottles, strollers) into animal areas.
- Do not eat food or drink beverages in animal areas or where animals are allowed to roam.

Section 24.3

How to Stay Healthy around Pet Fish

This section includes text excerpted from "Fish,"
Centers for Disease Control and Prevention (CDC),
October 1, 2015. Reviewed March 2020.

Healthy Habits
Handwashing Recommendations

The Centers for Disease Control and Prevention (CDC) recommends washing your hands before and after you work with aquariums or handle fish.

- Always wash your hands thoroughly with soap and running water before and after handling or cleaning aquariums and feeding fish. Be sure to help children wash their hands properly. Thoroughly washing your hands will reduce your risk of getting sick from a disease spread to you by your fish.

- To protect your fish, rinse your hands extremely well to reduce any soap residue after you wash your hands.
  - Adults should supervise handwashing for young children.
  - Use hand sanitizer if soap and water are not readily available. Be sure to have hand sanitizer readily available near the aquarium to encourage guests and children to practice good hand hygiene after feeding fish or touching the aquarium.

- Do not let children younger than five years old handle or touch aquariums or aquarium water or feed fish without supervision. Children younger than five years old are more likely to get sick from exposure to germs like *Salmonella*.

Tips for Preventing the Spread of Diseases from Fish and Aquariums

Before Choosing a Fish

- Find out what types of fish and aquariums are suitable for your family. Certain types of fish require more extensive care and supplies than others.
- Learn about the different types of aquariums and their maintenance needs. Work with pet-store staff to decide if a fresh or saltwater tank is right for you.
- Match the size of the tank to the space available in your home and to the amount of time you have to maintain it. Consider purchasing a second aquarium to be used when you are cleaning your first tank, or to house new fish before you place them in your established tank. Having a second tank to temporarily house fish may help reduce their stress and disease.
- Once you have decided what type of aquarium you want, learn how to set it up properly. Consider the following:
  - Tank size
  - Gravel type
  - Plants
  - Water temperature
  - Lighting (UV, etc.)
  - Aquarium filters and pumps
  - Methods to treat the water (chemically, etc.)
  - Frequency of tank cleaning and maintenance
  - Equipment and accessories
- Ask your veterinarian about the proper setup of your aquarium, the types of fish you should keep, as well as the food, care, and environmental requirements of your fish.
- Before you bring your fish home, make sure your aquarium is ready. Ask your veterinarian about "cycling a tank" to get the bacteria and nitrogen levels balanced.

Choosing Aquarium Fish

- Learn which fish can go in the aquarium you have. Most fish live exclusively in either saltwater or freshwater, not both. Consider the number of fish to keep in your tank; a good standard is 1 inch of fish per gallon of water. Also, evaluate which species of fish can be in the same tank together and what types of food they will need.

- Some types of fish, like male betta fish, cannot be in the same aquarium together because they will fight. However, having multiple female betta fish in the same aquarium is not a problem.
- Pick fish that are active in their tanks in the pet store. Compare the fish to those of the same type around it. Is it acting like the others or is it off by itself? Is it able to swim normally?
- Do not select fish from a tank that has a high number of dead fish.
- Healthy fish should have smooth, sleek, shiny scales that are free from discoloration. Their bodies should not have any bumps, and their fins should be intact.
- When bringing a new fish home, it is very important to acclimate it to your aquarium water. Purchased fish will often be given to you in a clear bag with water from their tank at the store. This water will be at a different temperature than your aquarium water at home. To acclimate your fish:
  - Place the entire bag, still intact, in your aquarium to float at the surface for about 30 minutes to an hour to acclimate the fish to the temperature of the tank.
  - Then, carefully open and gradually pour the bag to release the fish into your tank.
    - Do not remove the fish from the bag with a small net as this may injure the fish.
    - Try not to pour too much water from the bag into your aquarium at home because of the possible germs it may contain.

Cleaning and Maintaining Your Aquarium
- Be aware that fish and their aquariums may carry germs.
  - Wash your hands before and after cleaning or maintaining the aquarium or aquarium water. Plan to wear gloves when working with rough rocks or spiny fish to avoid injury.
- If you have any cuts or wounds on your hands, wear gloves or wait until your wounds are fully healed before working with your fish or aquarium water to avoid possible infection.

- Avoid cleaning fish aquariums in areas where people with weak immune systems may be affected.
- Do not allow children younger than five years of age or people with weak immune systems to clean aquariums.
- Do not use kitchen sinks to dump aquarium water into or to wash aquariums. If you use a bathtub to dump aquarium water into or to wash aquariums, clean the tub thoroughly afterward, and use a commercial disinfectant like bleach according to the manufacturer's instructions. Do not mix bleach with other cleaners, especially ammonia.

Monitor Your Pet's Health

- Monitor your fish daily for signs of illness. Symptoms may include abnormal swimming; appearance of red, brown, or white splotches; lack of appetite; or swelling.
- If a fish in your tank ever looks sick, it is best to remove it and place it in a tank by itself. This will help prevent other fish in your main aquarium from getting sick.
- Getting a diagnosis from a veterinarian experienced in fish medicine.
- Promptly remove any dead fish from your aquarium to decrease the risk of spreading disease to your other fish.
- Even though fish appear healthy, they may still spread germs to humans. If you become sick shortly after purchasing new fish or cleaning your aquarium, make sure to tell your healthcare provider that you have a pet fish.

What to Do If You No Longer Want Your Pet Fish

- Do not release your pet outdoors. Most fish released into ponds or rivers will die, and some grow to become a threat to natural wildlife populations.
- Find a new home for your pet:
  - Contact a nearby pet store for advice or for possible returns.
  - Consider giving your pet to another fish hobbyist.
  - Contact a local aquarium, school, or zoo to see if they would accept your pet.
  - Talk to your veterinarian. They may be able to help you find a new home for your pet.

Fish-Fin Scratches

Some larger fish have sharp points in their fins that could scratch or damage your skin when you are cleaning or working in the tank. This is an unusual occurrence, but germs can spread from fin scratches or scrapes from the gravel or rocks in the tank, even when the wound does not seem deep or serious.

Some fish are dangerous and even venomous and may not be safe to keep. Just because you can buy a fish does not mean that it is safe or legal to own. Some fish, like lionfish and some types of catfish, have venoms they can release to protect themselves. Most fish do not have teeth that can cause damage to skin, but some, like piranhas, have very sharp teeth that can cause serious harm.

- If you are scratched or bitten by a fish, you should:
  - Wash your wounds with soap and water immediately.
- Seek medical attention:
  - If the wound becomes red, painful, warm, or swollen, or
  - If the wound is serious (uncontrolled bleeding, loss of function, extreme pain, or there is muscle or bone exposure)
- If you seek medical attention, make sure to tell your healthcare provider you have had contact with fish and aquariums.

Section 24.4

Tips for Preventing the Spread of Diseases from Backyard Poultry and Waterfowl

This section includes text excerpted from "Backyard Poultry," Centers for Disease Control and Prevention (CDC), December 13, 2018.

Recommendations for Keeping Live Poultry

- Always wash your hands thoroughly with soap and water:
  - After handling poultry
  - After handling poultry food and water dishes or other equipment
  - After cleaning poultry coops, or anything in enclosures such as perches or other equipment
  - After being in areas near poultry, even if you did not touch the birds
  - Before you eat, drink, or smoke
- Adults should supervise handwashing for children under 5 years of age.
- Use hand sanitizer if soap and water are not readily available. Be sure to have an alcohol-based hand sanitizer that contains at least 60 percent alcohol near the poultry enclosure to encourage guests and children to clean their hands after handling poultry.
- Do not let children younger than 5 years of age handle or touch chicks, ducklings, or other live poultry without supervision. Children younger than 5 years of age are more likely to get sick from exposure to germs like *Salmonella*.
  - Do not give live baby chicks and ducklings to young children as gifts or Easter presents. Because their immune systems are still developing, children are more likely to get sick from germs commonly associated with live baby poultry, such as *Salmonella, Campylobacter,* and *E. coli.*
  - Make sure that your children and anyone who is visiting your home follow these rules as well.

- Do not let live poultry inside the house, in bathrooms, or especially in areas where food or drink is prepared, served, or stored, such as kitchens or outdoor patios.
- Do not eat or drink in the area where the live poultry live or roam.
- Do not snuggle, kiss, or touch your mouth to live baby poultry.
- Set aside a pair of shoes to wear while taking care of poultry and keep those shoes outside of the house.
- Stay outdoors when cleaning any equipment or materials—such as cages, feeds, or water containers—used to raise or care for live poultry.

Safe Egg Handling

- Always wash your hands with soap and water after handling eggs, chickens, or anything in their environment.
- Collect eggs often. Eggs that spend a significant amount of time in the nest can become dirty or break. Cracked eggs should be thrown away because bacteria on the shell can more easily enter the egg through a cracked shell.
- Refrigerate eggs after collection both to maintain freshness and to slow bacterial growth.
- Eggs with dirt and debris can be cleaned with fine sandpaper, a brush, or cloth. Do not wash warm, fresh eggs because colder water can pull bacteria into the egg.
- Cook eggs until both the yolk and white are firm. Egg dishes should be cooked to an internal temperature of 160°F (71°C) or hotter. Raw and undercooked eggs may contain *Salmonella* bacteria that can make you sick.

Bird Bites and Scratches

Backyard poultry and waterfowl do not have teeth, but their bills and beaks can still cause a lot of damage if they bite you. Germs can spread from poultry bites or pecking and scratches, even when the wound does not seem deep or serious.

- Avoid bites and scratches from your backyard poultry or waterfowl. This will prevent injury and reduce the risk of your poultry spreading germs to you.

- If you are bitten or scratched by poultry, you should:
  - Wash wounds thoroughly with soap and water immediately—hand sanitizer is not as effective at removing germs as washing your hands with soap and water
  - Seek medical attention and tell your doctor you were bitten or scratched by a bird, especially if:
    - The poultry appears sick
    - The wound is serious (uncontrolled bleeding, loss of function, extreme pain, or deep wound with the muscle or bone exposed)
    - The wound becomes red, painful, warm, or swollen
    - It has been more than 5 years since your last tetanus shot

Section 24.5

Protect Yourself from Wildlife

This section includes text excerpted from "Wildlife,"
Centers for Disease Control and Prevention (CDC),
October 22, 2018.

Wildlife should always be enjoyed from a distance. If you are close enough that the animal changes its behavior (for example, stops eating or runs away), you are too close! Wild animals can carry diseases despite not appearing to be sick at all, so staying away is the safest way to enjoy viewing wildlife. Follow these simple tips to help protect your family and pets from getting diseases from wildlife.

Protect Your Home

- Keep windows and doors closed or screened and cover any holes or openings to prevent bats, rodents, or other wild animals from entering your home, church, school, or other buildings.

- Clean up trash around your home and keep your garbage cans closed. Garbage and trash can attract unwanted visits from wildlife.
- Do not leave food (bait) outside to attract animals to your backyard. This brings the animals closer together and close to you, and this makes it easier for a disease to spread.
- Keep compost and woodpiles at least 100 feet away from buildings to help reduce rodent infestations in the building.
- Make sure pets do not have access to stagnant water sources (ponds, birdbaths, etc.) that are also used by wildlife.

Do Not Handle Wildlife

- Teach children to never handle unfamiliar animals, wild or domestic, even if they appear friendly or harmless.
- Do not touch or pick up dead animals with your bare hands. Consider calling animal control to remove any dead animals.
- Never adopt wild animals or bring them into your home. Do not try to save or rescue wild animals.
- If an animal appears sick or hurt, call animal control to help. Do not touch young animals that appear to be abandoned. Often their parents are close by waiting for you to leave before they return to their young.
- Protect wildlife in your national parks and local recreational areas by staying on trails and following visitor guidelines, including those for trash disposal.

Protect Yourself from Disease

- Make washing your hands a routine practice before eating or drinking and whenever you return from outside.
- Take care of bites and scratches:
  - Wash wounds well with soap and running water.
  - Contact your healthcare provider right away.
  - If you seek medical attention, make sure to tell them if you have had exposure to wildlife

- Keep bugs away:
  - Use a mosquito and tick repellent when spending time outdoors.
  - Use a monthly flea and tick preventive on your pets.
- Ask your veterinarian about how to protect your pets from wildlife diseases such as rabies, leptospirosis, and *Giardia*.
- Call animal control right away if an animal, wild or domestic, is acting strangely or out of character.

CHAPTER 25
Protecting Yourself from Disease Vectors

Chapter Contents

Mosquito Control: An Integrated Approach

This section includes text excerpted from "Success in Mosquito Control: An Integrated Approach," U.S. Environmental Protection Agency (EPA), October 11, 2016. Reviewed March 2020.

Controlling Mosquitoes Effectively Requires a Comprehensive Approach That Has Been Scientifically Tested and Proven

The Centers for Disease Control and Prevention (CDC) and U.S. Environmental Protection Agency (EPA) collaborate on mosquito-control activities throughout the United States to control diseases. By looking at biological information about the life and reproduction of the mosquito and epidemiological information about disease, the two organizations have developed a methodology on how best to control mosquitoes. Both the CDC and the EPA are helping Puerto Rico apply this methodology to develop a successful, sustainable program and approach to controlling mosquitoes that transmit Zika, dengue, chikungunya, and other diseases.

Successful mosquito management requires intervening at some point during the mosquito's life cycle before they bite and infect a human.

The best approach to controlling mosquitoes takes advantage of every life stage of a mosquito to achieve control, using a unified approach to integrated pest management (IPM).

Integrated Pest Management

The EPA and the CDC encourage all communities and mosquito-control districts, including those in territories such as Puerto Rico, to strictly adhere to integrated pest management (IPM). The IPM is a science-based, commonsense approach for managing pests and vectors, such as mosquitoes. The IPM uses a variety of pest-management techniques that focus on pest prevention, pest reduction, and the elimination of conditions that lead to pest infestations. The IPM programs also rely heavily on resident education and pest monitoring.

A successful IPM strategy can use pesticides. The IPM uses a combination of ways to control mosquito populations with decisions based on surveillance, such as keeping track or count of the numbers and types of mosquitoes in an area. Surveillance is a critical component to any successful IPM program because the results from the surveillance will help determine the appropriate response to an infestation. Extensive infestations, or those where the disease is present, merit a different response than will lower levels of infestations.

Both the CDC and the EPA recognize a legitimate and compelling need for the use of chemical interventions, under certain circumstances, to control adult mosquitoes. This is especially true during periods of mosquito-borne disease transmission or when source reduction and larval control have failed or are not feasible. Puerto Rico has been actively working to control mosquitoes that transmit Zika (and dengue and chikungunya) for some time; however, mosquito populations are increasing and additional methods are needed to control the mosquitoes during their adult stage.

A successful integrated mosquito-control strategy includes several tactics to eliminate mosquitoes and their habitat. Four critical tactics include:

- Remove mosquito habitats
- Use structural barriers
- Control mosquitoes at the larval stage
- Control adult mosquitoes

Remove Mosquito Habitats

An important part of mosquito control around homes is making sure that mosquitoes do not have a place to lay their eggs. Because mosquitoes need water for two stages of their life cycle, it is important to monitor standing-water sources.

- Get rid of standing water in rain gutters, old tires, buckets, plastic covers, toys, or any other container where mosquitoes can breed.
- The CDC provides a large amount of funding to purchase tire shredders for Puerto Rico. This is important because used or waste tires can collect standing water that attracts mosquitoes and leads to increased mosquito breeding.
- Empty and change the water in birdbaths, fountains, wading pools, rain barrels, and potted-plant trays at least once a week to eliminate potential mosquito habitats.
- Drain temporary pools of water or fill with dirt.
- Keep swimming-pool water treated and circulating.

Use Structural Barriers

Because *Aedes* mosquitoes frequently bite indoors, using structural barriers is an important way to reduce the incidence of bites. Examples of structural barriers include:

- Install window and door screens if they are not already in place.
- Cover all gaps in walls, doors, and windows to prevent mosquitoes from entering.
- Make sure window and door screens are "bug tight."
- Completely cover baby carriers and beds with netting. Nets can be especially important for protecting a sick person from getting more mosquito bites, which could transmit the disease to other people.

Control Mosquitoes at the Larval Stage

The greatest impact on mosquito populations will occur when they are concentrated, immobile, and accessible. This emphasis focuses on habitat management and controlling the immature stages (egg, larva, and pupa) before the mosquitoes emerge as adults. This approach maximizes the effectiveness of pesticide application and minimizes the use of widespread pesticide application. Larvicides target larvae in the breeding habitat before they can mature into adult mosquitoes and disperse. Larvicide treatment of breeding habitats helps reduce the adult mosquito population in nearby areas.

Egg and larva interventions are generally the most effective and least costly, way to control mosquitoes. However, these interventions are unlikely to be 100 percent effective, especially for mosquitoes such as the *Aedes aegypti* that breed in varied and scattered locations. In these cases, eliminating or treating all or even most standing water can be nearly impossible. Successful control efforts will need to supplement habitat removal with other means of control.

There are a number of EPA-registered active ingredients used in larvicides. Choosing which larvicide to use in a given area is best done by experts and will depend on a variety of factors, including potential human or environmental risk, cost, resistance, and ease of use.

Control Adult Mosquitoes

Using EPA-registered pesticide is one of the fastest and best options to combat an outbreak of mosquito-borne disease being transmitted by adult mosquitoes. The pesticides registered for this use are known as "adulticides." Adulticides are applied either using aerial applications by aircraft or on the ground by truck-mounted sprayers.

Aerial-spraying techniques can treat large areas with only small amounts of pesticide and have been used safely for more than 50 years. These aerial sprays are fully evaluated by the EPA and do not pose risks to people or the environment when used according to the directions on the label.

Mosquito adulticides are applied as ultra-low-volume (ULV) sprays. ULV sprayers dispense extremely small droplets. The naled insecticide, for example, uses 80 microns or less, which means hundreds of thousands of droplets could fit inside something as small as one pea. When released from an airplane, these tiny droplets are intended to stay airborne as long as possible and drift through an area above the ground, killing the mosquitoes in the air on contact. The small droplet size makes the pesticide more effective, which means less pesticide is used to better protect people and the environment.

Section 25.2

Tips for Preventing Mosquito Bites

This section includes text excerpted from "Prevent Mosquito Bites," Centers for Disease Control and Prevention (CDC), April 22, 2019.

Prevent Mosquito Bites

The most effective way to avoid getting sick from viruses spread by mosquitoes when at home and during travel is to prevent mosquito bites.

Mosquito bites can be more than just annoying and itchy. They can spread viruses that make you sick or, in rare cases, cause death. Although most kinds of mosquitoes are just nuisance mosquitoes, some kinds of mosquitoes in the United States and around the world spread viruses that can cause disease.

Mosquitoes bite during the day and night, live indoors and outdoors, and search for warm places as temperatures begin to drop. Some will hibernate in enclosed spaces, such as garages, sheds, and under (or inside) homes, to survive cold temperatures. Except for the southernmost states in North America, mosquito season starts in the summer and continues into fall.

Prevention

- **Use insect repellent:** Use EPA-registered insect repellent with one of the following active ingredients:
  - DEET
  - Picaridin
  - IR3535
  - Oil of lemon eucalyptus (OLE)
  - Para-menthane-diol (PMD)
  - 2-undecanone
- **Cover up:** Wear long-sleeved shirts and long pants.

- **Keep mosquitoes outside:** Use air conditioning, or window and door screens. If you are not able to protect yourself from mosquitoes inside your home or hotel, sleep under a mosquito bed net.

Planning a Trip

- Make a checklist of everything you will need for an enjoyable vacation and use the following resources to help you prepare.
- Learn about destination-specific health risks and recommendations.
- Pack a travel health kit. Remember to pack insect repellent and use it as directed to prevent mosquito bites.
- See a healthcare provider familiar with travel medicine, ideally four to six weeks before your trip.

Before Traveling

For most viruses spread by mosquitoes, there are no vaccines or medicines available. However, vaccines are available for viruses such as Japanese encephalitis and yellow fever. Travelers to areas with risk of those viruses should get vaccinated.

After Traveling

- Even if they do not feel sick, travelers should prevent mosquito bites for three weeks after their trip so they do not spread viruses such as dengue, Zika, or chikungunya to uninfected mosquitoes.
- If you have been traveling and have symptoms including fever, headache, muscle and joint pain, and rash, see your healthcare provider immediately and be sure to share your travel history.

Section 25.3

Using Insect Repellents Safely and Effectively

This section includes text excerpted from "Insect Repellents Help Prevent Malaria and Other Diseases Spread by Mosquitoes," Centers for Disease Control and Prevention (CDC), June 25, 2019.

Insect Repellents Help Prevent Malaria and Other Diseases Spread by Mosquitoes

Every year, millions of U.S. residents travel to countries where malaria and other diseases spread by mosquitoes are found. These diseases can cause serious illness and death in some cases. Preventing mosquito-borne infections is very important to staying well when you travel.

Why Do You Need to Use an Insect Repellent When You Travel to an Area with Malaria?

An insect repellent will help protect you from mosquitoes that spread malaria and other diseases, such as dengue, chikungunya, and yellow fever. You can use insect repellent on your skin and clothes to keep away insects. Your doctor may also prescribe a medication to prevent malaria (antimalarial drug). Although antimalarial drugs are very effective, they are not 100 percent effective in preventing malaria. This is why you need to also use an insect repellent and take other steps to keep mosquitoes from biting you (mosquito avoidance). In some areas where only a few cases of malaria occur, the Centers for Disease Control and Prevention (CDC) recommends mosquito avoidance as the only way to prevent malaria.

Are Insect Repellents Safe?

Most insect repellents that can be put on the skin must be registered by the U.S. Environmental Protection Agency (EPA) before they can be sold in stores. EPA registration means the insect repellent has been tested and approved for human safety and is effective when used according to directions on the label. Before you buy an insect repellent, be sure to look on the label for EPA approval.

Which Insect Repellents Will Give You Long-Lasting Protection against Mosquitoes?

For hours of long-lasting protection, look for insect repellents with the following active ingredients:
- DEET
- IR3535
- Oil of lemon eucalyptus (OLE)*
- Picaridin (KBR 3023)

Some brand names of repellents include:
- **DEET products:** Off!, Cutter, Sawyer, Ultrathon
- **IR3535 products:** Skin So Soft Bug Guard Plus Expedition, SkinSmart
- **OLE products:** Repel, Off! Botanicals
- **Picaridin products** (Autan, Bayrepel and icaridin outside the United States): Cutter Advanced, Skin So Soft Bug Guard Plus

"Pure" oil of lemon eucalyptus (essential oil) is not recommended. It has not been tested by the EPA for safety and effectiveness.

Are Insect Repellents Safe?

Most insect repellents that can be put on the skin must be registered by the EPA before they can be sold in stores.

EPA registration means the insect repellent has been tested and approved for human safety and is effective when used according to directions on the label. Before you buy an insect repellent, be sure to check on the label for EPA approval.

How Do You Use an Insect Repellent?
- Always follow directions on the label.

- Spray or rub the insect repellent onto your skin that is not covered by your clothes. Do not use under clothing.
- Use just enough insect repellent to cover your skin not covered by clothing. Heavy use of insect repellent or pouring it all over your body is not necessary.
- Never use insect repellents over cuts, wounds, or irritated skin.
- Do not spray insect repellents directly on your face—spray it onto your hands first and then pat the insect repellent onto your face.
- Do not spray or put insect repellents on your eyes or mouth, and put only a little around your ears.
- Use separate sunscreen and insect-repellent products. Put the sunscreen on first, then spray on the insect repellent.
- After returning indoors, wash the insect-repellent off your skin with soap and water or take a bath. This is especially important when you use insect repellents daily.
- Wash any clothes you treated with insect repellent before wearing them again.

Can You Use an Insect Repellent If You Are Pregnant or Breastfeeding?

Yes. Pregnant and breastfeeding women can use EPA-approved insect repellents. Always follow directions on the label.

Can You Put Insect Repellent on Your baby?

- Do not put insect repellent on babies younger than 2 months of age.
- Protect small babies under the age of 2 months by placing a fitted mosquito net around their infant seat or carrier.

How Do You Put Insect Repellent on a Child?

- Follow directions on the label.
- Use no more than 30 percent DEET on a child.
- Do not use insect repellent with lemon eucalyptus on children under the age of three years.

What Other Things Can You Do to Prevent Mosquito Bites?

- Wear a long-sleeved shirt, long pants, and a hat when you are outdoors.
- Spray insect repellent on your clothes for extra protection or buy a product with permethrin to treat your clothes and bed net to repel insects.
- Sleep in a well-screened or air-conditioned room, or sleep under a permethrin-treated bed net. This is because malaria mosquitoes mostly bite at night (dusk until dawn). Stay indoors during the times biting mosquitoes are most active.

What Should You Do If You Develop a Rash or Reaction to the Insect Repellent?

- Stop using insect repellent and wash the area with soap and water.
- If you see a doctor about the reaction, take the repellent container with you. You can also call the Poison Help Hotline at 800-222-1222.

Can You Put Insect Repellent on Your Baby?

- Do not put insect repellent on babies younger than 2 months of age.
- Protect small babies under the age of 2 months by placing a fitted mosquito net around their infant seat or carrier.

Section 25.4
Avoiding Tick Bites

This section includes text excerpted from
"Avoiding Ticks," Centers for Disease Control and
Prevention (CDC), January 10, 2019.

Preventing Tick Bites

Tick exposure can occur year-round, but ticks are most active during warmer months (April to September).

Before You Go Outdoors

- Know where to expect ticks.
- Treat clothing and gear with products containing 0.5 percent permethrin.
- Use the U.S. Environmental Protection Agency (EPA)-registered insect repellents containing DEET, picaridin, IR3535, Oil of Lemon Eucalyptus (OLE), para-menthane-diol (PMD), or 2-undecanone.
- Avoid contact with ticks.

After You Come Indoors

Check your clothing for ticks. Ticks may be carried into the house on clothing. Any ticks that are found should be removed. Tumble dry clothes in a dryer on high heat for 10 minutes to kill ticks on dry clothing after you come indoors. If the clothes are damp, additional time may be needed. If the clothes require washing first, hot water is recommended. Cold and medium temperature water will not kill ticks.

- Examine gear and pets.
- Shower soon after being outdoors.
- Check your body for ticks after being outdoors. Check these parts of your body and your child's body for ticks:
  - Under the arms
  - In and around the ears

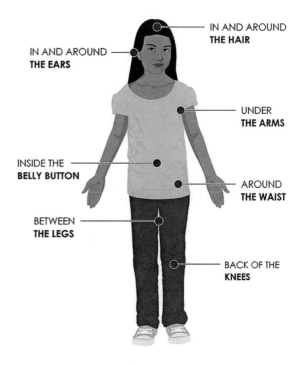

Figure 25.1. Tick Checkpoints

- Inside belly button
- Back of the knees
- In and around the hair
- Between the legs
- Around the waist

Preventing Ticks on Your Pets

Dogs are very susceptible to tick bites and tick-borne diseases. Vaccines are not available for most of the tick-borne diseases that dogs can get, and they do not keep the dogs from bringing ticks into your home. For these reasons, it is important to use a tick-preventive product on your dog.

Tick bites on dogs may be hard to detect. Signs of tick-borne disease may not appear for 7 to 21 days or longer after a tick bite, so watch your

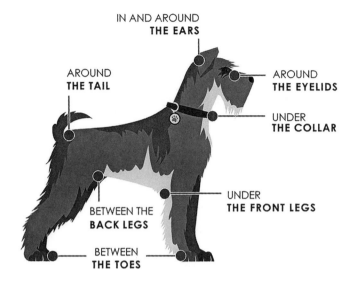

IN AND AROUND
THE EARS

AROUND
THE TAIL

AROUND
THE EYELIDS

UNDER
THE COLLAR

UNDER
THE FRONT LEGS

BETWEEN THE
BACK LEGS

BETWEEN
THE TOES

Figure 25.2. Tick Checkpoint for Pets

dog closely for changes in behavior or appetite if you suspect that your pet has been bitten by a tick.

Talk to your veterinarian about:

- The best tick-prevention products for your dog
- Tick-borne diseases in your area

To further reduce the chances that a tick bite will make your dog sick:

- Check your pets for ticks daily, especially after they spend time outdoors
- If you find a tick on your pet, remove it right away
- Reduce tick habitat in your yard

Preventing Ticks in the Yard
Apply Pesticides Outdoors to Control Ticks

Use of pesticides can reduce the number of ticks in treated areas of your yard. However, you should not rely on spraying to reduce your risk of infection.

When using pesticides, always follow label instructions. Before spraying, check with local health or agricultural officials about:
- The best time to apply pesticide in your area
- The best type of pesticide to use
- Rules and regulations regarding pesticide application on residential properties

Create a Tick-Safe Zone to Reduce Blacklegged Ticks in the Yard

Here are some simple landscaping techniques that can help reduce blacklegged tick populations:
- Remove leaf litter.
- Clear tall grasses and brush around homes and at the edge of lawns.
- Place a three-foot-wide barrier of wood chips or gravel between lawns and wooded areas to restrict tick migration into recreational areas.
- Mow the lawn frequently.
- Stack wood neatly and in a dry area (discourages rodents).
- Keep playground equipment, decks, and patios away from yard edges and trees.
- Discourage unwelcome animals (such as deer, raccoons, and stray dogs) from entering your yard by constructing fences.
- Remove from the yard old furniture, mattresses, or trash that may give ticks a place to hide.

Section 25.5

What to Do after a Tick Bite

This section includes text excerpted from "Tick
Bite: What to Do," Centers for Disease Control and
Prevention (CDC), August 29, 2019.

Tick Bite: What to Do

Ticks bites can make people sick. Here are some steps that you can take
after a tick bite to reduce your chances of getting sick and information on
how to get treatment promptly if you do get sick.

Remove the Tick as Soon as Possible

1. Use fine-tipped tweezers to grasp the tick as close to the skin as you can.
2. Pull upward with steady, even pressure. Do not twist or jerk the tick.
3. After removing the tick, clean the bite area and your hands with rubbing
   alcohol or soap and water.
4. Dispose of the tick by flushing it down the toilet. If you would like to
   bring the tick to your healthcare provider for identification, put it in
   rubbing alcohol or place it in a sealed bag/container.

Consider Calling Your Healthcare Provider

In general, the Centers for Disease Control and Prevention (CDC) does not
recommend taking antibiotics after tick bites to prevent tick-borne diseases.
However, in certain circumstances, a single dose of doxycycline after a
tick bite may lower your risk of Lyme disease. Consider talking to your
healthcare provider if you live in an area where Lyme disease is common.

Watch for Symptoms for 30 days

Call your healthcare provider if you get any of the following:
- Rash
- Fever

- Fatigue
- Headache
- Muscle pain
- Joint swelling and pain

Treatment for tick-borne diseases should be based on symptoms, history of exposure to ticks, and in some cases, blood-test results. Most tick-borne diseases can be treated with a short course of antibiotics.

Common Questions after a Tick Bite
Should You Get the Tick Tested for Germs?

Some companies offer to test ticks for specific germs. The CDC strongly discourages using results from these tests when deciding whether to use antibiotics after a tick bite.

- Results may not be reliable. Laboratories that test ticks are not required to meet the same quality standards as laboratories used by clinics or hospitals for patient care.
- Positive results can be misleading. Even if a tick contains a germ, it does not mean that you have been infected by that germ.
- Negative results can also be misleading. You might have been bitten unknowingly by a different infected tick.

Can You Get Sick from a Tick That Is Crawling on You, but Has Not Yet Attached?

Ticks must bite you to spread their germs. Once they attach to you, they will feed on your blood and can spread germs. A tick that is crawling on you, but is not attached could not have spread germs. However, if you have found a tick crawling on you, it is a sign there may be others, so do a careful tick check.

How Long Does a Tick Need to Be Attached before It Can Spread Infection?

Depending on the type of tick and germ, a tick needs to be attached to you for different amounts of time (minutes to days) to infect you with that germ.

Your risk for Lyme disease is very low if a tick has been attached for fewer than 36 hours. Check for ticks daily and remove them as soon as possible.

Section 25.6

Preventive Methods and Pesticides

This section includes text excerpted from "Pesticides and Public Health," U.S. Environmental Protection Agency (EPA), December 13, 2017.

Pesticides and Public Health

This section focuses on public-health problems caused by pests and the role that preventive measures and pesticides may play in protecting people from these health problems.

Why be concerned: Pests such as insects, rodents, and microbes can cause and spread a variety of diseases that pose a serious risk to public health.

Public-Health Issues and Pests

Debilitating and deadly diseases that can be caused or spread by pests such as insects, rodents, and microbes pose a serious risk to public health. Examples of significant public-health problems that are caused by pests include:

- **Vector-borne diseases** — Infectious diseases such as West Nile virus, Lyme disease, and rabies can be carried and spread by vector (disease-carrying) species such as mosquitoes, ticks, and rodents. The U.S. Environmental Protection Agency (EPA) registers several pesticide products, including repellents, that may be used to control the vectors that spread these diseases.
- **Asthma and allergies** — Indoor household pests such as cockroaches can contribute to asthma and allergies. In addition to registering

products to control these pests, the EPA provides information to the public about safely using these products in homes and schools.

- **Microbial contamination** — Various microorganisms, including bacteria, viruses, and protozoans, can cause microbial contamination in hospitals, public-health clinics, and food-processing facilities. The EPA registers antimicrobial products intended to control these microorganisms and help prevent the spread of numerous diseases.

- **Avian flu** — Avian flu, sometimes called "bird flu," is an infection that occurs naturally and chiefly in birds. Infections with these viruses can occur in humans, but the risk is generally low for most people. The EPA works to register and make available antimicrobial pesticide products (sanitizers or disinfectants) that may be used on inanimate surfaces to kill avian influenza virus and to help prevent the spread of avian flu viruses. These products are typically used by the poultry industry to disinfect their facilities.

- **Prions** — Certain proteins found in cells of the central nervous system of humans and animals may exist in abnormal, infectious forms called "prions." Prions share many characteristics of viruses, and may cause fatal diseases. In 2004, the EPA determined that prions are considered to be a pest under the Federal Insecticide, Fungicide, and Rodenticide Act (FIFRA) and that products used to control prions are subject to EPA regulation.

- **Anthrax** — Biological agents such as *Bacillus anthracis* spores can cause a threat to public health and national security. The EPA has issued emergency exemptions for several pesticides that were used in anthrax spore-decontamination efforts, including (but not limited to) bleach, chlorine dioxide, ethylene oxide, hydrogen peroxide and peroxyacetic acid, methyl bromide, paraformaldehyde, and vaporized hydrogen peroxide.

Safely Control Pests and Protect Your Health

The EPA, along with the Centers for Disease Control and Prevention (CDC) and many pest-control professionals, believes that prevention is the most effective way to control disease-carrying pests and their associated public-health risks. The combination of preventive measures and reduced-risk treatment methods to reduce reliance on, and therefore, corresponding risk from, the use of chemical pesticides is generally known as "integrated pest management" (IPM).

Prevent Pests

Pests such as cockroaches, rodents, and mosquitoes need food, water, and shelter. Often, problems involving these pests can be solved just by removing a few key items. Some actions you can take to reduce or prevent pest problems include:

- Making sure food and food scraps are tightly sealed and garbage is regularly removed from the home
- Not leaving pet food and water out overnight. Also, if you apply pesticides, pet food and water should be removed from the area.
- Fixing leaky plumbing and looking for other sources of water, such as trays under house plants
- Eliminating standing water in rain gutters, buckets, plastic covers, birdbaths, fountains, wading pools, potted-plant trays, or any other containers where mosquitoes can breed
- Keeping swimming-pool water treated and circulating, and draining temporary pools of water or filling them with dirt
- Closing off entryways and hiding places (e.g., caulking cracks and crevices around cabinets or baseboards)
- Making sure window and door screens are "bug tight"
- Replacing your outdoor lights with yellow "bug" lights, which tend to attract fewer mosquitoes than ordinary lights. However, the yellow lights are not repellents.

Safely Use Pesticide Products

In addition to preventive measures, traps, bait stations, and other pesticide products (including repellents) can be used to control some pests. These can be used with low risk of exposure to the pesticide, as long as they are kept out of the reach of children and pets and used according to label directions.

Pesticides with public-health uses are intended to limit the potential for disease, but in order to be effective, they must be properly applied. By their nature, many pesticides may pose some risk to humans, animals, or the environment because they are designed to kill or otherwise adversely affect living organisms. Safely using pesticides depends on using the appropriate pesticide and using it correctly.

The pesticide label is essential to using a pesticide safely and effectively. It contains important information that must be read and followed when using a pesticide product.

Tips for Hiring a Pest-Control Professional

If you have a pest issue that you are uncomfortable dealing with yourself, you may wish to hire a pest-control professional.

- Choose a pest-control company carefully. Firms offering pest-control services must be licensed by your state.
- The EPA's *Citizen's Guide to Pest Control and Pesticide Safety*, available for download at https://www.epa.gov/sites/production/files/2017-08/documents/citizens_guide_to_pest_control_and_pesticide_safety.pdf, offers more tips on how to choose a pest-control company.

Regulation of Pesticides with Public-Health Uses

The EPA is responsible under the FIFRA and the Food Quality Protection Act (FQPA) for regulating pesticides with public-health uses, as well as ensuring that these products do not pose unintended or unreasonable risks to humans, animals, and the environment.

- **Registration**—Through registration, the EPA evaluates pesticides to ensure that they can be used effectively without posing unreasonable risks to human health and the environment.
- **Reregistration**—Under reregistration and tolerance reassessment, the EPA reviewed older pesticides (those registered before November 1984) to ensure that they meet current scientific and regulatory standards and completed this reregistration in 2008.
- **Registration review**—Through registration review, the EPA plans to review all registered pesticides approximately every 15 years to ensure that they meet current scientific and regulatory standards.

- **Emergency exemptions and special local needs** — In cases where unexpected public-health issues arise, the EPA works to make pesticides available to states or federal agencies for emergency and special local-need uses.

Although pesticides with public-health use follow the same regulatory process as agricultural chemicals, the EPA recognizes that there may be some differences, including:

- **Exposure** — Pesticide use as part of a public-health program may lead to increased exposure for large segments of the population, including exposure to a sensitive subpopulation. The EPA carefully evaluates human and ecological risks from exposure to pesticides, including bystander and occupational exposure. The EPA places special emphasis on children's health in making regulatory decisions about all pesticides, including pesticides with public-health uses.
- **Efficacy** — The EPA requires scientific evidence that registered products sold to control pests that are known to carry West Nile virus, Lyme disease, and other vector-borne public-health threats are effective against the target pest.
- **Benefits** — The EPA considers the benefits from public-health pesticides when making regulatory decisions. The CDC is an important source of benefits information for public-health pesticides and the EPA and CDC entered into an agreement in 2000 to formalize this relationship.

CHAPTER 26

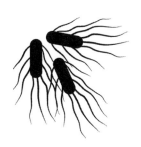

How to Protect Yourself and Your Family from Foodborne Illnesses and Diseases

Chapter Contents

Food Safety at Home

This section includes text excerpted from "Food Safety at Home," U.S. Food and Drug Administration (FDA), May 29, 2019.

Four Basic Steps for Food Safety

Each year millions of people get sick from food illnesses which can cause you to feel like you have the flu. Food illnesses can also cause serious health problems, even death. Follow these four steps to help keep you and your family safe.

Clean

Always wash your food, hands, counters, and cooking tools.

- Wash hands in warm soapy water for at least 20 seconds. Do this before and after touching food.
- Wash your cutting boards, dishes, forks, spoons, knives, and countertops with hot soapy water. Do this after working with each food item.
- Rinse fruits and veggies.
- Clean the lids on canned goods before opening.

Separate (Keep Apart)

Keep raw foods to themselves. Germs can spread from one food to another.

- Keep raw meat, poultry, seafood, and eggs away from other foods. Do this in your shopping cart, bags, and fridge.
- Do not reuse marinades used on raw foods unless you bring them to a boil first.
- Use a special cutting board or plate for raw foods only.

Cook

Foods need to get hot and stay hot. Heat kills germs.

- Cook to safe temperatures:
  - Beef, pork, lamb 145°F
  - Fish 145°F
  - Ground beef, pork, lamb 160°F
  - Turkey, chicken, duck 165°F
- Use a food thermometer to make sure that food is done. You cannot always tell by looking.

Chill

Put food in the fridge right away.

- 2-Hour Rule. Put foods in the fridge or freezer within 2 hours after cooking or buying from the store. Do this within 1 hour if it is 90 degrees or hotter outside.
- Never thaw food by simply taking it out of the fridge. Thaw food:
  - In the fridge
  - Under cold water
  - In the microwave
- Marinate foods in the fridge.

Think You Have a Food Illness?

Call your doctor and get medical care right away.

- Save the food package, can, or carton. Then report the problem.
- Call the U.S. Department of Agriculture (USDA) at 888-674-6854 if you think the illness was caused by meat, poultry, or eggs.
- Call the U.S. Food and Drug Administration (FDA) at 866-300-4374 for all other foods.
- Call your local health department if you think you got sick from food you ate in a restaurant or from an other food seller.

Who Is at Risk?

Anyone can get sick from eating spoiled food. Some people are more likely to get sick from food illnesses.

- Pregnant women
- Older adults
- People with certain health conditions, such as cancer, human immunodeficiency virus (HIV)/acquired immunodeficiency syndrome (AIDS), diabetes, and kidney disease

Some foods are more risky for these people. Talk to your doctor or other health provider about which foods are safe for you to eat.

Section 26.2
Food Safety in the Kitchen

This section includes text excerpted from "Food Safety in the Kitchen," Centers for Disease Control and Prevention (CDC), February 6, 2020.

Use these tools and tips to help prevent food poisoning every time you prepare food in the kitchen. Your kitchen is filled with food safety tools that, when used properly, can help keep you and your loved ones healthy. Learn how to make the most of these tools so that your kitchen is your home's food-safety headquarters.

Kitchen Sink
- Handwashing is one of the most important things you can do to prevent food poisoning. Wash your hands for 20 seconds with soap and running water. Scrub the backs of your hands, between your fingers, and under your nails.
- Wash fruits and vegetables before peeling. Germs can spread from the outside to the inside of fresh produce as you cut or peel.
- Do not wash raw meat, poultry, or eggs. Washing these foods can actually spread germs because juices may splash onto your sink or counters.

Cutting Board and Utensils

- Use separate cutting boards, plates, and knives for produce and for raw meat, poultry, seafood, and eggs.
- Clean with hot, soapy water or in dishwasher (if dishwasher-safe) after each use.

Thermometer

Use a food thermometer to make sure food cooked in the oven or on the stove top or grill reaches a temperature hot enough to kill germs.

Safe Minimum Cooking Temperatures

- All poultry, including ground: 165°F
- Ground beef, pork, lamb, and veal: 160°F
- Beef, pork, lamb, and veal chops, roasts, and steaks: 145°F (let rest 3 minutes before serving)
- Fish: 145°F

Microwave

- Know your microwave's wattage. Check inside the door, owner's manual, or manufacturer's website. Lower wattage means longer cooking time.
- Follow recommended cooking and standing times, to allow for additional cooking after microwaving stops. Letting food sit for a few minutes after microwaving allows cold spots to absorb heat from hotter areas and cook more completely.
- When reheating, use a food thermometer to make sure that microwaved food reaches 165°F.

Refrigerator

- Keep your refrigerator between 40°F and 32°F, and your freezer at 0°F or below.
- Refrigerate fruits, vegetables, milk, eggs, and meats within 2 hours. (Refrigerate within 1 hour if the temperature outside is above 90°F.)

- Divide warm foods into several clean, shallow containers so they will chill faster.
- Store raw meat on the bottom shelf away from fresh produce and ready-to-eat food.
- Throw out foods left unrefrigerated for over 2 hours.
- Thaw or marinate foods in the refrigerator.

Computer or Mobile Devices

- Look for tips to keep food safe at www.cdc.gov/foodsafety and www.foodsafety.gov.
- Stay up-to-date on food recalls at foodsafety.gov/recalls-and-outbreaks.

Section 26.3
Keep Food Safe

This section includes text excerpted from "Keep Food Safe," Foodsafety.gov, U.S. Department of Health and Human Services (HHS), April 26, 2019.

Healthy eating means more than managing calories or choosing a balanced diet of nutrient-rich foods. The best healthy eating plans also involve safe food handling, cooking, and storage practices that help prevent food poisoning and foodborne illness.

This year, an estimated one in six Americans will get sick from food poisoning. Find out what you can do to keep you and your family safe.

- **Check your steps.** Following four simple steps—clean, separate, cook, and chill—can help protect your family from food poisoning at home.
- **Keep food safe by type of food.**

- Keep food safe by type of events and seasons.
- Food safety in a disaster or emergency.
- FoodKeeper app.

Section 26.4

Eating Out

This section includes text excerpted from "Food Safety and Eating Out," Centers for Disease Control and Prevention (CDC), February 5, 2020.

Going out to eat? Look for a restaurant that keeps food safety on the menu. Here are tips to stay healthy and protect yourself from food poisoning while dining out.

Food Safety Tips for Eating at Restaurants

- **Check inspection scores.** Check a restaurant's score at your health department's website, ask the health department for a copy of the report, or look for it when you get to the restaurant.
- **Look for certificates that show kitchen managers have completed food-safety training.** Proper food-safety training can help improve practices that reduce the chance of spreading foodborne germs and illnesses.
- **Look for safe food-handling practices.** Sick food workers can spread their illness to customers. Most kitchens are out of the customer's sight, but if you can see food being prepared, check to make sure workers are using gloves or utensils to handle foods that will not be cooked further, such as deli meats and salad greens.
- **Order food that is properly cooked.** Certain foods, including meat, poultry, and fish, need to be cooked to a temperature high enough to kill harmful germs that may be present. If you are served undercooked meat,

poultry, seafood, or eggs, send them back to be cooked until they are safe to eat.

- **Avoid food served lukewarm.** Cold food should be served cold, and hot food should be served hot. If you are selecting food from a buffet or salad bar, make sure that the hot food is steaming, and the cold food is chilled. Germs that cause food poisoning grow quickly when food is in the danger zone, between 40°F and 140°F.
- **Ask your server if they use pasteurized eggs in foods, such as Caesar salad dressing, custards, or hollandaise sauce.** Raw or undercooked eggs can make you sick unless they are pasteurized to kill germs.
- **Take care of your leftovers quickly.** Refrigerate within 2 hours of eating out. If it is above 90°F outside, refrigerate leftovers within 1 hour. Eat leftovers within 3 to 4 days. Throw them out after that time.

If you think you or someone you know got sick from food, even if you do not know what food it was, please report it to your local health department. Reporting an illness can help public-health officials identify a foodborne disease outbreak and keep others from getting sick.

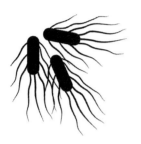

CHAPTER 27
Guide to Safe Water Systems

Chapter Contents

Section 27.1

Preventing Contamination of Drinking-Water Resources

This section includes text excerpted from "Preventing Contamination of Drinking Water Resources," U.S. Environmental Protection Agency (EPA), January 10, 2017.

All must work together to prevent contamination of drinking water. Many pollutants are put into the ground and into lakes, rivers, and streams every day. The disposal of wastes into ground and surface waters can cause contamination of water that is used for drinking and that is expected to be of excellent quality. It takes many years and it is very costly to remove contamination affecting water supplies. Often the damage is irreparable and the water resource can never be used as a drinking-water source again. Preventing pollution of drinking-water sources assures the availability of future drinking-water supplies. A protected source of drinking water combined with proper water-quality monitoring, treatment, maintenance and distribution, is necessary to provide safe, affordable drinking water to residents, businesses, and visitors.

The U.S. Environmental Protection Agency (EPA) has primary responsibility for ensuring the activities required by the Safe Drinking Water Act (SDWA), and many other environmental laws, are carried out. The EPA oversees several programs aimed at protecting drinking water resources:

- Groundwater discharges (underground injection-control program)
- Source Water Assessment Program (SWAP)
- Wellhead Protection Program
- Sole Source Aquifer Program

The EPA works closely with state drinking-water programs to carry out its drinking-water protection programs. In addition, many other organizations assist the EPA and the states to protect our nation's drinking-water sources.

In an effort to educate citizens and businesses about the value of their drinking water and how to protect it against contamination, the EPA is working with other organizations to help communities and water suppliers develop protection programs, technical-assistance documents and videos, classroom materials for schools, and a business honors program for drinking-water source protection. The EPA has developed many outreach documents and videos which may be used to educate people about drinking water. Many of these documents are available from the EPA's national website. Others may be available by contacting the Drinking Water Hotline at 800-426-4791.

Section 27.2

Community and Household Water Treatment

This section includes text excerpted from "Water Treatment," Centers for Disease Control and Prevention (CDC), January 20, 2015. Reviewed March 2020.

Community Water Treatment

Drinking-water supplies in the United States are among the safest in the world. However, even in the United States, drinking-water sources can become contaminated, causing sickness and disease from waterborne germs such as *Cryptosporidium, E. coli, Hepatitis A, Giardia intestinalis,* and other pathogens.

Drinking-water sources are subject to contamination and require appropriate treatment to remove disease-causing agents. Public drinking-water systems use various methods of water treatment to provide safe drinking water to the communities. The most common steps in water treatment used by community water systems (mainly surface-water treatment) include:

- **Coagulation and flocculation.** Coagulation and flocculation are often the first steps in water treatment. Chemicals with a positive charge are added to the water. The positive charge of these chemicals neutralizes the negative charge of dirt and other dissolved particles in the water. When this occurs, the particles bind with the chemicals and form larger particles, called "floc."
- **Sedimentation.** During sedimentation, floc settles to the bottom of the water supply, due to its weight. This settling process is called "sedimentation."
- **Filtration.** Once the floc has settled to the bottom of the water supply, the clear water on top will pass through filters of varying compositions (sand, gravel, and charcoal) and pore sizes, in order to remove dissolved particles, such as dust, parasites, bacteria, viruses, and chemicals.
- **Disinfection.** After the water has been filtered, a disinfectant (for example, chlorine, chloramine) may be added in order to kill any remaining parasites, bacteria, and viruses, and to protect the water from germs when it is piped to homes and businesses.

Water may be treated differently in different communities, depending on the quality of the water that enters the treatment plant. Typically, surface water requires more treatment and filtration than groundwater because lakes, rivers, and streams contain more sediment and pollutants and are more likely to be contaminated than groundwater.

Some water supplies may also contain disinfectant byproducts, inorganic chemicals, organic chemicals, and radionuclides. Specialized methods for controlling formation or removing them can also be part of water treatment.

Water Fluoridation

Community water fluoridation prevents tooth decay safely and effectively. Water fluoridation has been named one of 10 great public-health achievements of the 20th century.

Consumer Confidence Reports

Every community water supplier must provide an annual report, sometimes called a "Consumer Confidence Report," or "CCR," to its customers. The report provides information on your local drinking-water quality, including the water's source, contaminants found in the water, and how consumers can get involved in protecting drinking water.

- View the Centers for Disease Control and Prevention's (CDC) guide to Understanding Consumer Confidence Reports (www.cdc.gov/ healthywater/drinking/public/understanding_ccr.html)
- See if your CCR is posted online (www.epa.gov/ ground-water-and-drinking-water/local-drinking-water-information)

Household Water Treatment

Even though the U.S. Environmental Protection Agency (EPA) regulates and sets standards for public drinking water, many Americans use a home water treatment unit to:

- Remove specific contaminants
- Take extra precautions because a household member has a compromised immune system
- Improve the taste of drinking water

Household water-treatment systems are composed of two categories: point-of-use (POU) and point-of-entry (POE). POE systems are typically installed after the water meter and treat most of the water entering a residence. POU systems are systems that treat water in batches and deliver water to a tap, such as a kitchen or bathroom sink or an auxiliary faucet mounted next to a tap.

The most common types of household water-treatment systems consist of:

- **Filtration systems.** A water filter is a device which removes impurities from water by means of a physical barrier, chemical, and/or biological process.
- **Water softeners.** A water softener is a device that reduces the hardness of the water. A water softener typically uses sodium or

potassium ions to replace calcium and magnesium ions, the ions that create "hardness."

- **Distillation systems.** Distillation is a process in which impure water is boiled and the steam is collected and condensed in a separate container, leaving many of the solid contaminants behind.
- **Disinfection.** Disinfection is a physical or chemical process in which pathogenic microorganisms are deactivated or killed. Examples of chemical disinfectants are chlorine, chlorine dioxide, and ozone. Examples of physical disinfectants include ultraviolet light, electronic radiation, and heat.

Section 27.3
Drinking Water FAQs

This section includes text excerpted from "Drinking Water FAQ," Centers for Disease Control and Prevention (CDC), June 29, 2012. Reviewed March 2020.

The drinking water that is supplied to our homes comes from either surface water or groundwater. Surface water collects in streams, rivers, lakes, and reservoirs. Groundwater is water located below the ground where it collects in pores and spaces within rocks and in underground aquifers. Groundwater is obtained by drilling wells and pumping it to the surface.

Public water systems provide water from both surface and ground water for public use. Water-treatment systems are either government or privately held facilities. Surface water systems withdraw water from the source, treat it, and deliver it to people's homes. Groundwater systems also withdraw and deliver water, but they do not always treat it.

A private well uses ground water as its water source. Owners of private wells and other individual water systems are responsible for ensuring that their water is safe from contaminants.

Public Water Systems
What Type of Health Issues Can Be Related to Water Quality?

The presence of certain contaminants in water can lead to health issues, including gastrointestinal illness, reproductive problems, and neurological disorders. Infants, young children, pregnant women, the elderly, and immunocompromised people may be especially at risk for becoming ill after drinking contaminated water. For example, elevated levels of lead can cause serious health problems, especially for pregnant women and young children. Federal law requires that systems reduce certain contaminants to set levels, in order to protect human health.

How Do You Know That the Water in Your Home Is Safe to Drink?

The EPA is responsible for making sure that public water supplies within the United States are safe. In 1974, Congress passed the Safe Drinking Water Act (SDWA). This law sought to protect the nation's public drinking-water supply by giving the EPA authority to set the standards for drinking-water quality and oversee the states, localities, and water suppliers who implement those standards. In 1986 and 1996, the law was amended to protect drinking water and its sources, which include rivers, lakes, reservoirs, springs, and groundwater wells.

How Do Contaminants (Germs and Chemicals) Get into the Drinking Water?

There can be many sources of contamination of our water systems. Here is a list of the most common sources of contaminants:

- Naturally occurring chemicals and minerals (for example, arsenic, radon, uranium)
- Local land-use practices (fertilizers, pesticides, livestock, concentrated animal-feeding operations)
- Manufacturing processes
- Sewer overflows

- Malfunctioning wastewater treatment systems (for example, nearby septic systems)

Many contaminants that pose known human health risks are regulated by the EPA. The EPA makes sure that water meets certain standards, so you can be sure that high levels of contaminants are not in your water.

How Often Does Our Public Water System Test Drinking Water?

The frequency of drinking-water testing depends on the number of people served, the type of water source, and the types of contaminants. Certain contaminants are tested more frequently than others, as set forth by the Safe Drinking Water Act. You can find out about levels of regulated contaminants in your treated water for the preceding calendar year in your annual Consumer Confidence Report (CCR).

What Common Contaminants Are Included in This Testing?

The EPA sets standards and regulations for the presence and amount of over 90 different contaminants in public drinking water, including *E.coli*, *Salmonella*, and *Cryptosporidium* species. More information regarding the specific contaminants and maximum contaminant levels can be found on the EPA's website (Drinking Water Contaminant Candidate List and Regulatory Determinations (www.epa.gov/ccl)).

What Should You Do If You Want Your Household Water Tested?

The United States has one of the safest public-water supplies in the world. However, if you are concerned about contaminants in your home's water system, contact your state drinking-water certification officer to obtain a list of certified laboratories in your state. Depending on how many contaminants you wish to test for, a water test can cost from $15 to hundreds of dollars. The Safe Drinking Water Hotline at 800-426-4791 can give you information on testing methods.

Who Should You Contact If Your Water Has a Funny Smell, Taste, or Appearance?

A change in your water's taste, color, or smell is not necessarily a health concern. However, sometimes changes can be a sign of problems. If you notice a change in your water, call your public water-system company.

If you want to test your water, your local health department should assist in explaining any tests that you need for various contaminants. If your local health department is not able to help, you can contact a state certified laboratory to perform the test. To find a state certified laboratory in your area call the Safe Drinking Water Hotline at 800-426-4791 or visit the State Certified Drinking Water Laboratories list (www.epa.gov/dwlabcert).

How Can You Find Out If There Has Been a Violation in Your Public Water Standard?

When water-quality standards have not been met, your public water system must notify you through the media (television or radio), mail, or other means. Your annual CCR is another way to find out about the water quality in your area. The CCR provides information regarding contaminants, possible health effects, and the water's source.

How Do You Find Out If There Is a Boil Water Advisory or Other Water Advisory in Your Community?

Your public water system is responsible for notifying residents if the water quality does not meet EPA or state standards or if there is a waterborne disease emergency. The EPA sets guidelines for when residents must be notified, depending on the seriousness of a contamination event.

You should be notified by the media (TV, radio), mail, or other means.

There are three levels of public notification. A Tier 1 notification pertains to the most serious and acute contamination events. Notification must be broadcast by local media within 24 hours. Tier 2 allows for a 30-day notification. Tier 3 provides notification through the annual CCR.

If There Is a Boil Water Advisory in Your Community, How Do You Disinfect Your Drinking Water?

In order to disinfect your drinking water during a boil water advisory, you should boil your water at a rolling boil for at least 1 minute (at altitudes greater than 6,562 feet (> 2000 meters), boil water for 3 minutes). Boiling your water for at least 1 minute at a rolling boil will inactivate all harmful bacteria, parasites, and viruses from drinking water.

Chemicals (for example, bleach) are sometimes used for disinfecting small volumes of drinking water for household use. The parasite *Cryptosporidium* can survive a long time, even after the water is treated with chlorine or iodine. *Cryptosporidium* can be removed from water by filtering through a reverse osmosis filter, an "absolute one micron" filter, or a filter certified to remove *Cryptosporidium* under NSF International Standard #53 for either "cyst removal" or "cyst reduction." Filtering does not remove bacteria and viruses. Ultraviolet light treatment of water is not effective against *Cryptosporidium* at normally used levels.

Wells
What Are the Main Types of Groundwater Wells?

According to the EPA, there are three basic types of private drinking wells: dug, drilled, and driven. Proper well construction and continued maintenance are keys to the safety of your water supply. It is important to know what type of well you have. Well type affects how likely your water is to become contaminated and what kinds of maintenance procedures you should follow. You may be able to determine the type of well you have by looking at the outer casing and cover of the well.

As a Private Well Owner, Should You Have Your Well Tested?

Yes, as a private well owner, you are responsible for testing your well to ensure that your well water is safe to drink. The EPA is responsible for making sure that the public water supply within the United States is safe. However, the EPA does not monitor or treat private well drinking water.

How Do Contaminants (Germs and Chemicals) Get into Your Well Water?

A private well uses groundwater as its water source. There are many sources of contamination of groundwater. Here is a list of the most common sources of contaminants:

- Naturally occurring chemicals and minerals (for example, arsenic, radon, uranium)
- Local land use practices (fertilizers, pesticides, livestock, animal feeding operations, biosolids application)
- Manufacturing processes
- Sewer overflows
- Malfunctioning wastewater treatment systems (for example, nearby septic systems)

The EPA does not regulate private wells. You are responsible for testing your well water and making sure it is safe.

Your Well Water Has a Funny Smell or Taste; Should You Worry about Getting Sick?

Any time you notice a significant change in your water quality, you should have it tested. A change in your water's taste, color, or smell is not necessarily a health concern. However, sometimes changes can be a sign of problems.

What Germs and Chemicals Should You Test for in Your Well?

Several water quality indicators (WQIs) and contaminants that should be tested for in your water are listed below. A WQI test is a test that measures the presence and amount of certain germs in water. In most cases, WQIs do not cause sickness; however, they are easy to test for and their presence may indicate the presence of sewage and other disease-causing germs from human and/or animal feces.

Water Quality Indicators

- Total coliforms
- Fecal coliforms/*Escherichia coli* (*E. coli*)
- pH

Contaminants

- Nitrate
- Volatile organic compounds (VOCs)

Other germs or harmful chemicals that you should test for will depend on where your well is located on your property, which state you live in, and whether you live in an urban or rural area. These tests could include testing for lead, arsenic, mercury, radium, atrazine, and other pesticides. You should check with your local health or environmental department to find out if any of these contaminants are a problem in your region.

Please remember that if your test results say that there are germs or chemicals in your water, you should contact your local health or environmental department for help in interpreting the test, receive guidance on how to respond to the contamination, and test your water more often.

When Should You Have Your Well Tested?

You should have your well tested once each year for total coliform bacteria, nitrates, total dissolved solids, and pH levels. If you suspect other contaminants, you should test for those as well. However, spend time identifying potential problems as these tests can be expensive. You should also have your well tested if:

- There are known problems with well water in your area
- You have experienced problems near your well (i.e., flooding, land disturbances, and nearby waste disposal sites)
- You replace or repair any part of your well system
- You notice a change in water quality (i.e., taste, color, and odor)

Who Should Test Your Well?

State and local health or environmental departments often test for nitrates, total coliforms, fecal coliforms, volatile organic compounds, and pH. Health or environmental departments, or county governments should also have a list of the state-certified (licensed) laboratories in your area that test for a variety of WQIs and contaminants.

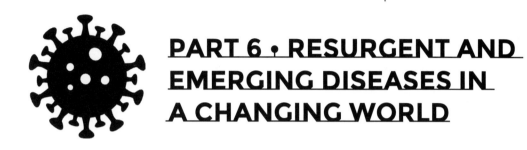

PART 6 · RESURGENT AND EMERGING DISEASES IN A CHANGING WORLD

CHAPTER 28
Major Factors in the Emergence of Infectious Disease

Chapter Contents

Impact of Travel and Migration on Disease Emergence

This section includes text excerpted from "Travel and the Emergence of Infectious Diseases," Centers for Disease Control and Prevention (CDC), December 22, 2010. Reviewed March 2020.

Many factors contribute to the emergence of infectious diseases. Those frequently identified include microbial adaptation and change, human demographics and behavior, environmental changes, technology and economic development, breakdowns in public-health measures and surveillance, and international travel and commerce. This section examines the pivotal role of global travel and movement of biologic life in the emergence of infectious diseases. It also examines the ways in which travel and movement are inextricably tied at multiple levels to other processes that influence the emergence of disease.

Travel is a potent force in disease emergence and spread. The volume, speed, and reach of travel are unprecedented. The consequences of migration extend beyond the traveler to the population visited and the ecosystem. Travel and trade set the stage for mixing diverse genetic pools at rates and in combinations previously unknown. Massive movement and other concomitant changes in social, political, climatic, environmental, and technological factors converge to favor the emergence of infectious diseases.

Disease emergence is complex. Often several events must occur simultaneously or sequentially for a disease to emerge or reemerge. Travel allows a potentially pathogenic microbe to be introduced into a new geographic area; however, to be established and cause disease a microbe must survive, proliferate, and find a way to enter a susceptible host. Any analysis of emergence must look at a dynamic process, a sequence of events, a milieu, or ecosystem.

Movement, changing patterns of resistance and vulnerability, and the emergence of infectious diseases also affect plants, animals, and insect vectors. Analysis of these species can hold important lessons about the dynamics of human disease.

To assess the impact of travel on disease emergence, it is necessary to consider the receptivity of a geographic area and its population to microbial introduction. Most introductions do not lead to disease. Organisms that survive primarily or entirely in the human host and are spread through sexual contact, droplet nuclei, and close physical contact can be readily carried to any part of the world. For example, AIDS, tuberculosis, measles, pertussis, diphtheria, and hepatitis B are easily carried by travelers and can spread in a new geographic area; however, populations protected by vaccines resist introduction. Organisms that have animal hosts, environmental limitations, arthropod vectors, or complicated life cycles become successively more difficult to "transplant" to another geographic area or population. Epidemics of dengue fever and yellow fever cannot appear in a geographic area unless competent mosquito vectors are present. Schistosomiasis cannot spread in an environment unless a suitable snail intermediate host exists in that region. Organisms that survive only under carefully tuned local conditions are less likely to be successfully introduced. Even if an introduced parasite persists in a new geographic area, it does not necessarily cause human disease. In the United States, humans infected with *Taenia solium*, the parasite that causes cysticercosis, infrequently transmit the infection because sanitary disposal of feces, the source of the eggs, is generally available. In short, the likelihood of transmission involves many biological, social, and environmental variables.

Movement of People

Travel for business and pleasure constitutes a small fraction of total human movement. People migrating individually or in groups may be immigrants, refugees, missionaries, merchant marines, students, temporary workers, pilgrims, or Peace Corps workers. Travel may involve short distances or the crossing of international borders. Its volume, however, is huge. In the early 1990s more than 500 million people annually crossed international borders on commercial airline flights. An estimated 70 million people. mostly from developing countries, work either legally or illegally in other countries. Movement may be temporary or seasonal, as with nomadic populations and migrant workers who follow the crops. Military maneuvers worldwide employ and move huge populations. The consequences of armed conflict and political unrest displace millions. In the early 1990s, there were an estimated 20 million refugees and 30 million displaced people worldwide.

One type of travel relevant to disease emergence is the shift of populations to urban areas. It is estimated that, by the year 2010, 50 percent of the world's population will be living in urban areas. It is projected that, by the year 2000, the world will comprise 24 "megacities"—sprawling metropolitan areas with populations exceeding 10 million. These areas will have the population density to support persistence of some infections and contribute to the emergence of others. Many of these areas are located in tropical or subtropical regions, where the environment can support a diverse array of pathogens and vectors. Also developing are huge peri-urban slums, populated with people from many geographic origins. Poor sanitation allows breeding of arthropod vectors, rodents, and other disease-carrying animals. Crowded conditions favor the spread of diseases that pass from person to person, including sexually transmitted infections. Travel between peri-urban slum areas and rural areas is common, paving the route for the transfer of microbes and disease. Transfer of resistance genes and genetic recombination may also occur in and spread from crowded environments of transients.

Acute disturbances, whether climatic or political, lead to interim living arrangements, such as refugee camps and temporary shelters, that provide ideal conditions for the emergence and spread of infections. Temporary living quarters often share similarities with peri-urban slums: crowding, inadequate sanitation, limited access to medical care, lack of clean water and food, dislocation, multiethnic composition, and inadequate barriers from vectors and animals. An example is the movement of 500,000 to 800,000 Rwandan refugees into Zaire in 1994. Almost 50,000 refugees died during the first month as epidemics of cholera and *Shigella dysenteriae* type 1 swept through the refugee camps.

Movement into a rural environment poses different risks and often places new rural populations in contact with pathogens that are in the soil and water or are carried by animals or arthropods. Some of these pathogens such as *Guanarito* and *Sabià* viruses in South America were recognized as capable of infecting humans.

Consequences of Movement

Human migration favors the emergence of infectious diseases through many mechanisms. When people migrate, they carry their genetic makeup, their accumulated immunologic experience, and much more. They may carry pathogens in or on their bodies and may also transport disease vectors, such as lice. Their technology (agricultural and industrial), methods for treating disease, cultural traditions, and behavioral patterns may influence their risk for infection in a new environment and their capacity to introduce disease into the new region. Their social standing and resources may affect their exposure to local infections and their access to adequate nutrition and treatment. People also change the environment in many ways when they travel or migrate—they plant, clear land, build, and consume.

Travel is relevant in the emergence of disease if it changes an ecosystem. The following examples show the many ways in which migration can influence the emergence of disease in a new area. Humans may carry a pathogen in a form that can be transmitted, then or later, directly or indirectly to another person. The pathogen may be silent (during the incubation period, chronic carriage, or latent infection) or clinically evident. Examples include hepatitis B virus, human immunodeficiency virus (HIV), *Mycobacterium tuberculosis*, *M. leprae*, *Salmonella typhi*, and other *Salmonella*. Disease may be especially severe when a pathogen is introduced into a population that has no previous exposure to the infection. How long the consequences of migration persist varies with the specific infection. The two most critical characteristics are the duration of survival of the pathogen in a potentially infective form and its means of transmission. Epidemic cholera in Africa spread along the West African coast and, when the disease moved inland, followed fishing and trading routes.

Markets, funerals, refugee camps that involve the migration of people and large gatherings with close contact—helped spread the infection. Humans may carry a pathogen that can be transmitted only if conditions are permissive. This permissiveness can pertain to human behavior, the environment, or the presence of appropriate vectors or intermediate hosts. For example, the ease with which HIV spreads in a population depends on sexual practices, condom use, the number of sex partners, and intravenous drug use, among other factors. Malaria requires specific mosquito vectors (with access to susceptible humans) to spread to new geographic regions. Schistosomiasis can be introduced into a new region only if the appropriate snail host is present and if the eggs excreted (in urine or feces, from an infected person) reach the snails in an appropriate environment.

Humans may carry a strain of microbe that has an unusual resistance pattern or virulence genes. A multiple-drug-resistant strain of *Klebsiella pneumoniae* appears to have been transferred by an asymptomatic woman from a hospital in Bahrain to Oxford, where it caused outbreaks in two British hospitals. People also carry their background flora in the intestinal tract, for example, which may contain plasmids and resistance genes that can interact with microbes in a new area. It is not just the classic pathogens that may be relevant to the emergence of a new disease, but the individual traveler's total microbiologic "baggage." Visitors to a region may lack immunity to locally endemic infections, such as hepatitis A and sandfly fever. Visitors may suffer severe or different manifestations of infection or disease at an age when the local population is immune to it. Resettlement of populations into malaria-endemic regions can lead to a high death rate from falciparum malaria. Kala-azar caused a deadly outbreak in remote villages in southern Sudan in 1994.

To determine the consequences of travel, both the traveler and the population visited must be considered. Migration may be in only one direction, though travel often involves returning to the point of origin, perhaps after the traveler has made many stops along the way. The changes in the various ecosystems as a consequence of the migration guide the emergence of diseases; therefore, any study that simply focuses on the traveler is too narrow.

Shipping and Commerce

The biomass of humans constitutes only a fraction of the matter moved about the earth. Humans carry and send a huge volume of plants, animals, and other materials all over the face of the globe. Much of this movement results from the planned transport of goods from one place to another, but some is an unintended consequence of shipping and travel. All has an impact on the juxtaposition of various species in different ecosystems. "Hitchhikers" include all manner of biologic life, both microscopic and macroscopic. Animals can carry potential human pathogens and vectors. The globalization of markets brings fresh fruits and vegetables to dinner tables thousands of miles from where they were grown, fertilized, and picked. Examples of introduced species include plants and animals — insects, microbes, and marine organisms. Ships convey marine organisms on their hulls and in their ballast water. For example, 367 different species were identified in the ballast water of ships traveling between Japan and Coos Bay, Oregon.

Introductions have had devastating effects in some areas such as the Black and Azov seas, for example, where newly introduced jellyfish-like creatures called "ctenophores" have ruined local fishing. *Vibrio cholerae* may have been introduced to South America by shipping. Researchers isolated the organism in samples of ballast, bilge, and sewage from 3 of 14 cargo ships docked at Gulf of Mexico ports. The ships had last ports of call in Brazil, Colombia, and Chile. *V. cholerae O1*, serotype Inaba, biotype El Tor, indistinguishable from the Latin American epidemic strain, was found in oysters and oyster-eating fish from closed oyster beds in Mobile Bay, Alabama. *V. cholerae O139* has spread along waterways in Asia, although the people carried on the boats doubtless played a role. *Aedes albopictus* was introduced into the United States inside used tires shipped from Asia.

Exotic animals transported from their usual habitats are clustered in zoos; others are used in research laboratories where they have occasionally caused severe disease in humans. Two examples are B virus from primates and hemorrhagic fever with renal syndrome from rodents. The world trade and globalization of organs, tissues, blood, and blood products is growing. Researchers are considering animals as sources for tissues and organs for transplantation. Plants may not directly cause human disease, but they can alter an ecosystem and facilitate the breeding of a vector for human disease. This can also displace traditional crops that provide essential nutrition. Vertical transmission of plant pathogens (and spread of plant diseases) can result from seed movement. Carriage of seeds into new areas can introduce plant pathogens. Migration and altered environments have increased the so-called weedy species. These species migrate easily and have high rates of reproduction. If they lack local predators, they can displace other species and often upset local ecology.

Global Travel

Global travel and the evolution of microbes will continue. New infections will continue to emerge, and known infections will change in distribution, severity and frequency. Travel will continue to be a potent factor in disease emergence. The World circumstances juxtapose people, parasites, plants, animals, and chemicals in a way that precludes timely adaptation. The combination of movement at many levels and profound change in the physical environment can lead to unanticipated diseases spread by multiple channels. In many instances, the use of containment, or quarantine, is not feasible. Research and surveillance can map the global movement and evolution of microbes and guide interventions. Integration of knowledge and skills from many disciplines—the social, biological, and physical sciences—is needed. The focus should be on system analysis and the ecosystem rather than on a disease, microbe, or host.

Section 28.2

Link between Land-Use Patterns and Infectious Disease

This section includes text excerpted from
"Land Use," U.S. Environmental Protection
Agency (EPA), July 16, 2018.

Definition of Land Use

"Land use" is the term used to describe the human use of land. It represents the economic and cultural activities (e.g., agricultural, residential, industrial, mining, and recreational uses) that are practiced at a given place. Public and private lands frequently represent very different uses. For example, urban development seldom occurs on publicly owned lands (e.g., parks, wilderness areas), while privately owned lands are infrequently protected for wilderness uses.

Land *use* differs from land *cover* in that some uses are not always physically obvious (e.g., land used for producing timber, but not harvested for many years and forested land designated as wilderness will both appear as forest-covered, but they have different uses).

Effects of Land-Use Changes

Land-use changes occur constantly and at many scales, and can have specific and cumulative effects on air and water quality, watershed function, generation of waste, extent and the quality of wildlife habitat, climate, and human health.

The U.S. Environmental Protection Agency (EPA) is concerned about different land-use activities because of their potential effects on the environment and human health. Land development and agricultural uses are two primary areas of concern, with a wide variety of potential effects.

Land Development

- Land development creates **impervious surfaces** through the construction of roads, parking lots, and other structures. Impervious surfaces:

- Contribute to nonpoint source water pollution by limiting the capacity of soils to filter runoff
- Affect peak flow and water volume, which heighten erosion potential and affect habitat and water quality
- Increase stormwater runoff, which can deliver more pollutants to water bodies that residents may rely on for drinking and recreation. Storm runoff from urban and suburban areas contains dirt, oils from road surfaces, nutrients from fertilizers, and various toxic compounds.
- Affect groundwater aquifer recharge
- **Point source discharges** from industrial and municipal wastewater treatment facilities can contribute toxic compounds and heated water.
- Some **land-development patterns**, in particular dispersed growth such as "suburbanization," can contribute to a variety of environmental concerns. For example:
  - Increased air pollution due to vehicle use results in higher concentrations of certain air pollutants in developed areas that may exacerbate human health problems such as asthma.
  - Land development can lead to the formation of "heat islands," or domes of warmer air over urban and suburban areas that are caused by the loss of trees and shrubs and the absorption of more heat by pavement, buildings, and other sources. Heat islands can affect local, regional, and global climate, as well as air quality.

Agricultural Uses

- Agricultural land uses can affect the **quality of water and watersheds**, including:
  - The types of crops planted, tillage practices, and various irrigation practices can limit the amount of water available for other uses.
  - Livestock grazing in riparian zones can change landscape conditions by reducing stream bank vegetation and increasing water temperatures, sedimentation, and nutrient levels.
  - Runoff from pesticides, fertilizers, and nutrients from animal manure can also degrade water quality.

- Agricultural land use may also result in **loss of native habitats** or increased wind erosion and dust, exposing humans to particulate matter and various chemicals.
- Some land uses can accelerate or exacerbate the **spread of invasive species**. For example:
  - Certain agricultural land-use practices, such as overgrazing, land conversion, fertilization, and the use of agricultural chemicals, can enhance the growth of invasive plants. These plants can alter fish and wildlife habitats, contribute to decreases in biodiversity, and create health risks to livestock and humans.
  - Introduction of invasive species on agricultural lands can reduce water quality and water availability for native fish and wildlife species.

Research is beginning to elucidate the connections between land-use changes and infectious disease. For example, some studies indicate that spread of vector-borne disease may be influenced by land use and/or other environmental changes.

Other studies indicate that fragmentation of forest habitat into smaller patches separated by agricultural activities or developed land increases the "edge effect" and promotes interaction among pathogens, vectors, and hosts.

Section 28.3

Social Inequalities and Emerging Infectious Diseases

This section includes text excerpted from "Social Inequalities and Emerging Infectious Diseases," Centers for Disease Control and Prevention (CDC), December 21, 2010. Reviewed March 2020.

The past decade has been one of the most eventful in the long history of infectious diseases. There are multiple indexes of these events and of the rate at which the knowledge base has grown. The sheer number of relevant publications indicates explosive growth; moreover, new means of monitoring antimicrobial resistance patterns are being used along with the rapid sharing of information (as well as speculation and misinformation) through means that did not exist even 10 years ago. Then there are the microbes themselves. One of the explosions in question—perhaps the most remarked upon—is that of "emerging infectious diseases."

Among the diseases considered "emerging," some are regarded as genuinely new; AIDS and Brazilian purpuric fever are examples. Others have newly identified etiologic agents or have again burst dramatically onto the scene. For example, the syndromes caused by Hantaan virus have been known in Asia for centuries, but now seem to be spreading beyond Asia because of ecologic and economic transformations that increase contact between humans and rodents. Neuroborreliosis was studied long before the monikers "Lyme disease" and *"Borrelia burgdorferi"* were coined, and before suburban reforestation and golf courses complicated the equation by creating an environment agreeable to both ticks and affluent humans.

Hemorrhagic fevers, including Ebola, were described long ago, and their etiologic agents were in many cases identified in previous decades. Still, other diseases grouped under the "emerging" rubric are ancient and well-known foes that have somehow changed in pathogenicity or distribution. Multidrug-resistant tuberculosis (TB) and invasive or necrotizing Group A streptococcal infection are cases in point.

In studying emerging infectious diseases, many thus make a distinction between a host of phenomena directly related to human actions—from improved laboratory techniques and scientific discovery to economic "development," global warming, and the failures of public health—and another set of phenomena, much less common and related to changes in the microbes themselves. Close examination of microbial mutations often shows that, again, human actions have played a large role in enhancing pathogenicity or increasing resistance to antimicrobial agents. In one long list of emerging viral infections, for example, only the emergence of Rift Valley fever is attributed to a possible change in virulence or pathogenicity, and this only after other social factors for which there is better evidence. No need, then, to call for a heightened awareness of the sociogenesis, or "anthropogenesis," of emerging infections. Some bench scientists in the field are more likely to refer to social factors and less likely to make immodest claims of causality about them than are behavioral scientists who study disease. Yet a critical epistemology of emerging infectious diseases is still in its early stages of development; a key task of such a critical approach would be to take existing conceptual frameworks, including that of disease emergence, and ask, What is obscured in this way of conceptualizing disease? What is brought into relief? A first step in understanding that the "epistemological dimension" of disease emergence involves developing "a certain sensitivity to the terms we are used to."

Heightened sensitivity to other common rubrics and terms shows that certain aspects of disease emergence are brought into relief while others are obscured. When thinking of "tropical diseases," malaria comes quickly to mind. In the Ohio River Valley, according to a researcher's 1850 study, thousands died in seasonal epidemics. During the second decade of the 20th century, when the population of 12 southern states was approximately 25 million, an estimated million cases of malaria occurred each year. Malaria's decline in this country was "due only in small part to measures aimed directly against it, but more to agricultural development and other factors some of which are still not clear." These factors include poverty and social inequalities, which led, increasingly, to differential morbidity with the development of improved housing, land drainage, mosquito repellents, nets, and electric fans—all well beyond the reach of those most at risk for malaria. In fact, many "tropical" diseases predominantly affect the poor; the groups at risk for these diseases are often bound more by socioeconomic status than by latitude.

Emerging How and to What Extent? The Case of Ebola

Hemorrhagic fevers have been known in Africa since well before the continent was dubbed "the white man's grave," an expression that, when deployed in reference to a region with high rates of premature death, speaks volumes about the differential valuation of human lives. Ebola itself was isolated fully two decades ago. Its appearance in human hosts has at times been insidious, but more often takes the form of explosive eruptions. In accounting for outbreaks, it is unnecessary to postulate a change in filovirus virulence through mutation. The Institute of Medicine lists a single "factor facilitating emergence" for filoviruses: "virus-infected monkeys shipped from developing countries via air."

Other factors are easily identified. Like that of many infectious diseases, the distribution of Ebola outbreaks is tied to regional trade networks and other evolving social systems. And, like those of most infectious diseases, Ebola explosions affect, researchers aside, certain groups (people living in poverty, healthcare workers who serve the poor), but not others in close physical proximity. Take, for example, the 1976 outbreak in Zaire, which affected 318 persons. Although respiratory spread was speculated, it has not been conclusively demonstrated as a cause of human cases.

Most expert observers thought that the cases could be traced to failure to follow contact precautions, as well as to improper sterilization of syringes and other paraphernalia—measures that in fact, once taken, terminated the outbreak. On closer scrutiny, such an explanation suggests that Ebola does not emerge randomly: in Mobutu's Zaire, one's likelihood of coming into contact with unsterile syringes is inversely proportional to one's social status. Local élites and sectors of the expatriate community with access to high-quality biomedical services (viz., the European and American communities and not the Rwandan refugees) are unlikely to contract such a disease.

The changes involved in the disease's visibility are equally embedded in social context. The emergence of Ebola has also been a question of social consciousness. Modern communications, including print and broadcast media, have been crucial in the construction of Ebola—a minor player, statistically speaking, in Zaire's long list of fatal infections—as an emerging infectious disease. Through Cable News Network (CNN) and other television stations, Kikwit became, however, briefly, a household word in parts of Europe and North America. Journalists and novelists wrote bestselling books about small but horrific plagues, which in turn became profitable cinema. Thus, symbolically and proverbially, Ebola spread like wildfire—as a danger potentially without limit. It emerged.

Section 28.4
Emerging Infections: An Evolutionary Perspective

This section includes text excerpted from "New and Reemerging Diseases: The Importance of Biomedical Research," Centers for Disease Control and Prevention (CDC), December 14, 2010. Reviewed March 2020.

A generation ago, it was suggested that the threat of infectious diseases would soon become an artifact of history. Two pandemics of extraordinary impact: the global influenza pandemic of 1918 to 1919, which killed more than 20 million people worldwide, and the HIV/AIDS pandemic, which began to accelerate in the early 1980s and continues unabated in some parts of the world. In addition, at least 30 other new and reemerging diseases and syndromes have been recognized since the 1970s, including liver disease due to hepatitis C virus, Lyme disease, foodborne illness caused by *Escherichia coli O157:H7* and *Cyclospora*, waterborne disease due to *Cryptosporidium*, hantavirus pulmonary syndrome, and human disease caused by the avian H5N1 influenza virus. Clearly, we remain vulnerable to new and reemerging diseases.

New diseases are superimposed on endemic diseases such as diarrheal diseases, malaria, tuberculosis (TB), and measles, which continue to exact a huge toll. Indeed, malaria and TB, among others, are reemerging in a drug-resistant form. Infectious diseases remain the leading cause of death worldwide and the third leading cause of death in the United States. Many pathogens are becoming increasingly resistant to standard antimicrobial drugs, making treatment difficult and, in some cases, impossible. Moreover, chronic conditions generally considered noninfectious actually have been found to have a microbial etiology.

Awareness of Emerging Infections

The challenges posed by infectious diseases are recognized by the public and the media, as well as by political leaders and policymakers at the highest levels of government. There is a growing awareness that we live in a global community, that diseases do not recognize borders, and that the United States public-health community has an important role to play in fostering global health.

The Importance of Research

The infectious-diseases community faces a difficult challenge: coping with ongoing problems, such as malaria and TB, while preparing for the inevitable emergence of diseases that are unknown or are recognized, but will reemerge in a more threatening form.

Within the federal government, the Centers for Disease Control and Prevention's (CDC) work in detecting and tracking pathogens is critical, especially with regard to diseases that have recently emerged or have the potential for emergence. Equally important, and complementary to the CDC's efforts, is basic and clinical research supported by the National Institutes of Health (NIH) and other agencies. Historically, basic research has led to important, often serendipitous, advances that have illuminated the etiology of sometimes mysterious diseases and facilitated the development of diagnostics, therapies, and vaccines.

At the National Institute of Allergy and Infectious Diseases (NIAID) at NIH, NIAID increased funding for emerging diseases from $39.3 million in fiscal year 1993 to an estimated (president's budget) $85.0 million in fiscal 1999. Approximately 21 percent of the NIAID non-AIDS infectious-diseases budget is devoted to emerging infectious diseases.

Among many studies domestically and internationally, the NIAID sponsors five international programs in tropical infectious diseases, most of which have components both in the United States and in the countries where the incidence of these diseases is greatest. It is essential to engage scientists in host countries and work with them collaboratively, both to tap their expertise and to help them build research infrastructure on their home soil.

Successful Partnerships

The public and private sectors, including government, academia, and industry, bring complementary skills and perspectives to the research endeavor. Cross-sector collaboration can yield extraordinary dividends. A cogent example is the development of protease inhibitors for the treatment of HIV disease.

After HIV was identified in 1983, researchers funded by the NIH and others began to intensively study the structural and regulatory genes of HIV and the role these genes and their products play in the replication cycle of the virus. This work led to an understanding of the importance of the HIV protease enzyme and methods to express, purify, and crystallize the enzyme. Building on these findings, researchers in the private sector designed and produced specific inhibitors of HIV protease and worked closely with the U.S. Food and Drug Administration (FDA), the NIH, and others to assess protease inhibitors in clinical trials.

Given in combination with at least two other antiretroviral drugs, protease inhibitors dramatically reduce levels of plasma viremia in a substantial proportion of patients with HIV.

Although drug combinations that include protease inhibitors have helped many patients, it is far too soon to become complacent or declare victory. Many patients have not benefited from the new drugs or cannot tolerate their side effects, and drug resistance will inevitably become more widespread. The development of the next generation of antiretroviral agents is crucial and will require the skills of investigators in both the public and private sectors.

Malaria Initiatives at the National Institutes of Health

Until relatively recently, AIDS was virtually the only emerging disease with global impact that was widely discussed in the United States; however, other diseases such as malaria and TB have actually caused more illnesses and deaths over the past two decades.

Malaria kills up to three million people each year, most of them children in sub-Saharan Africa. In the past year, the NIH worked with research organizations and donor agencies from around the world to form a coalition called the "Multilateral Initiative on Malaria." This unprecedented initiative enhances international collaborations, encourages the involvement in malaria research of scientists from malaria-endemic countries, and identifies additional malaria-research resources. In addition, the NIH has bolstered its long-term commitment to malaria research. NIH-supported malaria projects—many in collaboration with other government and international agencies—include (1) a new repository of materials available to researchers worldwide; (2) basic, field-based, and clinical research on all phases of malaria research; and (3) projects to determine the genetic sequences of important malaria species.

Responding to Avian H5N1 Influenza

A 1997 outbreak of avian H5N1 influenza in Hong Kong alarmed the medical community and the world. The multinational response to this outbreak involved the close collaboration of many organizations. As part of the NIH's long-standing research into respiratory viruses led to development of the specific antisera needed to quickly develop test kits that were used effectively by the CDC and others for detecting and tracking the virus. The rapid production of a recombinant vaccine against avian influenza virus for use in laboratory and healthcare personnel at risk was also initiated. Without a strong research base, the rapid response to this emergency would not have been possible.

Vaccine Development

With avian flu, malaria, AIDS, and other new and reemerging diseases, an important goal of the NIH is the development of vaccines. If just four vaccines (hepatitis B, rotavirus, *Haemophilus influenzae* type b, and acellular pertussis) were universally administered, more than three million deaths could be prevented each year.

Historically, scientific advances in microbiology and related disciplines have driven the development of new vaccines. For example, the identification of microbial toxins, as well as methods to inactivate them, allowed the development of some of the NIH's earliest vaccines, including those for diphtheria and tetanus. In the 1950s, tissue-culture techniques ushered in vaccines, including measles, mumps, and rubella. The NIH has seen rapid advances in understanding the immune system and host-pathogen interactions, as well as technical advances such as recombinant DNA technology, peptide synthesis, and gene sequencing. Each of these has facilitated the development of new vaccines and vaccine candidates for important pathogens.

Sequence information can be used in many ways and promises to be useful in identifying antigens to incorporate into vaccines, as well as determining the factors that influence the antigenicity or virulence of a microbe. More than 60 other sequencing projects for medically important pathogens, such as *Plasmodium* spp., *Mycobacterium* spp., *Chlamydia trachomatis*, *Vibrio cholerae*, and *Neisseria gonorrhoeae*, are under way.

CHAPTER 29
Emerging Infectious Diseases and Antimicrobial Resistance: A Global Threat

Chapter Contents

Section 29.1

About Microbial Resistance and the Fallout

This section includes text excerpted from "About Antibiotic Resistance," Centers for Disease Control and Prevention (CDC), February 10, 2020.

Antibiotic resistance happens when germs like bacteria and fungi develop the ability to defeat the drugs designed to kill them. That means the germs are not killed and continue to grow.

Infections caused by antibiotic-resistant germs are difficult, and sometimes impossible, to treat. In most cases, antibiotic-resistant infections require extended hospital stays, additional follow-up doctor visits, and costly and toxic alternatives.

Antibiotic resistance does not mean the body is becoming resistant to antibiotics; it is that bacteria have become resistant to the antibiotics designed to kill them.

Antibiotic Resistance Threatens Everyone

Antibiotic resistance has the potential to affect people at any stage of life, as well as the healthcare, veterinary, and agriculture industries, making it one of the world's most urgent public-health problems.

Each year in the United States, at least 2.8 million people are infected with antibiotic-resistant bacteria or fungi, and more than 35,000 people die as a result.

No one can completely avoid the risk of resistant infections, but some people are at greater risk than others (for example, people with chronic illnesses). If antibiotics lose their effectiveness, then we lose the ability to treat infections and control public-health threats.

Many medical advances are dependent on the ability to fight infections using antibiotics, including joint replacements, organ transplants, cancer therapy, and treatment of chronic diseases like diabetes, asthma, and rheumatoid arthritis.

Where Antibiotic Resistance Spreads
A Complex Web: Everything is Connected

Antibiotic-resistant germs can quickly spread across settings, including communities, the food supply, healthcare facilities, the environment (e.g., soil, water), and around the world. Antibiotic resistance is a One Health problem—the health of people is connected to the health of animals and the environment (soil, water).

It can affect our progress in healthcare, food production, and life expectancy. Antibiotic resistance is not only a United States problem—it is a global crisis. New forms of resistance emerge and can spread with remarkable speed between continents through people, goods, and animals.

Healthcare Facilities

Antibiotic-resistant germs, including new and emerging resistance, can spread within and between healthcare facilities. These germs can cause infections in patients, called "healthcare-associated infections," and can spread to the community or environment.

Community

Germs, including antibiotic-resistant germs, live and spread within our community and sometimes make people sick.

Environment

Human activity can introduce antibiotics and antibiotic-resistant germs into the environment, but it remains unclear how spread in the environment impacts human and animal health.

Food, Farms, and Animals

Animals, like people, carry germs in their gut, including antibiotic-resistant germs. The United States food supply is among the safest in the world, but these germs can get into the food supply and make people sick.

Section 29.2

The Burden of Microbial Resistance

This section includes text excerpted from "How
Antibiotic Resistance Happens," Centers for Disease
Control and Prevention (CDC), February 10, 2020.

Antibiotic Resistance

Antibiotics save lives but any time antibiotics are used, they can cause side effects and lead to antibiotic resistance.

Since the 1940s, antibiotics have greatly reduced illness and death from infectious diseases. However, as we use the drugs, germs develop defense strategies against them. This makes the drugs less effective.

Antimicrobials Treat Infections Caused by Microbes

Microbes are very small living organisms, like bacteria. Most microbes are harmless and even helpful to humans, but some can cause infections and disease. Drugs used to treat these infections are called "antimicrobials." The most commonly known antimicrobial is antibiotics, which kill or stop the growth of bacteria.

Two Types of Microbes

Bacteria cause illnesses such as strep throat and food poisoning. Bacterial infections are treated with drugs called "antibiotics" (such as penicillin).

Fungi cause illnesses like athlete's foot and yeast infections. Fungal infections are treated with drugs called "antifungals."

How Germs Become Resistant and Spread

Germs (bacteria and fungi) are everywhere. Some help us. Some make people, crops, or animals sick. Some of those germs are resistant to antibiotics.

Antibiotics kill germs that cause infections. But antibiotic-resistant germs find ways to survive. Antibiotics also kill good bacteria that protect the body from infection.

Antibiotic-resistant germs can multiply. Some resistant germs can also give their resistance directly to other germs.

Once antibiotic resistance emerges, it can spread into new settings and between countries.

Germ Defense Strategies

Antibiotics fight germs (bacteria and fungi). But germs fight back and find new ways to survive. Their defense strategies are called "resistance mechanisms." Bacteria develop resistance mechanisms by using instructions provided by their DNA. Often, resistance genes are found within plasmids, small pieces of DNA that carry genetic instructions from one germ to another. This means that some bacteria can share their DNA and make other germs become resistant.

Restrict Access of the Antibiotic

Germs restrict access by changing the entryways or limiting the number of entryways.

Example: Gram-negative bacteria have an outer layer (membrane) that protects them from their environment. These bacteria can use this membrane to selectively keep antibiotic drugs from entering.

Get Rid of the Antibiotic

Germs get rid of antibiotics using pumps in their cell walls to remove antibiotic drugs that enter the cell.

Example: Some Pseudomonas aeruginosa bacteria can produce pumps to get rid of several different important antibiotic drugs, including fluoroquinolones, beta-lactams, chloramphenicol, and trimethoprim.

Change or Destroy the Antibiotic

Germs change or destroy the antibiotics with enzymes, proteins that break down the drug.

Example: Klebsiella pneumoniae bacteria produce enzymes called "carbapenemases," which break down carbapenem drugs and most other beta-lactam drugs.

Bypass the Effects of the Antibiotic

Germs develop new cell processes that avoid using the antibiotic's target.

Example: Some Staphylococcus aureus bacteria can bypass the drug effects of trimethoprim.

Change the Targets for the Antibiotic

Many antibiotic drugs are designed to single out and destroy specific parts (or targets) of a bacterium. Germs change the antibiotic's target so the drug can no longer fit and do its job.

Example: *Escherichia coli* bacteria with the *mcr-1* gene can add a compound to the outside of the cell wall so that the drug colistin cannot latch onto it.

Section 29.3
Combat Strategies to Prevent Microbial Resistance

This section includes text excerpted from "U.S. Action to Combat Antibiotic Resistance," Centers for Disease Control and Prevention (CDC), November 4, 2019.

National Priority

Antibiotic resistance is a national priority, and the United States government has taken ambitious steps to fight this threat. For example, it established a U.S. National Strategy for Combating Antibiotic-Resistant

Bacteria (National Strategy) and an accompanying U.S. National Action Plan for Combating Antibiotic-Resistant Bacteria (National Action Plan).

Federal agencies are working together to:
- Respond to new and ongoing public-health threats
- Strengthen detection of resistance
- Enhance efforts to slow the emergence and spread of resistance
- Improve antibiotic use and reporting
- Advance development of rapid diagnostics
- Enhance infection control measures
- Accelerate research on new antibiotics and antibiotic alternatives

U.S. National Action Plan for Combating Antibiotic-Resistant Bacteria

The National Action Plan directs federal agencies to accelerate response to antibiotic resistance, and has pushed transformative improvements across the country that strengthen and expand the ability to prevent, identify, and respond to these threats.

Although the main purpose is to guide U.S. government activities, the National Action Plan is also designed to guide action by public health, healthcare, and veterinary partners in a common effort to address urgent and serious antibiotic-resistant threats that affect people in the United States and around the world.

The National Action Plan was developed by the Interagency Task Force for Combating Antibiotic-Resistant Bacteria in response to Executive Order 13676. It details specific steps and milestones to implement the U.S. National Strategy for Combating Antibiotic-Resistant Bacteria while also addressing the policy recommendations from the President's Council of Advisors on Science and Technology.

Five-Year Plan

The National Action Plan provides a five-year plan to reduce antibiotic resistance by:
- Encouraging innovation and research for new prevention strategies

- Increasing and enhancing surveillance
- Adopting of evidence-based stewardship strategies

Main Goals

The National Action Plan supports the five main goals identified in the National Strategy to guide collaborative action taken by the U.S. government:

- Slow the emergence of resistant bacteria and prevent the spread of resistant infections.
- Strengthen national One Health surveillance efforts to combat resistance.
- Advance development and use of rapid and innovative diagnostic tests for identification and characterization of resistant bacteria.
- Accelerate basic and applied research and development for new antibiotics, other therapeutics, and vaccines.
- Improve international collaboration and capacities for antibiotic resistance prevention, surveillance, control, and antibiotic research and development.

Anticipated Results

The National Action Plan will result in the following:

- Improved antibiotic stewardship in healthcare settings
- Prevention of the spread of antibiotic-resistant threats
- Elimination of the use of medically-important antibiotics for growth promotion in food-producing animals
- Expanded surveillance for antibiotic-resistant bacteria in humans and animals
- Creation of a regional public-health laboratory network
- Establishment of a specimen repository and sequence database that can be accessed by industrial and academic researchers
- Development of new diagnostic tests

The CDC is addressing its role in accomplishing these goals through its Antibiotic Resistance Solutions Initiative.

A Global Problem and Priority

Antimicrobial resistance has been found in all regions of the world. Modern travel of people, animals, and goods means antimicrobial resistance can easily spread across borders and continents.

Fighting this threat is a public-health priority. It requires a collaborative global approach across sectors to detect, prevent, and respond to these threats when they occur.

Global Strategies to Fight Resistance

Every country can take steps to slow antimicrobial resistance. Commit to setting goals across multiple sectors, including:

- Healthcare
- Food
- Communities (local and global)
- Environment (soil and water)

Create and implement a comprehensive plan with a One Health approach to achieve those goals, and track progress.

Every country plan can consider the following actions to prevent resistant infections and their spread:

- Implement infection prevention and control practices.
- Improve antibiotic use, including ensuring access.
- Implement data and tracking systems to track resistance, guide prevention strategies, and report results at the local and global level.
- Improve lab capacity to identify resistant bacteria.

In addition to these important actions, it is also critical to join the global effort to develop new drugs, diagnostics, vaccines, and therapeutics to treat infections.

The Global Action

The CDC shares expertise and deploys scientists to investigate and contain resistance outbreaks, and assists other countries in:

- Contributing to the development and implementation of national action plans

- Implementing programs in healthcare settings to prevent the spread of resistance (infection prevention and control programs) and support the appropriate use of antimicrobials (antimicrobial stewardship programs)
- Enhancing laboratory capacity to detect and report resistance that have global health implications
- Establishing or strengthening national tracking systems to respond rapidly to outbreaks, identify emerging pathogens, and track trends
- Supporting a national network of travel clinics to better understand the spread of resistance across the U.S. to ultimately improve the health of international travelers

In addition, the CDC collaborates in global activities, including:

- Participating in and acts as secretariat for the Transatlantic Taskforce on Antimicrobial Resistance (TATFAR), a collaborative effort between Canada, the European Union, Norway, and the U.S. to address antimicrobial resistance together
- Hosting a World Health Organization (WHO) Collaborating Center, part of the Antibiotic Resistance Surveillance and Quality Assessment Collaborating Centres Network that support countries in building capacity to track antimicrobial resistance by strengthening international collaboration and improving coordination
- Supporting WHO's tracking platforms, including the Global Antibiotic Resistance Surveillance System (GLASS), which provides a standardized approach to the collection, analysis, and sharing of global antimicrobial resistance data; ultimately, GLASS will alert countries worldwide when new resistance emerges

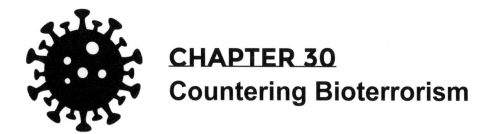

CHAPTER 30
Countering Bioterrorism

Chapter Contents

Bioterrorism as a Public-Health Threat

This section contains text excerpted from the following sources: Text in this section begins with excerpts from "Bioterrorism as a Public-health Threat," Centers for Disease Control and Prevention (CDC), December 20, 2010, Reviewed March 2020; Text beginning with the heading "Threat of Biological Warfare" is excerpted from "Epidemiology of Bioterrorism," Centers for Disease Control and Prevention (CDC), December 13, 2010. Reviewed March 2020.

In addition to meeting the continuing threat of new and reemerging infectious diseases, public-health officials must also prepare for the possible use of infectious agents as weapons by terrorists to further personal or political agendas.

The potential spectrum of bioterrorism ranges from hoaxes and use of non-mass-casualty devices and agents by individuals and small groups to state-sponsored terrorism that employs classic biological-warfare agents and can produce mass casualties. The agents of anthrax, plague, brucellosis, smallpox, viral encephalitides, and viral hemorrhagic fevers are of particular concern: they are relatively easy and inexpensive to produce, cause death or disabling disease, and can be aerosolized and distributed over large geographic areas. If released under ideal environmental circumstances, these agents can infect hundreds of thousands of people and cause many deaths. Such scenarios would present serious challenges for patient management and for prophylaxis of exposed people; environmental contamination could provide a continuing threat to the population (especially those exposed at the beginning of the crisis) and generate panic in the community.

Bioterrorist attacks could be covert or announced and could be caused by virtually any pathogenic microorganism. The case of the Rajneeshee religious cult in The Dalles, Oregon, is an example. The cult planned to infect residents with *Salmonella* on election day to influence the results of county elections. To practice for the attack, they contaminated salad bars at restaurants with *S. Typhimurium* on several occasions before the election. A community-wide outbreak of salmonellosis resulted; at least 751 cases were documented in a county that typically reports fewer than five cases per year. Although bioterrorism was considered a possibility when the outbreak was being investigated by public-health officials, it was considered unlikely. The source of the outbreak became known only when the Federal Bureau of Investigation (FBI) investigated the cult for other criminal violations. A vial of *S. Typhimurium* identical to the outbreak strain was found in a clinical laboratory on the cult's compound, and members of the cult subsequently admitted to contaminating the salad bars and putting *Salmonella* into a city water-supply tank. This incident, among other events, underscores the importance of improving preparedness at all levels.

A bioterrorist attack may be difficult to distinguish from a naturally occurring infectious-disease outbreak. Investigators must first examine the etiology and epidemiology of an outbreak to identify its source, mode of transmission, and people at risk. Certain clues may indicate whether an outbreak is the result of the purposeful release of microorganisms. Naturally occurring diseases are endemic to certain areas and involve traditional cycles of transmission; some diseases occur seasonally, and sentinel cases are not uncommon. In contrast, a disease outbreak due to bioterrorism could occur in a nonendemic-disease area, at any time of year, without warning, and depending on the etiologic agent and mode of transmission, in large numbers—thousands of cases might occur abruptly. Public-health officials must be appropriately sensitized to the possibility of bioterrorism when investigating disease outbreaks. Suspected bioterrorism should be reported promptly to the FBI, which is responsible for coordinating interagency investigations of such episodes. FBI scientists are also well trained in forensic methods for criminal investigations and are prepared to react quickly and effectively.

Maintaining effective disease surveillance is an essential first step in preparedness and is important in helping law-enforcement officials to react swiftly. Ensuring adequate epidemiologic and laboratory capacity nationwide are prerequisites to effective surveillance systems. Preparations also must include plans for rapid identification and characterization of agents involved and for emergency distribution of large quantities of medical supplies, especially antibiotics and vaccines. Coordination and communication links also need to be strengthened to minimize response time, especially at first exposure, but asymptomatic persons may still be treated prophylactically. Also, when response time is shortened, the possibility of apprehending perpetrators increases. Education and training in bioterrorism and its potential consequences must become national priorities.

Many agencies and organizations must work collaboratively to ensure national preparedness against bioterrorist attacks. The Centers for Disease Control and Prevention (CDC) is well-positioned to provide leadership in several areas. In partnership with state health departments, the agency maintains infectious-disease surveillance systems and provides reference laboratory diagnosis and epidemiologic support, especially during outbreak investigations; disseminates public-health recommendations and other information, issues quarantine measures, and provides expert advice on worker health and safety; and is the logical bridge between the public-health community and the FBI's scientific and response capabilities. Enhancing the public-health infrastructure will improve U.S. ability to respond to any infectious-disease outbreak and provide added value in the event of a bioterrorist event.

The Threat of Biological Warfare

Since the discovery of Iraq's biological-weapons program, concern regarding the threat of biological warfare has increased. Anthrax immunizations; increased nuclear, biological, and chemical-defense training; improved detection systems and protective gear; and increased vigilance have been instituted to protect the military.

However, the military is not the only population at risk for biological attacks. To effectively counter the potentially devastating effects of an attack, humans need to understand the basic epidemiologic principles of biological agents used as weapons.

A biological agent is commonly portrayed as a genetically engineered organism resistant to all known vaccines and drugs, highly contagious, and able to harm thousands of people. However, alleged attacks by the Aum

Shinrikyo did not result in a single illness from a biological agent, and the successful 1984 contamination of salad bars in The Dalles, Oregon, by a religious cult involved a common *Salmonella* strain that was not lethal or contagious and was susceptible to antibiotics.

Therefore, the level of suspicion and diligence in identifying and reacting to a biological attack must remain high, since the attack may not follow an expected pattern. Furthermore, a small outbreak of illness could be an early warning of a more serious attack, and recognition and prompt institution of preventive measures (such as effective vaccines and antibiotics) could save thousands of lives.

To facilitate the rapid identification of a bioterrorist attack, all healthcare providers and public-health personnel should have basic epidemiologic skills and knowledge of what to expect in such a setting.

Differential Diagnosis

Any small or large outbreak of disease should be evaluated as a potential bioterrorist attack. This initial investigation does not have to be time-consuming or involve law enforcement. A look at the facts surrounding the outbreak to determine if anything seems unusual or indicative of bioterrorism should suffice. Since a disease outbreak can be the result of intentional contamination, the differential diagnosis of an outbreak should first be considered. The possibilities include a spontaneous outbreak of a known endemic disease, a spontaneous outbreak of a new or reemerging disease, a laboratory accident, or an intentional attack with a biological agent. Epidemiologic tools can assist in differentiating between these possibilities.

The cause of a disease or even the occurrence of something unusual may be very difficult to determine, especially if the initial cases are few. Surveillance needs to be more than routine. Not only unusually high rates of illness but also unusual diseases should signal a warning. For example, even one case of inhalation anthrax should cause immediate concern and action.

Unlike chemical terrorism, biological terrorism is not immediately obvious but may appear insidiously, with primary-care providers witnessing the first cases. However, it may not even be emergency-room personnel who first detect a problem. The first to notice could be a hospital laboratory seeing unusual strains of organisms, or the county epidemiologist keeping track of hospital admissions, or even pharmacists distributing more antibiotics than usual, 911 operators noticing an increase in respiratory distress calls, or funeral directors with increased business. All epidemiologic data should be tracked and aggressively followed to ensure the most rapid recognition and response.

Epidemiologic Approach

The basic epidemiologic approach in the evaluation of a potential bioterrorist or biowarfare attack is not different from any standard epidemiologic investigation. The first step is to use laboratory and clinical findings to confirm that a disease outbreak has occurred. A case definition should be constructed to determine the number of cases and the attack rate. The use of objective criteria in the development of a case definition is very important in determining an accurate case number, as both additional cases may be found and some may be excluded, especially as the potential exists for hysteria to be confused with the actual disease. The estimated rate of illness should be compared with rates during previous years to determine if the rate constitutes a deviation from the norm.

Once the case definition and attack rate have been determined, the outbreak can be characterized in the conventional context of time, place, and person. These data will provide crucial information in determining the potential source of the outbreak.

Epidemic Curve

Using data gathered on cases over time, an epidemic curve can be calculated. The disease pattern is an important factor in differentiating between a natural outbreak and an intentional attack. In most naturally occurring outbreaks, numbers of cases gradually increase as a progressively larger number of people come in contact with other patients, fomites, and vectors that can spread disease. Eventually, most of the population has been exposed and is immune to further disease, and the number of cases, or epidemic curve, gradually decreases. Conversely, a bioterrorism attack is most likely to be caused by a point source, with everyone coming in contact with the agent at approximately the same time. The epidemic curve, in this case, would be compressed, with a peak in a matter of days or even hours, even with physiologic and exposure differences. If the biological agent is contagious, it is possible to see a second curve peak after the first, as original cases expose originally unexposed people to the agent. The steep epidemic curve expected in a bioterrorism attack is similar to what would be seen with other point-source exposures, such as foodborne outbreaks. Therefore, the compressed epidemic curve is still not pathognomonic for an intentional bioterrorism attack.

If a specific group has been exposed, the epidemic curve may indicate the time of exposure. From this information, a possible incubation period can be calculated, which can assist in determining the potential cause of illness, as well as suggesting a possible intentional attack (if the incubation period is shorter than usual as a result of an unusually high inoculum or more effective exposure route). Calculating the incubation period may also help determine if the disease is spread from person to person, which is extremely important to effective disease-control measures.

Epidemiologic Clues

As steep epidemic curves can be seen in natural point-source exposures, additional characteristics of the outbreak should be investigated to determine whether it is the result of a biological attack. None of the following clues alone constitute proof of intentional use of a biological agent, but together they can assist greatly in determining if further investigation is warranted.

- The presence of a large epidemic, with greater caseloads than expected, especially in a discrete population
- More severe disease than expected for a given pathogen, as well as unusual routes of exposure, such as a preponderance of inhalational disease as was seen in Sverdlovsk after the accidental release of aerosolized *Bacillus anthracis* spores
- A disease that is unusual for a given geographic area, is found outside the normal transmission season or is impossible to transmit naturally in the absence of the normal vector for transmission

- Multiple simultaneous epidemics of different diseases
- A disease outbreak with zoonotic as well as human consequences, as many of the potential threat agents are pathogenic to animals
- Unusual strains or variants of organisms or antimicrobial resistance patterns disparate from those circulating
- Higher attack rates in those exposed in certain areas, such as inside a building if the agent was released indoors, or lower rates in those inside a sealed building if an aerosol was released outdoors
- Intelligence that an adversary has access to a particular agent or agents
- Claims by a terrorist of the release of a biologic agent
- Direct evidence of the release of an agent, with findings of equipment, munitions, or tampering

Even with the presence of more than one of the above indicators, it may not be easy to determine that an attack occurred through nefarious means. For example, it took months to determine that the outbreak of salmonellosis in Oregon was caused by intentional contamination of salad bars. Other outbreaks, such as the hantavirus outbreak in the Four Corners area of the United States, have been thought of as possible results of intentional contamination. Even if no conclusive answer can be derived quickly, the means employed in determining the cause of an attack will still provide medical personnel with information that may prevent illness and death.

Recommendations for Preparedness

Improved awareness and readiness should a bioterrorism attack occur include education of all medical personnel, especially primary-care providers and emergency personnel, who are first to see patients affected by a biological attack. Training should include basic epidemiologic principles as well as clinical information on diagnosing and treating agents that pose the highest threat. Training should be refreshed periodically to ensure the skills remain.

Improved surveillance efforts should be instituted with as close to real-time data gathering as possible. All facets of surveillance should be used, including emergency visits, laboratory data, pharmacy use, school absenteeism, or any other data that correlate with an increase in infectious disease. Robust surveillance systems are essential to detcting any emerging or reemerging disease. Quick recognition of any change in disease patterns will facilitate determining the source and preventing further exposure, which should be the key driving force behind any epidemiologic investigation.

Through strong epidemiologic training, close attention to disease patterns, and a healthy respect for the threat of biological terrorism, potential problems can be discovered rapidly, and actions can be taken to decrease the impact of the disease, regardless of its origin.

Section 30.2

High-Priority Pathogens as Agents of Bioterrorism

This section includes text excerpted from "Bioterrorism Agents/Diseases," Centers for Disease Control and Prevention (CDC), April 4, 2018.

Category A

The U.S. public-health system and primary healthcare providers must be prepared to address various biological agents, including pathogens that are rarely seen in the United States. High-priority agents include organisms that pose a risk to national security because they:

- Can be easily disseminated or transmitted from person to person
- Result in high mortality rates and have the potential for major public-health impact
- Might cause public panic and social disruption
- Require special action for public-health preparedness

Agents/Diseases

- Anthrax (*Bacillus anthracis*)
- Botulism (*Clostridium botulinum* toxin)
- Plague (*Yersinia pestis*)
- Smallpox (variola major)
- Tularemia (*Francisella tularensis*)
- Viral hemorrhagic fevers, including
  - Filoviruses (Ebola, Marburg)
  - Arenaviruses (Lassa, Machupo)

Category B

Second-highest-priority agents include those that are moderately easy to disseminate;

- Result in moderate morbidity rates and low mortality rates.
- Require specific enhancements of the Centers for Disease Control and Prevention (CDC's) diagnostic capacity and enhanced disease surveillance.

Agents/Diseases

- Brucellosis (*Brucella* species)
- Epsilon toxin of *Clostridium perfringens*
- Food safety threats (Salmonella species, *Escherichia coli* O157: H7, Shigella)
- Glanders (*Burkholderia mallei*)
- Melioidosis (*Burkholderia pseudomallei*)
- Psittacosis (*Chlamydia psittaci*)
- Q fever (*Coxiella burnetii*)
- Ricin toxin from *Ricinus communis* (castor beans)
- Staphylococcal enterotoxin B
- Typhus fever (*Rickettsia prowazekii*)
- Viral encephalitis (alphaviruses, such as eastern equine encephalitis, Venezuelan equine encephalitis, and western equine encephalitis)
- Water safety threats (*Vibrio cholerae*, *Cryptosporidium parvum*)

Category C

Third-highest-priority agents include emerging pathogens that could be engineered for mass dissemination in the future because of

- Availability
- Ease of production and dissemination
- Potential for high morbidity and mortality rates and major health impact

Agents

- Emerging infectious diseases, such as Nipah virus and hantavirus

Section 30.3

Syndromic Surveillance and Bioterrorism-Related Epidemics

This section includes text excerpted from "Syndromic Surveillance and Bioterrorism-Related Epidemics," Centers for Disease Control and Prevention (CDC), January 10, 2011. Reviewed March 2020.

Because of heightened concerns about the possibility of bioterrorist attacks, public-health agencies are testing new methods of surveillance intended to detect the early manifestations of illness that may occur during a bioterrorism-related epidemic. Broadly labeled "syndromic surveillance," these efforts encompass a spectrum of activities that include monitoring illness syndromes or events, such as medication purchases, that reflect the prodromes of bioterrorism-related diseases. The Centers for Disease Control and Prevention (CDC) estimates that, as of May 2003, health departments in the United States have initiated syndromic surveillance systems in approximately 100 sites throughout the country. The goal of these systems is to enable earlier detection of epidemics and a more timely public-health response, hours or days before disease clusters are recognized clinically, or before specific diagnoses are made and reported to public-health authorities. Whether this goal is achievable remains unproven.

Establishing a Diagnosis

Two pathways to establishing a diagnosis are described by the scenarios below, using single, clandestine dissemination of an anthrax aerosol as an example.

Detection through Syndromic Surveillance

The early signs of inhalational anthrax include nonspecific symptoms that may persist for several days before the onset of more severe disease. Patients with prodromal illnesses seek outpatient care and are assigned nonspecific diagnoses such as "viral syndrome." Data on patients fitting various syndromic criteria are transferred to the health department and tested for aberrant trends. This process "flags" that a statistical detection threshold has been exceeded. Epidemiologists conclude that a preliminary investigation is warranted and collect blood for culture from several patients. Within 18 hours, one culture yields a presumptive diagnosis of anthrax, prompting a full-scale response.

Detection through Clinician Reporting

Some people in whom inhalational anthrax develops will have short incubation periods and prodromes. Respiratory distress occurs in one such person, and he is hospitalized. Routine admission procedures include blood cultures. Within 18 hours, a presumptive diagnosis of anthrax is made. The patient's physician informs the local health department, prompting a full-scale response.

   In practice, how a bioterrorism attack might be detected and diagnosed will probably be more complex. Published descriptions of 11 people with inhalational anthrax in the United States in 2001 provide some insight into this issue, even though that epidemic was too small and geographically diffuse to be detectable by syndromic surveillance. For six patients with known dates of exposure, the median duration between exposure and symptom onset was 4 days (range 4–6 days). The median duration between onset and the initial healthcare visit was 3 days (range 1–7 days), and the median duration between onset of symptoms and hospitalization was 4 days (range 3–7 days). Two of the 11 patients visited emergency departments and were sent home with diagnoses of gastroenteritis or viral syndrome 1 day before admission. In one patient, a blood culture obtained in the emergency room was read as positive for gram-positive bacilli the following day, which prompted recall of the patient. The culture was subsequently confirmed as positive for *Bacillus anthracis*. Two other patients were seen by primary-care physicians and sent home with diagnoses of viral syndrome or bronchitis 2 to 3 days before admission, including one patient who was put on empiric antibiotic therapy. For seven other patients, initial emergency-room or hospital visits led directly to admission. In addition to the patient whose blood culture was obtained in an emergency room, seven others had not received prior antibiotic therapy, and *B. anthracis* was presumptively identified from the blood within 24 hours of culture. One of these seven patients was the index patient, in whom *B. anthracis* was also recognized in the cerebrospinal fluid within 7 hours of specimen collection. Three other patients had received antibiotics before blood cultures were taken (one as an outpatient and two at the time of hospital admission), requiring alternative diagnostic methods.

Despite the small number of patients, their experience offers four lessons for detecting an epidemic of inhalational anthrax. First, a key objective of syndromic surveillance is to detect early-stage disease, but fewer than half of these patients sought care before hospitalization was necessary, and the interval between such care and admission was relatively narrow (1–3 days). This finding suggests that syndromic surveillance data must be processed, analyzed, and acted upon quickly if such data are to provide a clue to the diagnosis in advance of late-stage disease. Second, emergency-room data are a common source for syndromic surveillance, but detecting an increase in visits coincident with hospital admission may not provide an early warning because the time needed to process surveillance data and investigate suspected cases would be at least as long as the time for admission blood cultures to be positive for *B. anthracis*. Blood cultures are likely to be routine for patients admitted with fever and severe respiratory illness, regardless of whether anthrax is considered as a diagnostic possibility, and *B. anthracis* grows readily in culture in the absence of prior antibiotic therapy, as observed in most of these patients. Thus, if emergency-room data are to be useful in early detection of an anthrax epidemic, those data would need to be for visits that occur before hospital care is required—a pattern observed in only two patients. Third, the four patients who received early care and were discharged to their homes were assigned three different diagnoses, which suggests that syndromic surveillance systems must address the potential variability in how patients with the same infection may be diagnosed during the prodrome phase. Fourth, rapid diagnosis after hospitalization was possible only in those patients who had not received antibiotics before cultures were taken. This finding emphasizes the importance of judicious use of antibiotics in patients with nonspecific illness.

In addition to the specific attributes of individual bioterrorism agents, multiple considerations will shape the recognition of a bioterrorism-related epidemic. Five of these attributes follow.

Size

Syndromic surveillance would not detect outbreaks too small to trigger statistical alarms. Size would be affected by the virulence of the agent, its potential for person-to-person transmission, the extent and mode of agent dissemination, whether dissemination occurs in more than one time or place, and population vulnerability.

Population Dispersion

How people change locations after exposure will affect whether disease occurs in a concentrated or wide area, and thus whether clustering is apparent to clinicians or detectable through syndromic surveillance at specific sites.

Healthcare

The more knowledgeable providers are about bioterrorism agents, the greater the likelihood of recognition. Routine diagnostic practices or access to reference laboratories may affect the timeliness of diagnosis for some diseases. Familiarity with reporting procedures would increase prompt reporting of suspected or diagnosed cases.

Syndromic Surveillance

Syndromic surveillance will be affected by the selection of data sources, timeliness of information management, the definition of syndrome categories, selection of statistical-detection thresholds, availability of resources for followup, experience with false alarms, and criteria for initiating investigations.

Season

A fifth key attribute is seasonality. An increase in illness associated with a bioterrorism attack may be more difficult to detect if it occurs during a seasonal upswing in naturally occurring disease.

Agent- and disease-specific attributes may be among the most important factors affecting detection and diagnosis. The incubation period and its distribution in the population will affect the rate at which new cases develop and thus how quickly an alarm threshold is exceeded or whether clinicians recognize a temporal and geographic cluster. If a disease has a short prodrome, the chances are increased that a patient would be hospitalized and a definitive evaluation initiated before an increase in cases triggered a surveillance alarm. Alternatively, if a disease has a relatively long prodrome, chances are greater that prediagnostic events (e.g., purchase of medications or use of outpatient care for nonspecific complaints) would accrue to levels that exceed syndromic surveillance thresholds before definitive diagnostic evaluations are completed among patients with more severe disease. Arousing clinical suspicion for a particular diagnosis will depend on the specificity of both the early and late stages of illness as well as the presence or absence of a typical feature such as mediastinal widening in inhalational anthrax, that should alert clinicians to the diagnosis. If a routinely performed test is apt to be diagnostic in a short time (e.g., the blood culture in anthrax), a rapid diagnosis is likely, even in the absence of clinical suspicion. If routine tests are unlikely to yield a rapid diagnosis (e.g., the blood culture for the cause of tularemia, *Francisella tularensis*, or if the diagnosis requires a special test (e.g., the hemorrhagic fever viruses), a diagnosis may be delayed if not immediately considered.

The public-health benefit resulting from early detection of an epidemic is likely to vary by disease. If a disease has a relatively wide distribution of potential onsets, early recognition provides greater opportunity to administer prophylaxis to exposed people. For example, based on data from the Sverdlovsk incident, researchers Brookmeyer and Blades estimated that the use of antibiotic prophylaxis during the 2001 anthrax outbreak prevented nine cases of inhalational disease among exposed persons. If the incubation period of the disease has a relatively narrow distribution, early recognition may offer little opportunity for postexposure prophylaxis, although a potential benefit would remain for alerting healthcare providers and informing their care of others with similar symptoms. This pattern of illness is apt to result from exposure to an *F. tularensis* aerosol, which would likely result in an explosive epidemic with an abrupt onset and limited duration.

Detecting Specific Bioterrorism Epidemics and Agents

The attributes of the CDC category A bioterrorism agents that affect their detection, as well as the benefits of early detection, are on the basis of potential bioterrorism-related epidemic profiles developed by experts. These profiles reflect the knowledge of these diseases; their epidemiology might differ if novel modes of dissemination or preparation were employed. Each disease has attributes that could increase or decrease the likelihood of early-outbreak recognition through either clinical diagnosis or syndromic surveillance.

Inhalational Anthrax

The distribution of the incubation period for inhalational anthrax can be relatively broad as observed in Sverdlovsk (2–43 days); most cases occur within 1 to 2 weeks after exposure. In the 2001 United States outbreak, the distribution of incubation periods was more limited, 4 to 6 days, although later-onset cases may have been averted by antibiotic prophylaxis. The nonspecific prodrome for anthrax may last from several hours to several days. Taken together, these data suggest that the initial slope of an epidemic curve may be comparatively gradual during the first week, leading to slower recognition through syndromic surveillance than for other infections caused by bioterrorist agents with pulmonary manifestations, such as tularemia or pneumonic plague.

In contrast, mediastinal widening on chest x-ray or computed tomographic scan or Gram stain of cerebrospinal or pleural fluid should lead an alert and knowledgeable physician to consider the diagnosis of anthrax, even though these tests may not be conducted until relatively late in the clinical course. *B. anthracis* is likely to be detected quickly in cultures, favoring clinical recognition. Retrospective analysis of data from 2001 showed that inhalational anthrax can be distinguished from influenzas such as illness or community-acquired pneumonia by using an algorithm that combines clinical and laboratory findings, although the practical utility of this approach is untested. In addition to permitting antibiotic use among ill persons, early recognition would enable postexposure antibiotic prophylaxis.

Tularemia

The typical incubation period for tularemia is relatively narrow after a person is exposed to aerosolized *F. tularensis*, with abrupt onset of nonspecific febrile illness, with or without respiratory symptoms, in 3 to 5 days (range 1–14 days), followed by rapid progression to life-threatening pneumonitis. This relatively narrow incubation period for most patients and rapid progression to severe disease would lead to a rapid increase in cases after a large and acute exposure. Finding a number of such cases in a short interval should trigger both syndromic surveillance alarms and clinical suspicion. *F. tularensis* is a slow-growing and fastidious organism and may take up to 5 days after inoculation to be detectable, if it is detected at all, in a routinely processed blood culture. The use of special laboratory techniques may be required, delaying the likelihood of detection in the absence of clinical suspicion. After an epidemic is recognized, specific antibiotic therapy is recommended for exposed people in whom a febrile illness develops.

Pneumonic Plague

Exposure to aerosolized *Yersinia pestis* results in the pneumonic plague, which has a typical incubation period of 2 to 4 days (range 1–6 days). The disease has a relatively short prodrome, followed by rapidly progressive pneumonia, which would lead to a rapid increase in cases at the onset of an epidemic. Standard clinical-laboratory findings are nonspecific, which alone might not prompt clinical suspicion, but microscopic examination of a sputum smear may show characteristic findings, which should prompt consideration of the diagnosis. Cultures of blood or sputum are apt to show growth within 24 to 48 hours, but routine procedures may misidentify *Y. pestis* unless the diagnosis is suspected and special attention is given to specimen processing. Confirming the diagnosis depends on special tests available through reference laboratories. Treatment the first day of symptoms is generally considered necessary to prevent death in the pneumonic plague, so early recognition of an aerosol plague attack would enable lifesaving use of antibiotics in febrile patients and prophylaxis of contacts.

Botulism

Foodborne botulism typically has a relatively narrow incubation period (12–72 hours), which may vary from 2 hours to 8 days, depending on the inoculum. For the three known cases of inhalational botulism attributed to relatively low exposure to aerosolized toxin, the incubation period was approximately 72 hours. The characteristic clinical picture of descending paralysis should prompt consideration of botulism, and this unique pattern among bioterrorism agents lends itself to a specific syndrome category. However, the illness may be misdiagnosed, as observed in a large foodborne outbreak of botulism in 1985; 28 people who had eaten at a particular restaurant and in whom botulism had developed were assigned other diagnoses before the geographically dispersed outbreak was recognized and publicized in the media. Symptoms of inhalation botulism, choking, dysphagia, and dysarthria dominating the clinical picture, may differ from those associated with the ingestion of toxin and complicate the recognition of the disease. Specialized testing for botulinum toxin is available at a limited number of state laboratories and the CDC. Postexposure prophylaxis is limited by the scarcity of, and potential for, allergic reactions to botulinum antitoxin, leading to recommendations that exposed persons be observed carefully for early signs of botulism, which should prompt antitoxin use. Antitoxin should be given as early as possible—another fact that highlights the importance of early detection. Depending on the level of exposure and the geographic dispersion of affected persons, syndromic surveillance for characteristic neurologic symptoms could aid outbreak detection, or the occurrence of an epidemic might be obvious to clinicians.

Smallpox

The incubation period of smallpox is usually 12 to 14 days but may range from 7 to 17 days. The early symptomatic phase includes a severe febrile illness and appearance of a nonspecific macular rash over a 2- to 4-day period, followed by evolution to a vesicular and then pustular rash over the next 4 to 5 days. Thus, the initial phase of smallpox may lend itself to detection through surveillance of a febrile-rash illness syndrome. Once smallpox is suspected, the virus can be rapidly detected by electron microscopic examination of vesicular or pustular fluid, if laboratory resources for electron microscopy are available, or by a polymerase chain reaction, if the necessary primers are available. Contacts can be protected by vaccination up to 4 days after exposure. Discourse is substantial about the relative merits of pre-event versus postevent vaccination. Syndromic surveillance may show an increase in febrile-rash illness, although once the characteristic rash appears, the diagnosis should be quickly established.

Viral Hemorrhagic Fevers

This category includes multiple infectious agents that range from having a relatively broad to narrow incubation period (e.g., Ebola, 2–21 days; yellow fever 3–6 days). These diseases present with nonspecific prodromes that may have an insidious or abrupt onset. In severe cases, the prodrome is followed by hypotension, shock, central nervous system dysfunction, and a bleeding diathesis. The differential diagnosis includes a variety of viral and bacterial diseases. Establishing the diagnosis depends on clinical suspicion and the results of specific tests that must be requested from the CDC or the U.S. Army Medical Research Institute of Infectious Diseases (USAMRIID). The value of postexposure prophylaxis with antiviral medications is uncertain, and (with the exception of yellow fever, for which a vaccine is available) response measures are limited to isolation and observation of exposed persons, treatment with ribavirin (if the virus is one that responds to that antiviral drug), and careful attention to infection-control measures. Patients seen with symptoms during the prodromal phase may not clearly fit into a single syndrome category, but syndromic surveillance focused on the early signs of a febrile bleeding disorder would be more specific.

One of the biggest concerns about syndromic surveillance is its potentially low specificity, resulting in the use of resources to investigate false alarms. Specificity for distinguishing bioterrorism-related epidemics from more ordinary illnesses may be low because the early symptoms of bioterrorism-related illness overlap with those of many common infections. Specificity for distinguishing any type of outbreak from random variations in illness trends may be low if statistical detection thresholds are reduced to enhance sensitivity and timeliness. The likelihood that a given alarm represents a bioterrorism event will be low, assuming that the probability of such an event is low in a given locality. Approaches used to increase specificity include requiring that aberrant trends be sustained for at least 2 days or that aberrant trends be detected in multiple systems. Another approach to enhancing specificity would be to focus surveillance on the severe phases of the disease, since the category A bioterrorism infections are more likely than many common infections to progress to life-threatening illness. For those diseases that are likely to progress rapidly, such as pneumonic plague, syndromic detection of severe disease (e.g., through emergency-room visits, hospital admissions, or deaths) may be more feasible than detection aimed at early indicators before care is sought (e.g., purchases of over-the-counter medications) or when illness is less severe (e.g., primary-care visits). Whether detection of syndromic late-stage disease offers an advantage over detection through clinical evaluation will depend on the attributes of the infections and diagnostic resources, as described above.

Predicting how the mix of relevant factors would combine in a given situation to affect the recognition of a bioterrorism-related epidemic is difficult, although mathematical models may provide further insight. The most important factors affecting early detection are likely to be the rate of accrual of cases at the outset of an epidemic, geographic clustering, the selection of syndromic surveillance methods, and the likelihood of making a diagnosis quickly in clinical practice.

Ongoing efforts to strengthen the public-health infrastructure and to educate healthcare providers about bioterrorism diseases and reporting procedures should strengthen the ability to recognize bioterrorism outbreaks. For example, in Trenton, New Jersey in 2001, reporting of two early cases of cutaneous anthrax was delayed until publicity about other anthrax cases prompted physicians to consider the diagnosis and notify the health department, suggesting that opportunities for earlier use of postexposure prophylaxis were missed. In addition, while the importance of diagnostic tools, including rapid tests, should be emphasized, the essential role of existing diagnostic techniques should not be overlooked. Clinical suspicion is critical, and a key prompt for arousing clinical suspicion may be the microscopic examination of a routinely collected specimen, as occurred in the index case of the 2001 anthrax outbreak, when a Gram stain of the cerebrospinal fluid led to the diagnosis. However, as is highlighted by the Institute of Medicine, the use of basic diagnostic tests has decreased because of efforts to reduce the costs of care, the increasing use of empiric broad-spectrum antibiotic therapy, and federal laboratory regulations, such as the Clinical Laboratory Improvement Amendments of 1988 (CLIA), which have discouraged laboratory evaluation in some clinical settings.

While focused on the role of syndromic surveillance in detecting a bioterrorism-related epidemic, other uses of syndromic surveillance include detecting naturally occurring epidemics, providing reassurance that epidemics are not occurring when threats or rumors arise, and tracking bioterrorism-related epidemics regardless of the mode of detection.

Syndromic surveillance is intended to enhance, rather than replace, traditional approaches to epidemic detection. Evaluation of syndromic surveillance to consider the spectrum of potential uses is essential. A certain level of false alarms, as the result of either syndromic surveillance or calls from clinicians, will be necessary to ensure that opportunities for detection are not missed. Efforts to enhance the predictive value of syndromic surveillance will be offset by costs in timeliness and sensitivity, and defining the right balance in practice, particularly in the absence of an accurate assessment of bioterrorism risk, will be essential.

Two committees of the National Academies have recommended a more careful evaluation of the usefulness of syndromic surveillance before it is more widely implemented. Because the epidemiologic characteristics of different bioterrorism agents may vary in ways that affect the detection of epidemics, these evaluations should address the epidemiology of specific bioterrorism agents. Efforts to detect bioterrorism epidemics at an early stage should not only address the development of innovative surveillance mechanisms, but also strengthen resources for diagnosis and enhance relationships between clinicians and public-health agencies—relationships that will ensure that clinicians notify public-health authorities if they suspect or diagnose a possible bioterrorism-related disease.

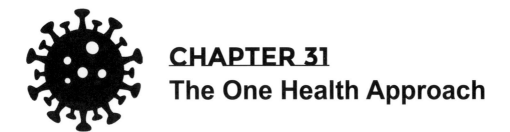

CHAPTER 31
The One Health Approach

Chapter Contents

Section 31.1
One Health Basics

This section includes text excerpted from "One Health Basics," Centers for Disease Control and Prevention (CDC), November 5, 2018.

One Health is a collaborative, multisectoral, and transdisciplinary approach—working at the local, regional, national, and global levels—with the goal of achieving optimal health outcomes by recognizing the interconnection between people, animals, plants, and their shared environment.

What Is One Health?

One Health is an approach that recognizes that the health of people is closely connected to the health of animals and our shared environment. One Health is not new, but the approach has become more important in recent years. This is because many factors have changed interactions between people, animals, plants, and our environment.

- Human populations are growing and expanding into new geographic areas. As a result, more people live in close contact with wild and domestic animals, both livestock and pets. Animals play an important role in our lives, whether for food, fiber, livelihoods, travel, sport, education, or companionship. Close contact with animals and their environments provides more opportunities for diseases to pass between animals and people.
- The earth has experienced changes in climate and land use, such as deforestation and intensive farming practices. Disruptions in environmental conditions and habitats can provide new opportunities for diseases to pass to animals.
- The movement of people, animals, and animal products has increased from international travel and trade. As a result, diseases can spread quickly across borders and around the globe.

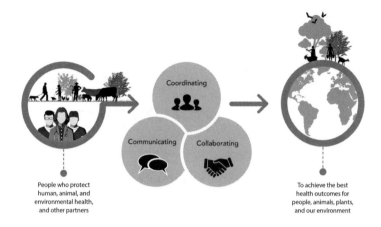

Figure 31.1. One Health

These changes have led to the spread of existing or known (endemic) and new or emerging zoonotic diseases, which are diseases that can spread between animals and people. Examples of zoonotic diseases include:

- Rabies
- *Salmonella* infection
- West Nile virus (WNV) infection
- Q Fever (*Coxiella burnetii*)
- Anthrax
- Brucellosis
- Lyme disease
- Ringworm
- Ebola

Animals also share our susceptibility to some diseases and environmental hazards. Because of this, they can sometimes serve as early warning signs of potential human illness. For example, birds often die of WNV before people in the same area get sick with WNV infection.

What Are Common One Health Issues?

One Health issues include zoonotic diseases, antimicrobial resistance, food safety and food security, vector-borne diseases, environmental contamination, and other health threats shared by people, animals, and the environment. Even the fields of chronic disease, mental health, injury, occupational health, and noncommunicable diseases can benefit from a One Health approach involving collaboration across disciplines and sectors.

How Does a One Health Approach Work?

One Health is gaining recognition in the United States and globally as an effective way to fight health issues at the human–animal–environment interface, including zoonotic diseases. The Centers for Disease Control and Prevention (CDC) uses a One Health approach by involving experts in human, animal, environmental health, and other relevant disciplines and sectors in monitoring and controlling public-health threats and to learn about how diseases spread among people, animals, plants, and the environment.

Successful public-health interventions require the cooperation of human, animal, and environmental health partners. Professionals in human health (doctors, nurses, public-health practitioners, epidemiologists), animal health (veterinarians, paraprofessionals, agricultural workers), environment (ecologists, wildlife experts), and other areas of expertise need to communicate, collaborate on, and coordinate activities. Other relevant players in a One Health approach could include law enforcement, policymakers, agriculture, communities, and even pet owners. No one person, organization, or sector can address issues at the animal–human–environment interface alone.

By promoting collaboration across all sectors, a One Health approach can achieve the best health outcomes for people, animals, and plants in a shared environment.

Section 31.2

Zoonoses and One Health

This section includes text excerpted from
"Perspectives: Zoonoses: The One Health Approach,"
Centers for Disease Control and Prevention (CDC),
June 24, 2019.

The One Health approach to zoonotic illnesses is predicated on the connection that exists between people, animals, and the environment. As a discipline, One Health includes specialists from multiple health sectors: human medicine and public-health, veterinary medicine, and environmental health; its areas of interest cover zoonotic diseases, antimicrobial resistance, food safety and security, vector-borne diseases, and other shared health threats at the human–animal–environment interface.

No single sector can address challenges at the human–animal–environment interface alone, but coordinated efforts to identify and manage animal or environmental sources of infection can prevent, detect, and respond to infectious-disease threats. For example, programs that use a One Health approach between medical and veterinary professionals have controlled rabies in animals; annual or biannual mass dog-vaccination campaigns prevent human rabies deaths.

Zoonotic Diseases

Diseases addressed by the One Health approach are typically zoonotic. Approximately 60 percent of all known human infectious-disease agents originate in animals, including brucellosis, anthrax, and salmonellosis. Most new or emerging infectious-diseases in humans, such as Ebola, Middle East respiratory syndrome (MERS), and highly pathogenic avian influenzaare zoonotic. Further, 80 percent of disease agents identified with bioterrorism potential are zoonotic.

One Health and Travel Medicine

International travelers may be at risk of zoonotic diseases through a variety of exposures not limited to wild or domestic animal contact or insect vectors. Contaminated environmental surfaces, freshwater sources (such as ponds and rivers), and food and beverages have also been implicated as sources of zoonotic illness in humans. Failure to identify sources of exposure associated with a traveler's destination, itinerary, and activities can delay correct diagnosis and treatment and potentially increase the risk for further transmission of disease.

Patients benefit when healthcare providers employ the One Health approach. In pretravel consultation, providers should make travelers aware of zoonotic and other infectious-disease risks in the areas where they travel and encourage them to take measures to reduce those risks (for example, through vaccinations or prophylactic medications). In the posttravel setting, providers should ask questions about interactions with animals (such as pets, free-roaming animals, livestock, and wildlife), including the apparent health of these animals and animal habitats encountered during travel. Occasionally, healthcare providers and veterinarians may need to consult together on a patient with a suspected zoonotic disease.

Zoonotic Transmission: Direct and Indirect Animal Contact

Travelers must remain aware of the risks associated with animal contact. Direct contact with the saliva, blood, urine, mucus, feces, or other body fluids of an infected animal increases the risk of exposure to zoonotic pathogens; common routes of contact include petting or handling animals and being bitten or scratched. Additionally, ecotourism ventures that involve riding animals such as horses, camels, or elephants pose a potential risk for injury or zoonotic diseases. However, it is difficult to know which animals could be carrying pathogenic organisms, especially since animal carriers can appear healthy. Contact with environmental surfaces where animals have been can also pose a risk of zoonotic-disease transmission. Travelers should avoid contact with animals and their secretions, and if animal contact cannot be avoided, travelers should ensure they are up-to-date with recommended vaccinations and seek medical care if bitten or scratched.

Zoonotic Transmission: Exposure to Disease Vectors

Rickettsial diseases, plague (*Yersinia pestis* infection), and yellow fever are all examples of zoonotic diseases transmitted by insect vectors. Travelers can minimize exposure to vectors by adhering to insect precautions and regularly performing tick checks on people and any traveling pets.

Zoonotic Transmission: Foodborne Exposure

Because many foodborne pathogens have an animal reservoir, consuming raw or undercooked animal parts or products exposes travelers to zoonotic pathogens. In many developing countries, for example, unpasteurized milk or dairy products (cheese, for example) made from unpasteurized milk carries the risk of *Brucella*, *Campylobacter*, *Cryptosporidium*, *Listeria*, and other zoonotic pathogens. Travelers should avoid eating bushmeat—raw, smoked, or partially processed meat from bats, nonhuman primates, rodents, or other wild animals. Advise travelers to eat only fully cooked meat, fish, shellfish, eggs, and other foods, and to drink only pasteurized milk and dairy products, to reduce the risk of foodborne illness while traveling.

Section 31.3

Working Together for One Health

This section includes text excerpted from "Working Together for One Health," Centers for Disease Control and Prevention (CDC), October 2, 2019.

One Health is the idea that the health of people is connected to the health of animals and our shared environment.

We Are All Connected

Did you know that animals and humans often can be affected by many of the same diseases and environmental issues? Some diseases, called zoonotic diseases, can be spread between animals and people. More than half of all infections people can get can be spread by animals—a few examples include coronavirus (currently, COVID-19), rabies, *Salmonella*, and West Nile virus (WNV). Environmental issues such as harmful algal blooms or lead contamination also can affect the health of both people and animals. Antimicrobial resistance is another emerging threat to the health of people and animals, and resistant germs often spread through our shared environment.

Animals can sometimes serve as early warning signals of potential human outbreaks. Tracking diseases in animals helps to keep domestic and wild animals healthy, and also can help prevent illnesses and disease outbreaks in people.

- *Salmonella* infections have been linked to contact with live poultry in backyard flocks, pet guinea pigs, reptiles such as lizards and turtles, as well as other pets. People can get sick with *Salmonella* by touching these animals or through contact with the animal's environment, including coops, cages, and other habitats.

- Wild water birds are hosts to many influenza A viruses that do not normally infect people but can infect and spread among domestic poultry. Some of these bird viruses can be passed to humans through contact with infected animals or virus-contaminated environments. Avian influenza A (H7N9) and H5N1 viruses are examples of bird flu viruses that are known to infect people. Other influenza A viruses also infect and spread in pigs, and there have been sporadic infections in people with these viruses.

- Rift Valley fever (RVF) is caused by a virus that is spread by mosquitoes, and has caused multiple outbreaks in Africa and the Middle East. People can get RVF from bites of infected mosquitoes, but more commonly people are infected through contact with blood, body fluids, or tissues of infected animals (mainly livestock). RVF can cause serious disease in both people and animals. Vaccinating animals can help protect people while also protecting the animals they rely on for food and as a source of income.

- Harmful algal bloom (HAB)-related illnesses can occur when algae and other plantlike organisms in water produce toxins. Algal blooms can occur in fresh, brackish, and saltwater, and they become HABs when the algae grow quickly. HABs can harm animals, people, or the environment.

One Health Involves Everyone

A One Health approach to public-health involves many experts working together to improve the health of people, animals—including pets, livestock, and wildlife—and the environment. Common types of professionals involved in One Health work include epidemiologists (disease detectives), laboratorians, human healthcare providers, veterinarians, physicians, nurses, scientists, ecologists, and policymakers. However, One Health issues can affect everyone, from pet owners, travelers, and farmers to anyone who buys and eats food or drinks or swims in water.

Partnerships and communication between experts in animal, human, and environmental health are an essential part of the One Health approach. A One Health approach can also include other partners and organizations working on shared health threats. Working together allows these experts to have the biggest impact on improving health for both people and animals. The Centers for Disease Control and Prevention (CDC) has partners in the United States and around the world, all working together to keep people healthy and educated about One Health. From researching sick sea otters in California to developing an app for farmers to track illness in animal herds, much of the One Health work being done around the world is dependent on agencies and organizations supporting each other and sharing resources and knowledge. All of this work can help to predict, prevent, and control zoonotic-disease outbreaks that threaten human and animal health, and can address other threats that affect humans, animals, and our shared environment.

How You Can Help

You can be a One Health hero by taking steps to prevent diseases spread between animals and people.

- Practice healthy pet habits
  - In the United States, pets and other animals such as backyard poultry are often the sources of disease outbreaks in people. To stay healthy, take steps to make sure your pet stays healthy and practice good hygiene around your pets.
- Keep wildlife wild
  - Enjoy wildlife from a distance to reduce the risk of illness and injury to you, your pets, and wild animals.
- Professionals in many fields, but especially human healthcare, veterinary medicine, public-health, animal health, and environmental health, can use a One Health approach.
  - Professionals should recognize the connection between human health, animal health, and the environment, and work together to achieve the best health for all.

CHAPTER 32
Strengthening Global Health Capacity against Infectious-Disease Threats

Chapter Contents

Global Disease Detection and Public-Health Research

This section includes text excerpted from "Global Disease Detection— Achievements in Applied Public Health Research, Capacity Building, and Public Health Diplomacy, 2001–2016," Centers for Disease Control and Prevention (CDC), December 2017.

Infectious Disease Outbreaks

Infectious disease outbreaks present a serious health threat that requires early detection and effective preventive action to avoid regional or even global spread. Such actions enhance global health security by protecting the health of people in the affected regions and in the United States. Epidemics, including severe acute respiratory syndrome (SARS) during 2002 to 2003, pandemic influenza A (H1N1) in 2009, Ebola virus disease (EVD) in 2014, and Zika virus infection during 2015 to 2016, as well as the current COVID-19 coronavirus pandemic, underscore this risk and highlight the critical need for building core global public-health capacity for detection and response.

In 2001, the Centers for Disease Control and Prevention (CDC) established the International Emerging Infections Program (IEIP) to conduct applied public-health surveillance and research aimed at preventing infectious-disease outbreaks with pandemic potential. IEIP placed CDC staff in key overseas locations to work with national public-health institutes and their partners to establish sentinel surveillance and conduct applied research on emerging infectious diseases. The program was modeled after the U.S. based Emerging Infections Program (EIP), a network of state health departments and their partners that conduct surveillance of certain infections and thereby provide a foundation for various epidemiologic studies to explore risk factors, a spectrum of disease, and prevention strategies. The IEIP had a similar objective, but on a global platform; namely, to conduct applied public-health research in strategic

507

global locations to prevent, detect, and control emerging and reemerging pathogens.

The CDC established the Global Disease Detection Program (GDD) in 2004 by using existing research programs within the IEIP as the scientific backbone of its GDD regional centers; this effort was made in response to data gaps identified during the SARS epidemic. The GDD Program's mission is to ensure that infectious diseases were detected and stopped at the source before crossing international borders. The GDD Program, like IEIP, set up a network of CDC technical experts stationed in GDD regional centers located in multiple countries across World Health Organization (WHO) regions. GDD regional centers were initially set up in countries with an IEIP presence (Thailand, Kenya, Guatemala, Egypt, China, and Kazakhstan). Subsequently, new GDD regional centers were established in Bangladesh, India, South Africa, and Georgia. These centers serve as regional resources for neighboring countries and are a framework for improving public health and global health security through close collaboration with local partners. To date, the 10 GDD regional centers have supported 90 countries around the world, including the United States. The GDD regional centers have assisted in the United States domestic public-health institutions in response to infectious diseases that affected international visitors while in the United States and the United States citizens while abroad.

The GDD Program promotes intersectoral public-health responses and applied epidemiologic research that includes ministries of health and agriculture, academic institutions, other United States government programs, and international and nongovernmental organizations (NGOs). These established and trusted relationships with national governments enable more effective prevention and detection of emerging infectious diseases. The GDD regional centers also provide an in-country infrastructure that enables the CDC to respond rapidly to public-health threats. A critical strength of the GDD Program is the long-term assignment (i.e., 2 to 6 years) of epidemiologists, laboratorians, statisticians, and other diverse technical staff at GDD regional centers in host countries. The GDD technical staff work alongside locally hired technical staff to foster close collaboration and bilateral knowledge transfer with host country partners. These strategically placed GDD technical staff can have localized information for early detection of unusual infectious disease events. During public-health emergencies, where time lost often equals lives lost, the ability to leverage trusted international public-health scientific partnerships is essential for life-saving action. The GDD field staff are often a first line of response during an epidemic. During the 2014 to 2016 West Africa Ebola outbreak, 30 GDD field-assigned staff, including United States and local personnel, deployed from GDD regional centers to assist with establishing diagnostic, contact-tracing, and data-analysis capacity. GDD field-staff experience in international settings was critical to the response and facilitated quick integration into ongoing response and prevention efforts. The GDD's sustained capacity-building efforts enabled these forward-deployed assets to respond quickly not only in their own regions, but also across the globe.

Activities and Accomplishments

The core activities of the GDD Program focus on applied public-health research, surveillance, laboratory, public-health informatics, and technical capacity building. "Applied public-health research" refers to activities that generate data to answer a research question, test a hypothesis, evaluate a program or programmatic element (e.g., a public-health practice, a surveillance system, data quality), or provide information for evidence-based decision making. "Surveillance" refers to activities that collect health-related data in a systematic manner over time to inform public health action. "Laboratory" refers to activities that collect specimens for laboratory analyses. "Informatics" refers to any activity that collects and aggregates data (paper-based or electronic) that could be used for further analysis. "Capacity building" refers to activities that increase the skills, infrastructure, or resources of individuals or partnering organizations. GDD program projects incorporate multiple core activities, with technical capacity building, laboratory, and public-health research being most common. These activities are essential for the identification of new health threats, monitoring and tracking of health threats over time, and for conducting applied research and pathogen discovery. At times, regional centers might conduct studies of noninfectious causes of illnesses because it is not always clear whether the etiologic agent is a pathogen, a toxin, or some other cause at the beginning of an outbreak. The GDD Program also provides a robust framework for public-health diplomacy and the development and implementation of coordinated multisite activities and studies.

Global Disease Detection by the Numbers

In 2015, the GDD Program performed a portfolio review of activities in the GDD regional centers for fiscal years 2015 and 2016 (October 1, 2014 to September 30, 2016). The unit of analysis was a GDD Program–funded project. Multiyear projects were counted once. Projects were not weighted by the size or scope of a project; thus, a small research study was equivalent to a large, multiyear, population-based surveillance project. The study excluded projects that listed HIV (n = 2) or noncommunicable disease (n = 1) as their primary focus. Projects were classified into core activity areas: technical capacity building, surveillance, applied public-health research, laboratory, and informatics. Activity areas were not mutually exclusive, so a project could be classified in multiple areas.

Overall, the 10 GDD regional centers engaged in 205 discrete projects from October 2014 to September 2016. The number of projects per GDD regional center ranged from 11 to 36. The variability in number of projects per center was attributable to a combination of factors, including the age of the center, the geographic region covered by the center, and funding and staffing resources available for the center. Capacity-building projects (n = 125) were most common. Technical projects were also classified into topical areas based on the key focus of the project. Topical areas were collated and categorized by major groupings. The variability in the range of topical areas was attributable to a combination of factors, including the epidemiology of the disease (nationally and globally), available funding, the technical capacity at the local level, and the changing priorities of the United States and local partners (e.g., ministries of health, national public-health institutes, and research institutes). Of 205 projects with a defined topical area, 24 percent (n = 50) were focused on acute respiratory illness, which is expected given that respiratory-disease surveillance has been a core function since the inception of the program. Health-system strengthening (n = 36), One Health (n = 30), and emerging infectious disease (n = 22) were the next most common topical areas. The increasing prevalence of these new topical areas indicates an expansion of the breadth of projects being conducted by GDD regional centers.

Global Disease Detection Core Activities
Applied Public-Health Research

The GDD Program has a broad portfolio of applied public-health research and special epidemiologic studies, ranging from ensuring infection-control practices for Nipah virus in Bangladesh to evaluating antimicrobial drug–resistant invasive salmonellosis in Thailand. Conducting applied public-health research and epidemiologic studies in international settings can address important knowledge gaps in infectious-disease issues. Many of these issues would be difficult to examine in the United States, primarily because of the low prevalence of many infectious-diseases. International public-health research studies contribute to the scientific knowledge base and help answer questions that can influence U.S. public-health policy.

Examples range from gathering data for the issuance of travel notices to conducting vaccine studies needed to guide domestic vaccination guidelines. The GDD regional centers work closely with international partners, often a ministry of health or national public-health institute, to identify common areas of research interests and national priorities. The data generated from these collaborations have been used by host governments to quantify the public-health issue and, ultimately, to guide and inform public-health policy. Implementing high-quality research studies also serves as a hands-on training mechanism for international partners. Projects are conducted in collaboration with in-country hosts, from developing the concept, writing the research protocol, implementing the study, analyzing and interpreting the data, to publishing the results. A tangible way that highlights the results of these collaborations is dissemination of findings in the scientific literature.

Surveillance

GDD regional centers partner with host countries to develop and strengthen surveillance for key illnesses and to limit the spread of disease to the point of origin. Projects integrate laboratory, clinical, and epidemiologic information that can guide public-health interventions and other control measures. GDD centers achieve this objective through several types of surveillance strategies, such as syndrome based, laboratory-based, population-based, and sentinel systems. Population-based surveillance provides a framework for applied public-health research that can help to characterize the burden, risk factors, and transmission characteristics of new or emerging infectious diseases and to assess the effectiveness of prevention strategies. Sentinel surveillance in a few key sites or facilities for specific or syndromic infectious diseases can help to identify emerging or reemerging pathogens.

Outbreaks of the severe acute respiratory syndrome (SARS) and avian influenza A (H5N1) highlighted the need to have systems in place for detecting emerging pathogens. Thus, establishing population-based infectious-disease surveillance for pneumonia and acute respiratory infections was a primary goal of the GDD Program. The resulting surveillance activities also provide a platform for other GDD core activities. Moreover, the GDD respiratory-surveillance research projects have helped quantify the burden of illness for pneumonia- and influenza-associated acute respiratory illness, especially among children, and a high incidence of several respiratory pathogens, including respiratory syncytial virus, parainfluenza, and adenoviruses.

As the GDD regional centers have matured, existing surveillance platforms have increasingly been adapted to include emerging pathogens, special noncommunicable-disease studies, and projects focused on the animal–human interface (i.e., zoonotic diseases). In 2014, the GDD regional centers began efforts to link common acute febrile illness (AFI) syndromic surveillance strategies across 5 regional sites (Egypt, Guatemala, India, Kenya, and Thailand) to gain a global perspective on AFI. Conducting AFI surveillance at GDD regional centers is of public-health importance because AFI represents a common clinical syndrome for multiple diseases of outbreak potential or emerging zoonotic infections and provides an opportunity to evaluate novel diagnostics. Unlike respiratory-illness syndromes such as severe acute respiratory illness and influenza-like illness, no international consensus case definition exists for AFI surveillance, although recommendations for improving methods have been proposed. In addition, very few published AFI etiology studies have been conducted in multiple countries. A literature review currently underway has found that, of 169 AFI studies aiming to identify etiology and published from 2005 to 2016, only 6 (4%) had enrolled cases in multiple countries.

A multisite research effort has the potential to catalyze historically disparate AFI syndromic-surveillance systems toward globally comparable data of high utility at all levels for public-health response. Network activities across different GDD regional centers that represent diverse disease risks enhanced the ability to study a range of infectious diseases for which a single country might not have the capacity or incidence of disease to study for evidence-based public-health decision making. The GDD effort, to date, has included consistent case-definition use with a focus on undifferentiated AFI, multipathogen detection of local and globally significant infectious diseases, use of standard and investigational diagnostics where feasible, and prospective sentinel health facility-based surveillance methods of >1 year in duration to evaluate seasonal epidemic trends. Barriers to launch and harmonization to a common research protocol have included variation in local priority pathogens, resource availability, and time required for integration into existing public-health surveillance and healthcare networks. Established enhanced AFI surveillance has thus far provided a useful platform for investigating emerging infections with a febrile-illness component, such as Zika virus and scrub typhus.

Laboratory

Effective public-health requires close collaboration between epidemiologists and laboratory scientists. The GDD works with partner countries to strengthen diagnostic technical capacity for priority diseases, evaluate new laboratory diagnostics, establish frameworks for national laboratories that include quality assurance and specimen referral systems, improve biosafety/biosecurity, and train laboratory personnel on benchtop skills, laboratory management, and public-health laboratory functions. These efforts have improved the capacity of GDD host countries and their regions to detect, and respond to emerging infectious-disease threats and to sustain these efforts through a strong cadre of laboratory scientists dedicated to improving the global public-health laboratory infrastructure.

Research at the GDD regional centers has assisted in the detection and identification of 12 novel strains and pathogens that were new to the world and 62 novel strains of pathogens that were new to the region where they were discovered. GDD laboratorians have helped implement capacity to conduct >380 new diagnostic tests in 59 countries, improving disease-detection capability and contributing to faster response times within the region.

Public-Health Informatics

Informatics is the application of public-health information systems to capture, manage, analyze, and use information to improve public-health practice. Examples of key activities include the use of electronic databases, either as the source of data or as a method to collate data, for expediting the time between data collection and use. At the GDD regional centers, public-health informatics is a crosscutting activity for disease surveillance, laboratory studies, and applied epidemiologic research to ensure that data are collected and managed in a systematic and reliable manner. Most GDD data-collecting projects currently underway have an informatics component.

Capacity Building

Strengthening local public-health capacity and workforces is key for improving detection and response to infectious diseases globally. The transfer of epidemiology, laboratory, and emergency-preparedness skills to local public-health professionals is necessary for sustainability, both nationally and across regions. Capacity building is another crosscutting activity at GDD regional centers and ranges from establishing or strengthening existing surveillance, laboratory, emergency preparedness, and health systems to conducting high-quality epidemiologic research studies to address knowledge gaps. This capacity is achieved through on-the-job training of local partners, providing technical expertise, conducting high-quality research studies, and collaborating on analysis of information to inform evidence-based decision making.

Public-Health Diplomacy

Scientific exchange can play a strong role in building bonds across countries. Because health is an area of concern for all nations, international projects that address a common threat, such as infectious diseases that easily cross borders, can open avenues of communication and ease tensions between the United States and other nations. GDD China serves as an example of how two strong national public-health institutes (one in China and one in the United States) can collaborate and benefit. During the West Africa Ebola outbreak in 2014, China CDC had the resources and willingness to respond, but not necessarily the U.S. CDC experience or technical expertise with Ebola outbreaks and response. Since 2006, Chinese laboratorians have worked alongside U.S. colleagues to build greater diagnostic-testing capacity throughout China. Because of this preexisting relationship, the two countries were able to forge a new type of collaboration in Sierra Leone; scientists from both countries worked together to offer critical training and resources to Sierra Leone to help stop the spread of the largest Ebola outbreak in history. By building strong partnerships and scientific systems, GDD protects the United States and countries around the world from threats to health, safety, and security.

Lessons Learned and the Future

The GDD Program promotes the prompt detection and mitigation of disease threats globally. GDD works with multiple countries to conduct applied public-health research and develop and enhance public-health capacity to rapidly detect, accurately identify, and promptly contain emerging and reemerging infectious diseases. The activities of the GDD Program are critical to helping countries improve their disease-surveillance networks and enhance laboratory capabilities for the detection of emerging pathogens. The program also has greatly expanded epidemiology-workforce networks to meet their commitment to global health security and the International Health Regulations 2005.

The activities of the GDD Program have developed needed technical capacity, advanced science, and provided critical information for policy change. Activities of the GDD regional centers have allowed a greater understanding of which infections or conditions are of concern in the countries and regions in which they work. They have increased awareness of the emergence of antimicrobial resistance and the growing threat of infections that can be acquired in healthcare settings. Strengthening disease surveillance, applied public-health research, and laboratory capacity have allowed for a better understanding of pathogens associated with illnesses that present with acute fever. The activities established serve as a base, or launch pad, for the rapid and timely implementation of surveillance for emerging infections such as Zika virus and applied epidemiologic-research studies to better understand which populations are being affected and to enumerate potential factors associated with infection and spread of illness.

As new laboratory techniques for the detection of pathogens are developed, the GDD regional centers have served as a platform to examine the performance of these new tests in multiple settings and promote the adoption of new techniques in multiple countries. Because of ongoing surveillance and routine collection of epidemiologic information, GDD regional centers and the countries they work with have the tools needed to best characterize pathogens that are circulating and explore potential reservoirs and sources associated with these infections. Increased informatics capacity is concurrently enabling the active linkage of information and interfacing of data housed in multiple data systems within the countries and regions.

GDD regional centers make critical contributions to global disease detection by improving infectious-disease detection capacity through integration of applied public-health research and laboratory capacity building, which in turn will generate quality data that can inform high-level policy. The GDD Program has matured and transformed over the past 10 years and continues to evolve. Further advancing the technical capacity that has already been developed is allowing the GDD Program to focus on needed research and generation of data to develop and evaluate interventions and inform policies needed to reduce the burden of multiple conditions worldwide. Examples of research activities needed include studies to understand the actual burden of conditions at play, assessments of the impact of multiple conditions on local and global populations, quantification of the societal and economic costs of illnesses, and evaluation of control measures.

Threats posed by emerging pandemics and other infectious diseases will remain a challenge to global health security, endangering economies and decreasing political stability. The GDD will continue to work with countries to strengthen core capacities and conduct applied public-health research so that emerging and reemerging diseases and conditions can be detected and stopped faster and closer to the source, thereby enhancing global health security.

Section 32.2
The Global Health Security Agenda

This chapter contains text excerpted from the following sources: Text in this section begins with excerpts from "Protecting Americans from the Threat of Infectious Disease," Centers for Disease Control and Prevention (CDC), September 16, 2019; Text beginning with the heading "Prevent: CDC-Supported Achievements in 17 Phase-1 Countries" is excerpted from "Preventing, Detecting, and Responding to Epidemics: CDC's Achievements," Centers for Disease Control and Prevention (CDC), September 23, 2019.

The Global Health Security Agenda (GHSA) was launched in 2014; it is an global effort to strengthen the world's ability to prevent, detect, and respond to infectious-disease threats, whether they are naturally occurring, or accidentally or intentionally released. The Centers for Disease Control and Prevention (CDC) plays a leading role in the implementation of the GHSA for the United States by working with countries to strengthen their capabilities to identify, track, and stop disease outbreaks and public-health emergencies as quickly as possible. Because of the nature of infectious diseases, everyone remains vulnerable, including people living in the United States, until every country in the world can rapidly identify and contain public-health threats.

Infectious Diseases Travel Faster and Farther than Before

New and reemerging diseases spread quickly across the globe, resulting in outbreaks that overwhelm health systems, jeopardize lives, and devastate economies. In a tightly connected world, a disease can be transported from a remote village to major cities on all continents in as little as 36 hours. The second largest Ebola outbreak is ongoing in the Democratic Republic of the Congo (DRC), in a resource-limited environment and armed conflict zone. This outbreak is another test of the world's preparedness for infectious-disease outbreaks and the collective capacity to respond rapidly to stop further spread. Global outbreaks not only cause illness and death, but also can lead to a decrease in demand for the U.S. services and exports, jeopardizing the economy and American jobs. When an uncontained outbreak becomes a regional or global epidemic, costs escalate, and national and regional economies suffer. Effective and functional global health security capabilities reduce the threat and economic consequence of infectious-disease outbreaks to the United States and the world.

Strategic Vision for Global Health Security

The Global Health Security Agenda (GHSA) is a multisectoral and multilateral effort that seeks to accelerate progress toward implementation of the International Health Regulations (IHR) (2005)–the legally binding instrument adopted by 196 countries that set requirements for preparedness and response to public-health emergencies. The strategic approach of GHSA is to build capacities across 11 technical areas spanning multiple

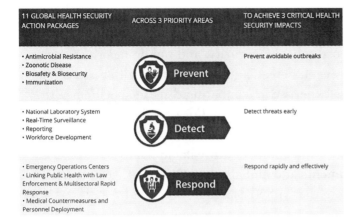

Figure 32.1. The Strategic Approach of the Global Health Security Agenda

sectors and disciplines, including animal and human health, agriculture, and security. While the international community has made significant progress in mitigating infectious-disease threats, challenges remain, which underscores the importance of the ongoing work to improve global health security. To address these challenges, the Centers for Disease Control and Prevention (CDC) works domestically and around the world to strengthen health security and expand the capacity to prevent, detect, and respond to public-health threats.

The CDC: A World Leader in Global Health Security

As the preeminent public-health agency of the United States, the Centers for Disease Control and Prevention (CDC) is committed to its mission to protect the health and safety of the American people. Global health security is a critical component of America's national security and the CDC has the responsibility, technical expertise, and unmatched experience to fulfill this mission that spans the globe. The CDC employs experts in all aspects of public health, including infectious and noninfectious diseases, violence and injury prevention, environmental health, and emergency response. The CDC plays a leading role in implementing the GHSA by utilizing its core strengths in disease surveillance and laboratory systems, workforce development, emergency management, border health security, and public-health science, to assist other nations to prevent, detect, and respond to health threats. The CDC maintains world-class expertise in combating disease-specific health threats, domestically and in its overseas offices. For decades, the CDC has used its technical expertise to combat threats across the globe, beginning with the response to smallpox and cholera outbreaks in 1958. The CDC is a trusted partner to governments and global institutions that work to limit health threats from coming to the United States from abroad.

The CDC Forges Partnerships to Combat Infectious Disease Threats

Under the GHSA, the United States committed to partnering with 17 Phase-1 countries (Bangladesh, Burkina Faso, Cameroon, Côte d'Ivoire, Guinea, Ethiopia, India, Indonesia, Kenya, Liberia, Mali, Pakistan, Senegal, Sierra Leone, Tanzania, Uganda, and Vietnam). These countries receive technical assistance and financial support from the CDC.

How the CDC Advances the Global Health Security Agenda

The CDC works government-to-government with ministries of health, ministries of agriculture, and other relevant ministries, and directly with partner organizations to build capacity to contain diseases and prevent outbreaks at their source before they spread. The CDC also leverages partnerships with nongovernmental organizations, academia, multilateral organizations, the private sector, and other stakeholders to support this mission with host governments. Public-health experts at the CDC contribute their unique scientific expertise to these partnerships to strengthen national public-health capacities, working hand-in-hand with countries to detect and contain global health threats and respond to epidemics. With its partners, the CDC has made great strides toward strengthening health security globally, focusing on the core technical areas of surveillance, laboratory, public-health

	Antimicrobial Resistance	Zoonotic Disease	Biosafety/Biosecurity	Immunization
Result	11 countries demonstrated successful detection and reporting of antimicrobial resistant pathogens in the last 6 months	9 countries shared surveillance data between human and animal health sectors for at least 80% of prioritized zoonotic diseases	5 countries improved security controls and electronic inventories for all dangerous pathogens and toxins in national laboratories	14 countries increased immunization coverage based on surveillance of disease burden at the community level
Why it Matters	Antimicrobial-resistant organisms have adapted to widespread use of antibiotics, decreasing our ability to treat diseases. Identifying Antimicrobial-resistant organisms allows us to react quickly when they spread	An estimated 6 out of 10 infectious diseases are zoonotic and spread between animals and humans. We quickly need to know about zoonotic disease outbreaks in animals to prepare for and prevent possible spread into human populations	Dangerous pathogens need to be handled carefully and stored securely to prevent them from accidentally or intentionally being released and harming the public	Effective immunization systems reduce illness and death from vaccine-preventable diseases and help limit the magnitude and number of infectious disease outbreaks

Figure 32.2. Prevent: CDC-Supported Achievements in 17 Phase-1 Countries

workforce development, and emergency management. The CDC's focus on these core capacities has already resulted in measurable progress in the 17 Phase-1 GHSA countries where the CDC has invested time and resources. The CDC works to ensure collaboration, increased engagement, and accountability across the GHSA community.

Prevent: CDC-Supported Achievements in 17 Phase-1 Countries
The CDC's Contributions toward Prevention

- Reduce factors that contribute to the development and spread of antimicrobial resistance, including improving infection prevention and control.
- Keep laboratory workers safe and reduce the risk of theft, loss, or mishandling of dangerous pathogens that could harm the public.
- Strengthen the prevention, detection, and response to zoonotic diseases and the development of national action plans to combat the spillover of disease from animals to humans.
- Establish and strengthen vaccination programs to protect people from highly contagious yet preventable diseases, and conduct vaccination-outbreak response measures.

	National Lab Systems	Real Time Surveillance	Reporting	Workforce Development
Result	11 countries can conduct laboratory tests to detect national priority pathogens that cause disease, outbreaks, or death	10 countries can connect disease surveillance data with laboratory data 7 countries have established event-based surveillance in communities and health care facilities 4 countries detected more than 3000 health events through this surveillance	13 countries established a web-based national database for surveillance	17 countries established or expanded their program to train disease detectives
Why It Matters	Confirming diagnosis with laboratories allows health workers to respond rapidly with the most effective treatment and prevention methods, reducing spread of disease and deaths	Effective disease surveillance with rapid laboratory diagnosis enables countries to quickly detect outbreaks and continuously respond to potential risks	Having a national database that is web-based helps countries detect, respond, and report potential outbreaks and allows experts to assess public health events and respond rapidly	To maintain global health security capabilities, countries need a disease detective workforce that can quickly investigate potential outbreaks and take swift action

Figure 32.3. Detect: CDC-Supported Achievements in 17 Phase-1 Countries

Challenges Persist

One example of a remaining challenge in preventing avoidable outbreaks is the exchange of surveillance data between the human and animal health sectors. The lack of information sharing between these sectors can leave countries vulnerable, creating barriers to collaborative action to prevent, detect, or respond to zoonotic diseases (e.g., rabies, influenza viruses, hemorrhagic fevers, and anthrax). To address this challenge, the CDC is working across ministries in partner countries to prioritize zoonotic diseases and to strengthen disease-surveillance systems that are able to share information rapidly between sectors for faster action.

Detect: CDC-Supported Achievements in 17 Phase-1 Countries
The CDC's Contributions in Prevention

- Establish monitoring systems that can predict and identify infectious-disease threats at various levels of the health system, including community, district, and national levels, as well as global monitoring through the CDC Global Disease Detection (GDD) Operations Center.

- Strengthen countries' ability to quickly and accurately collect, analyze, and use public-health information.
- Train disease detectives, laboratory scientists, veterinarians, and healthcare infection-prevention experts who are equipped to identify, track, and contain outbreaks in humans and animals before they spread.
- Build tiered laboratory networks at the local, regional, and national levels that can transport samples safely, increase the number of samples laboratorians are able to test, and transfer information securely between patients, responders, and policymakers.

Challenges Persist

One example of a persistent challenge in the early detection of health security threats is the lack of national, Web-based databases that link suspected cases of illness with laboratory confirmation. This leaves countries vulnerable, as they cannot accurately and quickly identify the presence of pathogens in order to minimize the spread of disease. To address this challenge, the CDC is sharing technical expertise with countries to strengthen disease detection through databases that are linked to laboratory results, enabling timelier and more coordinated outbreak detection and response.

Respond: CDC-Supported Achievements in 17 Phase-1 Countries
The CDC's Contributions in Prevention

- Establish public-health emergency operations centers (EOCs) to serve as centralized locations in partner countries to efficiently and effectively respond to a crisis.
- Develop technical expertise and the capacity needed for countries to lead their own effective responses to public-health threats.
- Train public-health emergency management fellows to lead and manage emergency responses.

	Emergency Operation Centers (EOCs)	Public Health and Law Enforcement	Medical Countermeasures	Border Health
Result	15 countries trained emergency management specialists and experts to support a well-functioning EOC	7 countries coordinated public health and security personnel to respond to infectious disease threats	11 countries improved their operating procedures and logistics systems to deploy staff, medicines, and/or supplies to combat infectious disease threats	13 countries enhanced their cross-border communication and collaboration
Why it Matters	EOCs bring together experts and stakeholders to efficiently and effectively coordinate response to an emergency or public health threat	Health and security personnel must often work closely together to combat infectious disease threats. First responders may be police officers or security personnel, not doctors. Close ties between health and security can help the sectors work together to detect, report, and limit the threat of infectious disease	During a public health emergency, countries need medications, vaccines, or personal protective equipment. Putting systems in place before an emergency strikes is critical to preventing delays in patient care	Because of the high influx of travelers through ports of entry (POE) and in porous border regions, it is important for countries to have systems in place to reliably detect and quickly respond to infectious disease threats at borders to prevent international spread

Figure 32.4. Respond: CDC-Supported Achievements in 17 Phase-1 Countries

- Establish and strengthen CDC rapid-response teams that can mobilize quickly to address the critical and diverse needs and priorities that arise from infectious-disease outbreaks.
- Develop, test, and train on protocols for the rapid identification of health threats at point of entries (POEs).

Challenges Persist

One example of a persistent challenge in responding rapidly and effectively to health security threats is the limited functionality of the Establish public-health emergency operations centers (EOC). Without well-functioning EOCs, countries' coordination during an outbreak is at risk. To address this challenge, the CDC is working with countries to develop EOC infrastructure, implement sustainable models for EOC operations, and assist with training current and new EOC staff to activate and manage emergency responses.

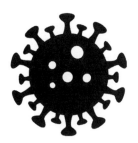

CHAPTER 33
Priority Pathogens:
Research and Development

Chapter Contents

Understanding Immunization and Infectious Diseases

This section includes text excerpted from "Immunization and Infectious Diseases," Office of Disease Prevention and Health Promotion (ODPHP), U.S. Department of Health and Human Services (HHS), March 15, 2010. Reviewed March 2020.

The increase in life expectancy during the 20th century is largely due to improvements in child survival; this increase is associated with reductions in infectious-disease mortality, due largely to immunization. However, infectious diseases remain a major cause of illness, disability, and death. Immunization recommendations in the United States currently target 17 vaccine-preventable diseases across the lifespan.

Healthy People 2020 goals for immunization and infectious diseases are rooted in evidence-based clinical and community activities and services for the prevention and treatment of infectious diseases. Objectives focus on technological advancements and ensuring that states, local public-health departments, and nongovernmental organizations (NGOs) are strong partners in the nation's attempt to control the spread of infectious diseases. Objectives for 2020 reflect a more mobile society and the fact that diseases do not stop at geopolitical borders. Awareness of disease and completing prevention and treatment courses remain essential components for reducing infectious-disease transmission.

Why Are Immunization and Infectious Diseases Important?

People in the United States continue to get diseases that are vaccine-preventable. Viral hepatitis, influenza, and tuberculosis (TB) remain among the leading causes of illness and death in the United States and account for substantial spending on the related consequences of infection.

The infectious-disease public-health infrastructure, which carries out disease surveillance at the federal, state, and local levels, is an essential tool in the fight against newly emerging and reemerging infectious diseases. Other important defenses against infectious-diseases include:

- Proper use of vaccines
- Antibiotics
- Screening and testing guidelines
- Scientific improvements in the diagnosis of infectious disease-related health concerns

Understanding Immunization and Infectious Diseases

Immunization

Vaccines are among the most cost-effective clinical preventive services and are a core component of any preventive-services package. Childhood immunization programs provide a very high return on investment. For example, for each birth cohort vaccinated with the routine immunization schedule (this includes DTap, Td, Hib, Polio, MMR, Hep B, and varicella vaccines), society:

- Saves 33,000 lives
- Prevents 14 million cases of disease
- Reduces direct healthcare costs by $9.9 billion
- Saves $33.4 billion in indirect costs

Despite progress, approximately 42,000 adults and 300 children in the United States die each year from vaccine-preventable diseases. Communities with pockets of unvaccinated and undervaccinated populations are at increased risk for outbreaks of vaccine-preventable diseases. In 2008, imported measles resulted in 140 reported cases—nearly a three-fold increase over the previous year. The emergence of new or replacement strains of vaccine-preventable disease can result in a significant increase in serious illnesses and death.

Surveillance

The nation's public-health goals focus on reducing illness, hospitalization, and death from vaccine-preventable diseases and other infectious diseases; expanding surveillance is crucial to those ends. Further efforts to improve disease surveillance will allow for earlier detection of the emergence and spread of diseases. Increased surveillance will save lives by allowing the maximum time possible for public-health responses, including vaccine production and development of evidence-based recommendations on disease prevention and control. Surveillance enables rapid information sharing and facilitates the timely identification of people in need of immediate treatment. Increasing laboratory capacity is essential for these efforts.

Respiratory Diseases

Acute respiratory infections, including pneumonia and influenza, are the eigth leading cause of death in the United States, accounting for 56,000 deaths annually. Pneumonia mortality in children fell by 97 percent in the last century, but respiratory infectious diseases continue to be leading causes of pediatric hospitalization and outpatient visits in the United States. On average, influenza leads to more than 200,000 hospitalizations and 36,000 deaths each year. The 2009 H1N1 influenza pandemic caused an estimated 270,000 hospitalizations and 12,270 deaths (1,270 of which were of people younger than age 18) between April 2009 and March 2010.

Hepatitis and Tuberculosis

Viral hepatitis and TB can be prevented, yet healthcare systems often do not make the best use of their available resources to support prevention efforts. Because the United States healthcare system focuses on treatment of illnesses, rather than health promotion, patients do not always receive information about prevention and healthy lifestyles. This includes advancing effective and evidence-based viral hepatitis- and TB- prevention priorities and interventions.

Emerging Issues in Immunization and Infectious Diseases

In the coming decade, the United States will continue to face new and emerging issues in the area of immunization and infectious diseases. The public-health infrastructure must be capable of responding to emerging threats. State-of-the-art technology and highly skilled professionals need to be in place to provide rapid response to the threat of epidemics. A coordinated strategy is necessary to understand, detect, control, and prevent infectious diseases. Below are some specific emerging issues.

- Providing culturally appropriate preventive healthcare is an immediate responsibility that will grow over the decade. As the demographics of the population continue to shift, public health and healthcare systems will need to expand their capacity to protect the growing needs of a diverse and aging population.
- New infectious agents and diseases continue to be detected. Infectious diseases must be looked at in a global context due to increasing:
  - International travel and trade
  - Migration
  - Importation of foods and agricultural practices
  - Threats of bioterrorism
- Inappropriate use of antibiotics and environmental changes multiply the potential for worldwide epidemics of all types of infectious diseases.

Infectious diseases are a critical public health, humanitarian, and security concern; coordinated efforts will protect people across the nation and around the world.

Section 33.2

Priority Emerging Infectious Diseases in Need of Research and Development

This section includes text excerpted from "World Health Organization Methodology to Prioritize Emerging Infectious Diseases in Need of Research and Development," Centers for Disease Control and Prevention (CDC), July 31, 2018.

Outbreaks of Ebola virus disease, Middle East respiratory syndrome, and Zika virus disease illustrate that emerging infectious diseases will continue to cause major public-health emergencies. Further work is needed to strengthen defenses with medical countermeasures (MCMs) and other protective interventions. Building on experiences and at the request of the World Health Assembly in May 2015, the World Health Organization (WHO) launched the research and development (R&D) Blueprint for action to prevent epidemics. This global strategy and preparedness plan is designed to ensure that targeted R&D will strengthen emergency response by accelerating availability of biomedical technologies to populations and patients during epidemics. The R&D Blueprint focuses on severe emerging diseases that pose a major risk for causing a public-health emergency and for which MCMs or substantial R&D initiatives and pipelines are insufficient or nonexistent.

Experts compiled an initial list of relevant diseases at an informal consultation in December 2015. A more robust methodology was needed, one that could be standardized and repeated regularly for reviewing and, if necessary, updating the list in the light of successful development of new interventions or the emergence of new disease threats.

The WHO settled on a three-pronged approach: (1) a methodology development and review process; (2) an annual review of a list of prioritized diseases; and (3) a decision instrument to guide decision-making on a novel disease. All three processes use a common set of weighted criteria and subcriteria, such as the human-to-human transmissibility of the disease or its potential societal impact. This process is inherently expert-driven because the R&D Blueprint addresses pathogens that are yet fully characterized and for which an understanding of how to diagnose, prevent, and treat the resulting diseases is incomplete. Further, these pathogens might behave differently on different occasions because of variation in the biologic, cultural, or environmental context. In such scenarios, decisions have to be made on the basis of partial information supplemented by expert opinion and with an awareness that any methodology will be prone to biases.

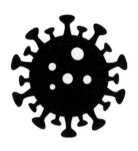

CHAPTER 34
Animal-Borne Pathogens

Chapter Contents

Priority Pathogens

This section includes text excerpted from "Emerging and Zoonotic Infectious Diseases," Centers for Disease Control and Prevention (CDC), June 13, 2017.

Responding to Outbreaks

Perhaps what the National Center for Emerging and Zoonotic Infectious Diseases (NCEZID) is best known for is responding to outbreaks of infectious disease. Here are a few large-scale responses that NCEZID has led since 2010:

- 1st outbreak of Zika virus in the Western Hemisphere, which was linked to birth defects.
- Largest Ebola epidemic in history, which killed more than 11,000 people.
- Fungal meningitis outbreak caused by contaminated steroid injections.
- The second-largest outbreak of West Nile virus infections that sickened 5,600 people in the United States.
- Outbreak of cholera in Haiti, which killed at least 10,000 people.

The NCEZID provides rapid assistance to states and foreign ministries of health through formal requests called "epidemic-assistance investigations," or Epi-Aids. Each year, NCEZID conducts almost half (~25) of all of the Centers for Disease Control and Prevention (CDC)'s Epi-Aid investigations of outbreaks—large and small, domestic and international. Examples of Epi-Aids and other outbreak investigations that NCEZID participated in include:

- *E. coli* (*Escherichia coli*) infections among children who visited a goat farm in Connecticut
- Emerging, drug-resistant fungal infections (*Candida auris*) that spread among patients in healthcare settings

- Rarely seen bloodstream infections (*Elizabethkingia*) in patients in Wisconsin
- Illness caused by *E. coli*-tainted flour that infected people in more than 20 states
- *Listeria* bacteria in packaged salads that hospitalized 19 people, killing 1

Innovating Solutions

Pathogens constantly evolve. Protecting Americans demands that the CDC develop better tools to keep humans one step ahead of emerging infectious diseases. Innovation is taking place across NCEZID.

What the National Center for Emerging and Zoonotic Infectious Diseases Is Doing

Examples of innovations worked on by NCEZID scientists include:

- Advanced Molecular Detection (AMD), which combines two powerful technologies (deoxyribonucleic acid (DNA) sequencing and advanced computing) to solve complex infectious disease mysteries— the who, what, where, when, and how of microbes harming people. Since the Office of Advanced Molecular Detection was established in 2014, AMD has played a pivotal role in:
  - Identifying the genetic makeup of Ebola and Zika during each of those outbreaks
  - Solving foodborne outbreaks involving Listeria infection faster by linking food sources to clusters of illness
- New diagnostics such as these are ensuring that diseases are accurately and quickly diagnosed and treated:
  - A test kit for yellow fever that used to take 2 days gives results in 4 hours now.
  - A new rapid and cost-effective *Candida*-identifying tool that screens for antifungal resistance when treating invasive candidiasis, the most common cause of healthcare-associated bloodstream infections in the United States
- Safer and more effective vaccines against rabies for use in people and animals

• An electronic platform called "Epathology" that allows physicians and scientists from anywhere in the world to electronically submit images and scanned pathology slides to CDC pathologists for evaluation. Doctors working in the most remote and resource-limited villages just need an Internet connection to share slides of their patient's specimens with pathologists at NCEZID.

Section 34.2

U.S. Government Approach to Animal-Borne Pathogens

This section includes text excerpted from "National Center for Emerging and Zoonotic Infectious Diseases Accomplishments 2015," Centers for Disease Control and Prevention (CDC), 2015. Reviewed March 2020.

Unraveling, Discovering, Linking

Innovation and discovery characterize much of the work in the National Center for Emerging and Zoonotic Infectious Diseases (NCEZID,) and the range of discoveries made in 2015 are far-reaching, including old mysteries solved, never-before-seen pathogens identified, and discovery of a new disease involving cancer cells that originate in a common tapeworm. Examples of notable work include:

• Poxvirus experts at the NCEZID unraveled a mystery, dating back to 2000, which involved a renal transplant patient from New York who developed a rash, the cause of which could not be identified. The patient made a full recovery, but infectious-disease specialists in New York and poxvirus experts at the Centers for Disease Control and Prevention (CDC) initially were stumped about the cause of illness. Years later, scientists in New York and in the CDC's Poxvirus

Lab combined pathological and chemical analysis and applied next-generation sequencing methods to discover this was a new poxvirus genus, similar to *Orthopoxvirus*.

- Across the continent, another new *Orthopoxvirus* was discovered in Alaska. Alaska public-health personnel contacted CDC poxvirus experts about a woman who had tested positive for an *Orthopoxvirus* that had not been seen before. The CDC used whole-genome sequencing to help them better characterize the new poxvirus.
- After a woman was bitten by a rabid fox in Lincoln County, New Mexico, the NCEZID's Rabies Lab was asked to help in the identification. Genetic sequencing done by the Rabies Lab showed that this was a rabies virus strain that had never before been identified. The new strain was related to other rabies strains found in bats.

NCEZID pathologists were amazed when they found a new disease that involves tapeworms growing inside a person essentially getting cancer that spreads to the person, causing tumors. The cancer cells that originate in a common tapeworm can take root in people with weakened immune systems. It is the first known case of a person becoming ill from cancer cells that arose in a parasite—in this case, *Hymenolepis nana*, the dwarf tapeworm, which is also the most common tapeworm in humans. The lead author of the study, published in the *New England Journal of Medicine,* acknowledged that this type of event is rare. However, the tapeworm is found worldwide and millions of people around the world suffer from conditions such as HIV that weaken their immune system and make them more vulnerable to this tapeworm. So there may be more cases that are unrecognized.

Why Does This Work Matter?

- Increasing numbers of people have developed *Orthopoxvirus* infections since routine vaccination against smallpox ended in the 1980s.
- The report about cancer cells originating in a common tapeworm raises the concern that similar cases may be misdiagnosed as human cancer, especially in less developed countries where this tapeworm and illnesses such as HIV are widespread.

Section 34.3

Zoonotic Disease Programs for Enhancing Global Health Security

This section includes text excerpted from "Zoonotic Disease Programs for Enhancing Global Health Security," Centers for Disease Control and Prevention (CDC), November 20, 2017.

Zoonotic disease pathogens such as rabies virus have been causing outbreaks in humans for thousands of years. In fact, most infectious diseases in humans originate in animals, and the frequency of such transmissions has been increasing over time. Taylor et al. identified that 75 percent of emerging infectious organisms pathogenic to humans are zoonotic in origin. Recently emerged zoonotic diseases include globally devastating diseases such as Ebola virus disease, Middle East respiratory syndrome, highly pathogenic avian influenza, severe acute respiratory syndrome, and bovine spongiform encephalopathy. These and other zoonotic diseases affect many countries, resulting in high morbidity and mortality rates in humans and animals; cause disruptions of regional and global trade; and strain national and global public-health resources. Newly emerging health threats are associated with substantial economic costs, including direct and indirect impacts on the healthcare system, costs associated with the actual response, and overall disruption of economic activity.

The World Bank estimated that 6 major zoonotic disease epidemics during 1997 to 2009 resulted in an economic loss of >$80 billion. Experiences from most outbreaks indicate that detecting and effectively responding to emerging epidemics requires a multisectoral approach. In 2010, recognizing the need for multidisciplinary collaboration to address health threats at the human-animal–ecosystem interface, the World Health Organization (WHO), Food and Agriculture Organization (FAO), and World Organisation for Animal Health (OIE) formalized their collaboration and identified 3 priority areas of work together, 2 of which are zoonotic diseases (rabies and zoonotic influenza). Endemic zoonotic diseases have the dual impact of causing illness and death in humans and animals as well as substantial economic loss in resource-poor societies where livestock farming is a major engine of economic growth at the household and national levels. Fortunately, proven control and prevention strategies exist for many zoonotic diseases that are most prevalent in affected communities. (e.g., rabies, anthrax, brucellosis) zoonotic diseases

To better prevent, detect, and respond to global infectious-disease threats, the U.S. government and other partners developed the Global Health Security Agenda (GHSA) with initial implementation in 17 phase-1 countries in Africa and Asia. The GHSA is charged with making progress in the implementation of WHO International Health Regulations, the OIE Veterinary Services Pathway, and other similar frameworks for achieving an adequate level of preparedness to tackle emerging health threats in animals and humans.

To build the necessary infrastructure and human capital, the U.S. government and its global partners allocated funds to advance 11 GHSA action packages that included zoonotic diseases. This section describes the specific steps taken to prevent, detect, and respond to endemic zoonotic diseases and explains how to leverage them to detect and effectively respond to emerging and reemerging zoonotic health threats, thereby enhancing global health security. Some of these steps have been implemented in several of these phase-1 countries.

Approaches for One Health Zoonotic Disease Program Implementation

Mitigating the impact of endemic and emerging zoonotic diseases of public-health importance requires multisectoral collaboration and interdisciplinary partnerships. Collaborations across sectors relevant to zoonotic diseases, particularly among human and animal (domestic and wildlife) health disciplines, are essential for quantifying the burden of zoonotic diseases, detecting and responding to endemic and emerging zoonotic pathogens, prioritizing the diseases of greatest public-health concern, and effectively launching appropriate prevention, detection, and response strategies.

Multisectoral approaches under a One Health umbrella are more expedient and effective and lead to efficient utilization of limited resources.

Prioritization of Zoonotic Diseases

Developing strategies to prevent, detect, and respond to zoonotic diseases is challenging in resource-poor settings where there are other competing public-health priorities. In addition, effective mitigation of their impact requires multisectoral collaborations and interdisciplinary partnerships that may take time to establish. Therefore, having all relevant sectors jointly identify zoonotic diseases of greatest concern is an essential first step for many countries. Multisectoral partnerships are easier to create if participants from multiple sectors, including humans, animals (domestic and wildlife), and environmental health develop a prioritized list of zoonotic diseases to work on together and commit to sharing public- and animal-health resources. Engagement of different sectors early in the process facilitates collaboration during program implementation and ensures program ownership. In addition, systems developed to address the prioritized diseases can be leveraged to tackle other zoonotic infections and emerging health threats.

To help identify high-priority zoonotic diseases for multisectoral engagement, the One Health office at the Centers for Disease Control and Prevention (CDC) developed the One Health Zoonotic Disease Prioritization tool, a semiquantitative tool for prioritization with equal input from represented sectors, irrespective of whether reliable surveillance data are available. The tool is designed to bring together a multidisciplinary team of professionals from the human, animal, and environmental health agencies and other relevant sectors with a common goal of developing country-specific criteria for ranking zoonotic diseases of greatest national concern. The tool has been used to select zoonotic diseases for further programmatic activity in multiple countries in the implementation of the zoonotic disease action package of GHSA.

Typically, the prioritization is performed by trained facilitators during a workshop with voting members from multiple ministries covering human, animal, and environmental health and from multinational organizations (e.g, the FAO, the WHO, the OIE), academic institutions, and other partners working in the area of zoonotic diseases (e.g., the CDC, the U.S. Agency for International Development). The country's government ministries should select participants. In countries that have conducted prioritization workshops, the CDC provided training to in-country workshop facilitators to promote country ownership of the process. Minimizing the role of external facilitators helps to retain objectivity in the process and allow decision making by host-country representatives.

Assessing the Burden of Zoonotic Diseases

Accurately estimating the burden of zoonotic diseases is a critical step in both identifying public- and animal-health priorities and assessing the impact of prevention and control strategies, including potential economic effects on the food supply, such as with avian and swine influenza viruses. Metrics for human zoonotic disease burden may include numbers of cases of illness, hospitalizations, deaths, disability, or quality-adjusted life years, and economic impacts such as healthcare-associated costs and lost productivity. Some of these metrics can also be used to assess animal-health burden. In countries where zoonotic disease data may not be readily available, the burden of different zoonotic diseases could be better ascertained by conducting studies in selected regions.

Such studies may focus on zoonotic diseases selected in the prioritization process or diseases that are deemed more prevalent on the basis of limited epidemiologic or clinical data. Estimation of disease burden should involve studies in humans and affected or implicated animal species. Conducting ecologic and wildlife studies may be necessary to define risk to humans from selected zoonotic pathogens in animal reservoirs or arthropod vectors. Investigators should consider using existing databases or laboratory specimens, such as banked sera collected as part of HIV indicator surveys, to quantify the potential risks to humans of some zoonotic diseases.

Zoonotic Disease Surveillance in Animals and Humans

A rapid and effective response to endemic and emerging zoonotic diseases relies heavily on timely and efficient surveillance and reporting systems. Surveillance in animals and humans is critical for early identification and possible prediction of future outbreaks, allowing for preemptive action. Components of effective surveillance include establishing event- and indicator-based surveillance, and adequate laboratory capacity in both public- and animal- health laboratory systems. Training epidemiologists and the establishment of effective laboratory systems are critical for a successful zoonotic disease surveillance program.

An effective surveillance system may require the following: standard case definitions for priority zoonotic diseases under surveillance, based on existing guidance from global human and animal health organizations such as the WHO, the CDC, the OIE, and the FAO; evaluation of existing national surveillance systems to determine their timeliness, effectiveness, and usefulness; new or refined surveillance and reporting systems and linkages to share data between public- and animal- health agencies and other relevant sectors; evaluation of potential electronic disease reporting mechanisms, including the use of smartphone technologies; establishment of surveillance data dissemination platforms to provide awareness and feedback to human and animal health agencies and other stakeholders; evaluation of available diagnostic tests and appropriate testing capabilities in central and regional public- and animal- health laboratories; and establishment of a national emergency-management system, such as an Emergency Operations Center (EOC), to assist in coordinated zoonotic-disease surveillance, response to zoonotic-disease outbreaks, and prevention and control efforts across relevant sectors.

Laboratory Systems

Timely, accurate, and reliable laboratory tests are critical for building outbreak response capacities, identifying etiologies of disease, and monitoring endemic and emerging zoonotic diseases in humans, domestic and food animals, and wildlife. Well-functioning and separate national public- and animal- health laboratory systems are essential to identify etiologic agents so that appropriate prevention, detection, and response strategies can be implemented. Laboratories should be an integral part of the public-health infrastructure with a system for rapid testing of prioritized samples and timely sharing of results. Successful and sustainable laboratory systems require strategic interagency planning across sectors and building on existing capacities in the country to standardize laboratory methods, prioritize laboratory resources, and develop information-sharing channels. A requirement for ensuring testing quality is commitment from the top levels of management to provide the necessary resources to sustain the functional roles of the laboratory in an environment that supports quality and safety. The roles and responsibilities of all human and animal laboratory staff need to be defined, documented, and communicated, and written policies and procedures should be available and understood. In addition, all laboratory staff should be trained on these policies and procedures to ensure they are executed in a consistent and reliable manner. Accurate and reliable test results depend on having a sample that has been collected, stored, and transported correctly; sample requirements vary by the disease and suspected pathogen. Laboratories should be designed to optimize workflow, support the quality of testing, and protect the safety of laboratory staff and the community. Regularly conducted proficiency testing helps to monitor the quality and performance of the laboratory.

Critical human and animal laboratory systems that countries need to establish or expand include central and regional laboratory capacity; specimen referral systems for rapid, safe, and reliable specimen transport; laboratory training programs that promote workforce development and retention; and affordable, flexible laboratory accreditation schemes to ensure lab quality. Opportunities for mentoring relationships with reference laboratories or private partnerships should be encouraged. Laboratories may assist in determining disease burden and characterization of human, animal, and ecologic drivers of disease spillover from animals to humans to optimize models for predicting disease emergence (e.g., risk mapping).

Outbreak Response Using One Health Approach

A successful zoonotic disease outbreak response requires (1) the ability to detect the outbreak using established surveillance systems, including event-based reporting; (2) adequate laboratory capability to confirm the outbreak etiology; (3) a workforce trained to respond and perform descriptive and analytical epidemiology for animal and human diseases; (4) the ability to implement appropriate control and prevention measures; and

(5) an outbreak and emergency-management system in place to coordinate multisectoral response activities at the national to subnational levels. The involvement of all relevant stakeholders is crucial, including those in human, animal, and environmental health sectors. Outbreak response activities are best supported by an overarching operations framework that clearly identifies the roles and responsibilities of key institutions and officials for all relevant sectors and provides direction for coordination of activities at the local and national levels. Countries should establish functional cross-sector coordination and communication pathways before an outbreak occurs. Multisectoral collaboration is easier during an emergency if agencies have already been collaborating in joint priority-setting and actively working together to address prioritized zoonotic diseases.

Early detection of an impending human outbreak may in some instances be achieved through the detection of an increase in disease in animal populations, such as livestock and wildlife. Detection of an outbreak or an increase in case count of a zoonotic disease by the wildlife, livestock, or public-health agency should trigger enhanced surveillance by the other agencies. This detection can only occur if there is effective communication between the different sectors. Outbreak-response protocols or national strategies should be developed for priority zoonotic diseases that specifically address coordination of activities, data sharing (including how to integrate animal, human, and environmental health information), trigger points or thresholds for action, and identified roles and responsibilities of each stakeholder. Establishing joint training opportunities for animal and human health workers will facilitate information sharing and enhance collaboration for effective prevention, detection, and response programs. When possible, joint simulation exercises can be conducted to demonstrate the proficiency of response and adequate interagency and multisectoral collaboration.

Prevention and Control of Zoonotic Diseases

The prevention and control strategies of zoonotic diseases will vary by disease and the availability of proven interventions. Some of the zoonotic diseases most prevalent in resource-limited areas are vaccine-preventable (e.g., rabies, brucellosis, anthrax). Therefore, the implementation of routine immunization programs may be needed for disease prevention. Depending on the disease, this may be primarily human vaccination or vaccination of livestock or other domestic animals. For some diseases, such as highly pathogenic avian influenza, prevention and control may involve large-scale culling and effective biosecurity programs. For diseases such as anthrax and rabies, preemptive vaccination of animals will prevent outbreaks in the animal population while at the same time protecting humans. In others (e.g., Rift Valley fever), disease outbreaks in animals may be the first signal to start the implementation of prevention programs such as ring vaccination of animals. Waiting until an outbreak is detected in humans can be costly to the lives of animals and humans and can strain limited public-health resources.

Effective human and animal disease-surveillance systems are critical for early detection and response, for planning prevention and control programs, and to evaluate the effectiveness of control and prevention strategies. Timely and effective communication and collaboration between human and animal health agencies are essential to developing disease prevention and control strategies involving both human and animal populations. As part of an effective response, countries should consider developing and evaluating communication strategies to educate human and animal healthcare providers and the general population on zoonotic disease transmission and prevention. Community education programs may include safe farming and biosecurity measures, animal-slaughtering practices, understanding animal contact and exposure risks, and the use of personal prevention measures to avoid or reduce exposure to vector-borne and other zoonotic diseases. Livestock and poultry are key sources of food and livelihood, and important economically for trade; prevention strategies that target zoonotic diseases associated with food animals must be compatible with the needs of the communities that are economically dependent on those animals.

Communicating effectively regarding prevention strategies will also enhance engagement in future outbreak control efforts because the communities will better understand the reasons behind any intervention. Similarly, a well-informed population can serve as an early alert system, notifying appropriate authorities about possible cases of disease in humans or animals. For zoonotic diseases with potential domestic and food animal reservoirs, important strategies in disease control can include animal vaccination, vector control, test and treat, or cull programs, as well as effective biosecurity measures. The development and implementation of cost-effectiveness and cost-benefit models to evaluate and refine disease prevention and control methods and programs will ensure effective use of resources. Development of these policies and models, however, should also evaluate the negative effects that culling and other measures may have on the societal well-being and livelihood of farmers.

CHAPTER 35
Insect-Borne Pathogens

Chapter Contents

Emerging Insect-Borne Pathogens

This section includes text excerpted from "Guarding against the Most Dangerous Emerging Pathogens: Insights from Evolutionary Biology," Centers for Disease Control and Prevention (CDC), December 21, 2010. Reviewed February 2020.

Vector-Borne Transmission

The most serious threat involved in vector-borne transmission comes from pathogens that can be maintained by human/mosquito cycles, but are absent from suitable areas because of historical accidents or past eradication campaigns. Dengue and malaria are members of this category; they have the potential to spiral out of control immediately upon release into areas with suitable vectors. Nonevolutionary analyses of emerging infections recognize the threat posed by these pathogens because their damaging effects on human populations are known.

Vector-borne pathogens that have not used humans as the primary vertebrate host, but may be capable of doing so represent less easily recognized threats. Evolutionary considerations heighten concern because such vector-borne pathogens are expected to become increasingly harmful as they become adapted to human/vector cycles of transmission.

Rift Valley fever virus provides an example. For most of this century, this virus was believed to infect humans only as dead-end hosts. Although the virus was vector-borne in ungulates, humans were considered to have acquired the infection either when involved in the slaughtering process or when bitten by mosquitoes that had acquired the infection from other vertebrates. Recent outbreaks have spread to an extent consistent with substantial human/mosquito cycling, but the existence of such cycling has not been conclusively documented. If human/mosquito cycling is occurring, the door is open for further adaptation to humans and for evolution of increased virulence in humans, increased efficiency of human/vector transmission, and increased spread through human populations. Rift Valley fever virus viremias seem sufficient for human/mosquito cycling, and the lethality of the largest outbreaks was particularly high, as one would expect if some evolution toward increased virulence accompanied a temporary establishment of human/mosquito cycles. To assess the long-term threat posed by Rift Valley fever virus and to block this virus should it prove to be particularly threatening, public-health policy needs to emphasize the following research priorities: (1) study the transmission of Rift Valley fever virus in human/mosquito cycles, (2) assess the potential for such transmission over extended periods, and (3) evaluate the effects of such transmission on virus virulence.

All emerging vector-borne pathogens need not be viewed as equally threatening. For example, *Borrelia burgdorferi*, the agent of Lyme disease (an emerging vector-borne pathogen in human populations in North America), does not need to be monitored to avoid its establishment as a human pathogen because once emerged, it does not threaten to spiral out of control; it is tick-borne, and ongoing human/tick cycles are not feasible because of the limited exposure of infected humans to susceptible tick populations of the appropriate instar (developmental stages of arthropods before sexual maturity is reached). Tick- and mite-borne Rickettsiae do not present a great threat for similar reasons.

Dangerous Emergences of the Past

Each of the organisms that caused devastating epidemics over the past 5 centuries would have been identified as an extremely dangerous pathogen by the criteria proposed here. *Y. pestis*, for example, is durable in the external environment and is vector-borne. Its threat is lower now than centuries ago when fleas and rats were abundant domiciliary inhabitants, but it still represents a threat where these hosts are present.

The periodic emergence of yellow fever in European and American cities during the 18th and 19th centuries took a heavy toll; the 1878 epidemic, for example, killed about a quarter of the population of Memphis, Tennessee. If yellow fever virus were first encountered today, it would be recognized as an important threat because it is vector-borne and can be transmitted indefinitely through human/mosquito cycles.

Resurgent Vector-Borne Diseases as a Global Health Problem

This section includes text excerpted from "Resurgent Vector-Borne Diseases as a Global Health Problem," Centers for Disease Control and Prevention (CDC), December 14, 2010. Reviewed February 2020.

Vector-borne infectious diseases are emerging or resurging as a result of changes in public-health policy, insecticide and drug resistance, shifts in emphasis from prevention to emergency response, demographic and societal changes, and genetic changes in pathogens. Effective prevention strategies can reverse this trend. Research on vaccines, environmentally safe insecticides, alternative approaches to vector control, and training programs for healthcare workers are needed.

In the 120 years since arthropods were shown to transmit human disease, hundreds of viruses, bacteria, protozoa, and helminths have been found to require a hematophagous (blood-sucking) arthropod for transmission between vertebrate hosts. Historically, malaria, dengue, yellow fever, plague, filariasis, louse-borne typhus, trypanosomiasis, leishmaniasis, and other vector-borne diseases were responsible for more human disease and death in the 17th through the early 20th centuries than all other causes combined. During the 19th and 20th centuries, vector-borne diseases prevented the development of large areas of the tropics, especially in Africa; it was not until these diseases were controlled that engineering feats such as the Panama Canal could be completed.

Not long after the 1877 discovery that mosquitoes transmitted filariasis from human to human, malaria (1898), yellow fever (1900), and dengue (1903) were shown to have similar transmission cycles. By 1910, other major vector-borne diseases such as African sleeping sickness, the plague, Rocky Mountain spotted fever, relapsing fever, Chagas disease, sandfly fever, and louse-borne typhus had all been shown to require a blood-sucking arthropod vector for transmission to humans.

Prevention and control programs were soon based on controlling the arthropod vector. Yellow fever in Cuba was the first vector-borne disease to be effectively controlled in this manner, followed quickly by yellow fever and malaria in Panama. Over the next 50 years, most of the important vector-borne public-health threats were effectively controlled. Most of these programs established vertically structured vector-control organizations that emphasized elimination of arthropod breeding sites (source reduction) through environmental hygiene, along with limited use of chemical insecticides. By the 1960s, vector-borne diseases were no longer considered major public-health problems outside Africa. Urban yellow fever and dengue, both transmitted by *Aedes aegypti*, were effectively controlled in Central and South America and eliminated from North America; malaria was nearly eradicated in the Americas, the Pacific Islands, and Asia. The discovery and effective use of residual insecticides in the 1940s, 1950s, and 1960s contributed greatly to these successes.

However, the benefits of vector-borne disease-control programs were short-lived. A number of vector-borne diseases began to reemerge in the 1970s, a resurgence that has greatly intensified in the past 20 years. Although the reasons for the failure of these programs are complex and not well understood, two factors played important roles: (1) the diversion of financial support and subsequent loss of public-health infrastructure, and (2) reliance on quick-fix solutions such as insecticides and drugs.

Section 35.3

Factors Involved in Vector-Borne Disease Emergence

This section includes text excerpted from "Resurgent Vector-Borne Diseases as a Global Health Problem," Centers for Disease Control and Prevention (CDC), December 14, 2010. Reviewed February 2020.

The factors responsible for the emergence/resurgence of vector-borne diseases are complex. They include insecticide and drug resistance, changes in public-health policy, emphasis on emergency response, de-emphasis of prevention programs, demographic and societal changes, and genetic changes in pathogens. Public-health policy decisions greatly decreased the resources for surveillance, prevention, and control of vector-borne diseases in the 1960s and 1970s, primarily because control programs had reduced the public-health threat from these diseases. Those decisions, the technical problems of insecticide and drug resistance, as well as too much emphasis on insecticide sprays to kill adult mosquitoes, contributed greatly to the resurgence of diseases such as malaria and dengue. Decreased resources for infectious diseases in general resulted in the discontinuation or merger of many programs and ultimately to the deterioration of the public-health infrastructure required to deal with these diseases.

Moreover, good training programs in vector-borne diseases decreased dramatically after 1970. Thus, in 1998, we faced a critical shortage of specialists trained to respond effectively to the resurgence of vector-borne diseases. A related problem is the lack of preventive medicine training in most medical schools. The curative approach and emphasis on high-tech solutions to disease control have led most physicians, health officials, and the public to rely on "magic bullets" to cure an illness or control an epidemic.

Major global demographic and societal changes of the past 50 years have directly affected the emergence/resurgence of vector-borne and other infectious diseases. Unprecedented population growth, mostly in developing countries, resulted in major movements of people, primarily to urban centers. This unplanned and uncontrolled urbanization (inadequate housing, deteriorating water, sewage, and waste-management systems) produced ideal conditions for increased transmission of mosquito-borne, rodent-borne, and waterborne diseases. The prospects for the future are not good; nearly all of the world's population growth in the next 25 years will occur in the urban centers of developing countries, many of them in tropical areas where vector-borne diseases occur most frequently.

Other societal changes, such as agricultural practices and deforestation, increase the risk for vector-borne disease transmission. Many irrigation systems and dams have been built in the past 50 years without regard to their effect on vector-borne diseases. Similarly, tropical forests are being cleared at an increasing rate, and agricultural practices such as rice production have also increased.

Consumer products make ideal breeding sites for domesticated mosquitoes. Packaged in nonbiodegradable plastics, cellophanes, and tin, these products tend to be discarded in the environment, where they collect rainwater. Discarded automobile tires, many in the domestic environment, make ideal mosquito breeding places as well as rat and rodent harborages. Container shipping and the global used-tire industry have contributed to the increased geographic distribution of selected mosquito species that lay their eggs in used tires.

Finally, the jet airplane has had a major influence on global demographics. The airplane provides the ideal mechanism for transporting pathogens between population centers. The result is a constant movement of viruses, bacteria, and parasites among cities, countries, regions, and continents.

Climate change (e.g., global warming and El Niño Southern Oscillation) is often cited as the cause for the emergence/resurgence of vector-borne diseases, especially malaria, dengue, and yellow fever. While meteorologic factors such as temperature, rainfall, and humidity influence the transmission dynamics of vector-borne diseases, climate change has not yet been scientifically proven to have caused the emergence/resurgence of any of the vector-borne diseases described above.

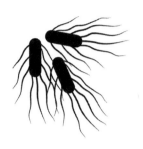

CHAPTER 36
Foodborne Pathogens

Chapter Contents

Food Vehicles of Transmission

This section includes text excerpted from "Emerging Foodborne Diseases: An Evolving Public Health Challenge," Centers for Disease Control and Prevention (CDC), December 21, 2010. Reviewed March 2020.

Along with new pathogens, an array of new food vehicles of transmission for disease have been implicated. Traditionally, the food implicated in a foodborne outbreak was undercooked meat, poultry, or seafood, or unpasteurized milk. Now, additional foods previously thought safe are considered hazardous. For example, for centuries, the internal contents of an egg were presumed safe to eat raw. However, epidemic *Salmonella* enteritidis infection among egg-laying flocks indicates that intact eggs may have internal contamination with this *Salmonella* serotype. Many outbreaks are caused by contaminated shell eggs, including eggs used in such traditional recipes as eggnog and Caesar salad, lightly cooked eggs in omelets and French toast, and even foods one would presume thoroughly cooked, such as lasagna and meringue pie. *E. coli* O157:H7 has caused illness through an ever-broadening spectrum of foods, beyond the beef and raw milk that are directly related to the bovine reservoir.

In 1992, an outbreak caused by apple cider showed that this organism could be transmitted through food with a pH level of less than 4.0, possibly after contact of fresh produce with manure. An outbreak traced to venison jerky suggests a wild deer reservoir, so both cattle and feral deer manure are of concern. Imported raspberries contaminated with *Cyclospora* caused an epidemic in the United States in 1996, possibly because contaminated surface water was used to spray the berries with fungicide before harvest.

Norwalk-like viruses, which appear to have a human reservoir, have contaminated oysters harvested from pristine waters by oystercatchers who did not use toilets with holding tanks on their boats and were themselves the likely source of the virus.

559

The new food vehicles of disease share several features. Contamination typically occurs early in the production process, rather than just before consumption. Because of consumer demand and the global food market, ingredients from many countries may be combined in a single dish, which makes the specific source of contamination difficult to trace. These foods, such as salt, sugar, or preservatives, have fewer barriers to microbial growth; and therefore, simple transgressions can make the food unsafe. Because the food has a short shelf life, it may often be gone by the time the outbreak is recognized; therefore, efforts to prevent contamination at the source are very important.

An increasing, though still limited, proportion of reported foodborne outbreaks is being traced to fresh produce. A series of outbreaks investigated by the Centers for Disease Control and Prevention (CDC) has linked a variety of pathogens to fresh fruits and vegetables harvested in the United States. The investigations have often been triggered by detection of more cases than expected of a rare serotype of *Salmonella* or *Shigella* or by diagnosis of a rare infection like cyclosporiasis. Outbreaks caused by common serotypes are more likely to be missed. Various possible points of contamination have been identified during these investigations, including contamination during production and harvest, initial processing and packing, distribution, and final processing. For example, fresh or inadequately composted manure is used agriculturally sometimes, although *E. coli* O157:H7 has been shown to survive for up to 70 days in bovine feces. Untreated or contaminated water seems to be a particularly likely source of contamination. Water used for spraying, washing, and maintaining the appearance of produce must be microbiologically safe. After two large outbreaks of salmonellosis were traced to imported cantaloupe, the melon industry considered a "Melon Safety Plan," focusing particularly on the chlorination of water used to wash melons and to make ice for shipping them. Although the extent to which the plan was implemented is unknown, no further large outbreaks have occurred. After two large outbreaks of salmonellosis were traced to a single tomato packer in the Southeast, an automated chlorination system was developed for the packing plant wash tank. Because tomatoes absorb water (and associated bacteria) if washed in water colder than they are, particular attention was also focused on the

Table 36.1. Foodborne Outbreaks Traced to Fresh Produce, 1990–1996

Yr.	Pathogen	Vehicle	Cases (No.)	States (No.)	Source
90	*S.* Chester	Cantaloupe	245	30	C.A.a
90	*S.* Javiana	Tomatoes	174	4	U.S.b
90	Hepatitis A	Strawberries	18	2	U.S.
91	*S.* Poona	Cantaloupe	>400	23	U.S./C.A
93	*E. coli* O157:H7	Apple cider	23	1	U.S.
93	*S.* Montevideo	Tomatoes	84	3	U.S.
94	*Shigella flexneri*	Scallions	72	2	C.A.
95	*S.* Stanley	Alfalfa sprouts	242	17	N.K.c
95	*S.* Hartford	Orange juice	63	21	U.S.
95	*E. coli* O157:H7	Leaf lettuce	70	1	U.S.
96	*E. coli* O157:H7	Leaf lettuce	49	2	U.S.
96	*Cyclospora*	Raspberries	978	20	C.A.
96	*E. coli* O157:H7	Apple juice	71	3	U.S.

Table 36.2. Events and Potential Contamination Sources during Produce Processing

Event	Contamination Sources
Production and harvest	
Growing, picking, bundling	Irrigation water, manure, lack of field sanitation
Initial processing	
Washing, waxing, sorting, boxing	Wash water, handling
Distribution	
Trucking	Ice, dirty trucks
Final processing	
Slicing, squeezing, shredding, peeling	Wash water, handling, cross-contamination

temperature of the water bath. No further outbreaks have been linked to southeastern tomatoes. Similar attention is warranted for water used to rinse lettuce heads in packing sheds and to crisp them in grocery stores as well as for water used in processing other fresh produce.

Section 36.2

Foodborne Pathogens: Outbreak Challenges

This section includes text excerpted from "Emerging Foodborne Diseases: An Evolving Public Health Challenge," Centers for Disease Control and Prevention (CDC), December 21, 2010. Reviewed March 2020.

A New Outbreak Scenario

Because of changes in the way food is produced and distributed, a new kind of foodborne outbreak has appeared. The traditional foodborne outbreak scenario often follows a church supper, family picnic, wedding reception, or other social event. This scenario involves an acute and highly local outbreak, with a high inoculum dose and a high attack rate. The outbreak is typically immediately apparent to those in the local group, who promptly involve medical and public-health authorities. The investigation identifies a food-handling error in a small kitchen that occurred shortly before consumption. The solution is also local. Such outbreaks still occur, and handling them remains an important function of a local health department.

However, diffuse and widespread outbreaks involving many counties, states, and even nations, are identified more frequently and follow an entirely different scenario. The new scenario is the result of low-level contamination of a widely distributed commercial food product. In most jurisdictions, the increase in cases may be inapparent against the background illness. The outbreak is detected only because of a fortuitous concentration of cases in one location, because the pathogen causing the outbreak is unusual, or because laboratory-based subtyping of strains collected over a wide area identifies a diffuse surge in one subtype. In such outbreaks, investigation can require coordinated efforts of a large team to clarify the extent of the outbreak, implicate a specific food, and determine the source of contamination. Often, no obvious terminal food-handling error is found. Instead, contamination is the result of an event in the industrial chain of food production. Investigating, controlling, and preventing such outbreaks can have industrywide implications.

These diffuse outbreaks can be caused by a variety of foods because fresh produce is usually widely distributed. Some of the largest outbreaks affected most states at once. For example, an outbreak of *Salmonella Enteritidis* infections caused by a nationally distributed brand of ice cream affected the entire nation. Although it caused an estimated 250,000 illnesses, it was detected only when vigorous routine surveillance identified a surge in reported infections with *S.* Enteritidis in one area of southern Minnesota. The consumers affected did not make food-handling errors with their ice cream, so food safety instruction could not have prevented this outbreak. The ice cream premix was transported after pasteurization to the ice-cream factory in tanker trucks that had been used to haul raw eggs. The huge epidemic was the result of a basic failure on an industrial scale to separate the raw from the cooked.

S. Enteritidis infections also illustrate why the surveillance and investigation of sporadic cases are needed. A diffuse increase in sporadic cases can occur well before a local or large outbreak focuses attention on the emergence of a pathogen. The isolation rate for *S.* Enteritidis began to increase sharply in the New England region in 1978; all cases were sporadic. In 1982, an outbreak in a New England nursing home was traced to eggs from a local supplier. However, the egg connection was not really appreciated until 1986, when a large multistate outbreak of *S.* Enteritidis infections was traced to stuffed pasta made with raw eggs and labeled "fully cooked." This outbreak, affecting an estimated 3,000 people in seven states, led to the documentation that *S.* Enteritidis was present on egg-laying farms and to the subsequent demonstration that both outbreaks and sporadic cases of infections were associated with shell eggs. Since then, enteritidis has become the most common serotype of *Salmonella* isolated in the United States, accounting for 25 percent of all *Salmonella* reported in the country and causing outbreaks coast to coast. Eggs remain the dominant source of these infections, causing large outbreaks when they are pooled and undercooked and individual sporadic cases among consumers who eat an individual egg. Perhaps focused investigation and control measures taken when the localized increase in sporadic *Salmonella* cases was just beginning might have prevented the subsequent spread.

Section 36.3
Changing Surveillance Strategies

This section includes text excerpted from "Emerging Foodborne Diseases: An Evolving Public Health Challenge," Centers for Disease Control and Prevention (CDC), December 21, 2010. Reviewed March 2020.

In the United States, surveillance for diseases of major public-health importance has been conducted for many years. The legal framework for surveillance resides in the state public-health epidemiology offices, which share data with the Centers for Disease Control and Prevention (CDC). The first surveillance systems depended on physician or coroner notification of specific diseases and conditions, with reports going first to the local health department, then to state and federal offices. Now electronic, this form of surveillance is still used for many specific conditions. In 1962, a second channel was developed specifically for *Salmonella,* to take advantage of the added public-health information provided by subtyping the strains of bacteria. Clinical laboratories that isolated *Salmonella* from humans were requested or required to send the strains to the state public-health laboratory for serotyping. Although knowing the serotype is usually of little benefit to the individual patient, it has been critical to protecting and improving the health of the public at large. Serotyping allows cases that might otherwise appear unrelated to be included in an investigation because they are of the same serotype. Moreover, infections that are close in time and space to an outbreak but are caused by non-outbreak serotypes and are probably unrelated can be discounted. Results of serotyping are now sent electronically from public-health laboratories and can be rapidly analyzed and summarized. *Salmonella* serotyping was the first subtype-based surveillance system and is a model for similar systems. Yet another source of surveillance data involves summary reports of foodborne disease-outbreak investigations from local and state health departments. About 400 such outbreaks are reported annually by a system that remains paper-based, labor-intensive, and slow.

Existing surveillance systems provide a limited and relatively inexpensive net for tracing large-scale trends in foodborne diseases under surveillance and for detecting outbreaks of established pathogens in the United States. However, they are less sensitive to diffuse outbreaks of common pathogens, provide little detail on sporadic cases, and are not easy to extend to emerging pathogens. In the future, changes in health delivery may impinge on the way that diagnoses are made and reported, leading to artifactual changes in reported disease incidence.

Therefore, the CDC, in collaboration with state health departments and federal food regulatory agencies, is enhancing national surveillance for foodborne diseases in several ways. For example, the role of subtyping in public-health laboratories continues to be expanded to encompass new molecular subtyping methods. Beginning in 1997, a national subtyping network for *E. coli* O157:H7 of participating state public-health department laboratories and the CDC began using a single standardized laboratory protocol to subtype strains of this important pathogen. The standard method, pulsed-field gel electrophoresis, can be easily adapted to other bacterial pathogens. In this network, each participating laboratory is now able to routinely compare the genetic gel patterns of strains of *E. coli* O157:H7 with the patterns in a national pattern bank. This enables rapid detection of clusters of related cases within the state and focuses investigative resources on the cases most likely to be linked. It also enables related cases scattered across several states to be linked so that a common source can be sought.

Another surveillance strategy, now implemented, is active surveillance in sentinel populations. Since January 1996, at five U.S. sentinel sites, additional surveillance resources have made it possible to contact laboratories directly for regular reporting of bacterial infections likely to be foodborne. In addition, surveys of the population, physicians, and laboratories measure the proportion of diarrheal diseases that are undiagnosed and unreported so that the true disease incidence can be estimated. This surveillance, known as "FoodNet," is the platform on which more detailed investigations, including case-control studies of sporadic cases of common foodborne infections, are being conducted.

Yet another surveillance initiative is the routine monitoring of antimicrobial resistance among a sample of *Salmonella* and *E. coli* O157:H7 bacteria isolated from humans. A cluster-detection algorithm is being applied routinely to surveillance data for *Salmonella* at the national level, making it possible to detect and flag possible outbreaks as soon as the data are reported. Implementation of such algorithms for other infections and at the state level will further increase the usefulness of routine surveillance.

Further enhancements are possible as active surveillance through FoodNet is extended to a wider spectrum of infections, including foodborne parasitic and viral infections. Active surveillance for *Cyclospora* began in FoodNet in 1997, for example, and quickly resulted in the detection of a diffuse outbreak among people who had been on a Caribbean cruise ship that made stops in Mexico and Central America (CDC, unpub. data). Application of standardized molecular-subtyping methods to other foodborne pathogens will continue to provide a more sensitive warning system for diffuse outbreaks of a variety of pathogens. To handle outbreaks in areas not covered by FoodNet, standard surveillance and investigative capacities in state health department epidemiology offices and laboratories should be strengthened. In addition, enhanced international consultation will be critical to better detect and investigate international or global outbreaks.

Section 36.4

New Approaches to the Prevention of Foodborne Disease

This section includes text excerpted from "Emerging Foodborne Diseases: An Evolving Public Health Challenge," Centers for Disease Control and Prevention (CDC), December 21, 2010. Reviewed March 2020.

Meeting the complex challenge of foodborne disease prevention will require the collaboration of regulatory agencies and industry to make food safe and keep it safe throughout the industrial chain of production. Prevention can be "built-in" to the industry by identifying and controlling the key points—from the field, farm, or fishing grounds to the dinner table—at which contamination can either occur or be eliminated. The general strategy, known as "Hazard Analysis and Critical Control Points" (HACCP) replaces the strategy of final product inspection. Some simple control strategies are self-evident once the reality of microbial contamination is recognized. For example, shipping fruit from Central America with clean ice or in closed refrigerator trucks, rather than with ice made from untreated river water, is common sense. Similarly, requiring oyster harvesters to use toilets with holding tanks on their oyster boats is an obvious way to reduce fecal contamination of shallow oyster beds. Pasteurization provides the extra barrier that will prevent *E. coli* O157:H7 and other pathogens from contaminating a large batch of freshly squeezed juice.

For many foodborne diseases, multiple choices for prevention are available, and the best answer may be to apply several steps simultaneously. For *E. coli* O157:H7 infections related to the cattle reservoir, pasteurizing milk and cooking meat thoroughly provide an important measure of protection but are insufficient by themselves. Options for better control include continued improvements in slaughter-plant hygiene and control measures under HACCP, developing additives to cattle feed that alter the microbial growth either in the feed or in the bovine rumen to make cows less hospitable hosts for *E. coli* O157, immunizing or otherwise protecting the cows so that they do not become infected in the first place, and irradiating beef after slaughter. For *C. jejuni* infections related to the poultry reservoir, future control options include modification of the slaughter process to reduce contamination of chicken carcasses by bile or by water baths, freezing chicken carcasses to reduce *Campylobacter* counts, chlorinating the water that chickens drink to prevent them from getting infected, vaccinating chickens, and irradiating poultry carcasses after slaughter.

Outbreaks are often fertile sources of new research questions. Translating these questions into research agendas is an important part of the overall prevention effort. Applied research is needed to improve the strategies of subtyping and surveillance. Veterinary and agricultural research on the farm is needed to answer the questions about whether and how a pathogen such as *E. coli* O157:H7 persists in the bovine reservoir, to establish the size and dynamics of a reservoir for this organism in wild deer, and to look at potential routes of contamination connecting animal manure and lettuce fields. More research is needed regarding foods defined as sources in large outbreaks in order to develop better control strategies and better barriers to contamination and microbial growth and to understand the behavior of new pathogens in specific foods. Research is also needed to improve the diagnosis, clinical management, and treatment of severe foodborne infections and to improve our understanding of the pathogenesis of new and emerging pathogens. To assess and evaluate potential prevention strategies, applied research is needed into the costs and potential benefits of each or of combinations.

In preparing for the 21st century, the Centers for Disease Control and Prevention (CDC) will continue to enhance our public-health food-safety infrastructure by adding new surveillance and subtyping strategies and strengthening the ability of public-health practitioners to investigate and respond quickly. The CDC will also encourage the prudent use of antibiotics in animal and human medicine to limit antimicrobial resistance. The CDC will further continue basic and applied research into the microbes that cause foodborne disease and into the mechanisms by which they contaminate our foods and cause outbreaks and sporadic cases.

Better understanding of foodborne pathogens is the foundation for new approaches to disease prevention and control.

Section 36.5

Emerging Foodborne Pathogens

This section includes text excerpted from "Emerging Foodborne Diseases: An Evolving Public Health Challenge," Centers for Disease Control and Prevention (CDC), December 21, 2010. Reviewed March 2020.

Substantial progress has been made in preventing foodborne diseases. For example, typhoid fever, extremely common at the beginning of the 20th century, is now almost forgotten in the United States. It was conquered in the preantibiotic era by disinfection of drinking water, sewage treatment, milk sanitation and pasteurization, and shellfish bed sanitation. Similarly, cholera, bovine tuberculosis, and trichinosis have also been controlled in the United States. However, new foodborne pathogens have emerged. Among the first of these were infections caused by nontyphoid strains of *Salmonella*, which have increased decade by decade since World War II.

In the last 20 years, other infectious agents have been either newly described or newly associated with foodborne transmission. *Vibrio vulnificus*, *Escherichia coli* O157:H7, and *Cyclospora cayetanensis* are examples of newly described pathogens that often are foodborne. *V. vulnificus* was identified in the bloodstream of people with underlying liver disease who had fulminant infections after eating raw oysters or being exposed to seawater; this organism lives in the sea and can be a natural summertime commensal organism in shellfish. *E. coli* O157:H7 was first identified as a pathogen in 1982 in an outbreak of bloody diarrhea traced to hamburgers from a fast-food chain; it was subsequently shown to have a reservoir in healthy cattle. *Cyclospora*, known previously as a cyanobacteria-like organism, received its current taxonomic designation in 1992 and emerged as a foodborne pathogen in outbreaks traced to imported Guatemalan raspberries in 1996. The similarity of *Cyclospora* to *Eimeria* coccidian pathogens of birds suggests an avian reservoir.

Some known pathogens have only recently been shown to be predominantly foodborne. For example, *Listeria monocytogenes* was long known as a cause of meningitis and other invasive infections in immunocompromised hosts. How these hosts became infected remained unknown until a series of investigations identified food as the most common source. Similarly, *Campylobacter jejuni* was known as a rare opportunistic bloodstream infection until veterinary diagnostic methods used on specimens from humans showed it was a common cause of diarrheal illness. Subsequent epidemiologic investigations implicated poultry and raw milk as the most common sources of sporadic cases and outbreaks, respectively. *Yersinia enterocolitica*, rare in the United States but a common cause of diarrheal illness and pseudoappendicitis in northern Europe and elsewhere, is now known to be most frequently associated with undercooked pork.

These foodborne pathogens share a number of characteristics. Virtually all have an animal reservoir from which they spread to humans; that is, they are foodborne zoonoses. In marked contrast to many established zoonoses, these new zoonoses do not often cause illness in the infected host animal. The chicken with lifelong ovarian infection with *Salmonella* serotype enteritidis, the calf carrying *E. coli* O157:H7, and the oyster carrying Norwalk virus or *V. vulnificus* appear healthy; therefore, public-health concerns must now include apparently healthy animals. Limited existing research on how animals acquire and transmit emerging pathogens among themselves often implicates contaminated fodder and water; therefore, public-health concerns must now include the safety of what food animals themselves eat and drink.

For reasons that remain unclear, these pathogens can rapidly spread globally. For example, *Y. enterocolitica* spread globally among pigs in the 1970s; *Salmonella* serotype Enteritidis appeared simultaneously around the world in the 1980s; and *Salmonella* Typhimurium Definitive Type (DT) 104 is now appearing in North America, Europe, and perhaps elsewhere;

therefore, public-health concerns must now include events happening around the world as harbingers of what may appear here.

Many emerging zoonotic pathogens are becoming increasingly resistant to antimicrobial agents, largely because of the widespread use of antibiotics in the animal reservoir. For example, *Campylobacter* isolated from human patients in Europe is now increasingly resistant to fluoroquinolones, after these agents were introduced for use in animals. *Salmonellae* have become increasing resistant to a variety of antimicrobial agents in the United States; therefore, public-health concerns must include the patterns of antimicrobial use in agriculture as well as in human medicine.

The foods contaminated with emerging pathogens usually look, smell, and taste normal, and the pathogen often survives traditional preparation techniques: *E. coli* O157:H7 in meat can survive the gentle heating that a rare hamburger gets; *Salmonella* Enteritidis in eggs survives in an omelet, and Norwalk virus in oysters survives gentle steaming. Hence, following standard and traditional recipes can cause illness and outbreaks. Contamination with the new foodborne zoonoses further eludes traditional food inspection, which relies on visual identification of hazards. These pathogens demand new control strategies, which would minimize the likelihood of contamination in the first place. The rate at which new pathogens have been identified suggests that many more remain to be discovered. Many of the foodborne infections of the future are likely to arise from the animal reservoirs from which we draw our food supply.

Once a new foodborne disease is identified, a number of critical questions need to be answered to develop a rational approach to prevention: What is the nature of the disease? What is the nature of the pathogen? What are simple ways to easily identify the pathogen and diagnose the disease? What is the incidence of the infection? How can the disease be treated? Which foods transmit the infection? How does the pathogen get into the food, and how well does it persist there? Is there an animal reservoir? How do the animals themselves become infected? How can the disease be prevented? Does the prevention strategy work?

The answers to these questions do not come rapidly. Knowledge accumulates gradually, as a result of detailed scientific investigations, often conducted during outbreaks. Better slaughter procedures and pasteurization of milk are useful control strategies for this pathogen in meat and milk, as irradiation of meat may be in the future. More needs to be learned: for example, it remains unclear how best to prevent this organism from contaminating lettuce or apple juice.

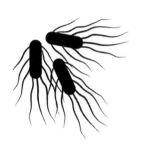

CHAPTER 37
Waterborne Pathogens

Chapter Contents

Dynamic Epidemiology

This section includes text excerpted from "A Human Health Perspective on Climate Change," National Institute of Environmental Health Sciences (NIEHS), April 22, 2010. Reviewed March 2020.

Waterborne Diseases

Waterborne diseases are caused by a wide variety of pathogenic microorganisms, biotoxins, and toxic contaminants found in the water we drink, clean with, play in, and are exposed to through other less-direct pathways such as cooling systems. Waterborne microorganisms include protozoa that cause cryptosporidiosis, parasites that cause schistosomiasis, bacteria that cause cholera and legionellosis, viruses that cause viral gastroenteritis, amoebas that cause amoebic meningoencephalitis, and algae that cause neurotoxicity.

In the United States, the majority of waterborne disease is gastrointestinal, though waterborne pathogens affect most human organ systems and the epidemiology is dynamic. A shift has been seen in waterborne disease outbreaks from gastrointestinal toward respiratory infections such as that caused by *Legionella*, which lives in cooling ponds and is transmitted through air-conditioning systems. In addition to diarrheal disease, waterborne pathogens are implicated in other illnesses with immunologic, neurologic, hematologic, metabolic, pulmonary, ocular, renal, and nutritional complications. The World Health Organization (WHO) estimates that 4.8 percent of the global burden of disease (as measured in disability-adjusted life years (DALYs)) and 3.7 percent of all mortality attributable to the environment is due to diarrheal disease.

Most of these diseases produce more serious symptoms and greater risk of death in children and pregnant women. For most waterborne pathogens in the United States, surveillance is spotty, diagnoses are not uniform, and a full epidemiological understanding of the impact of normal weather and climate variation on disease incidence, as well as illness and death burdens, is not firmly established. Impacts of any intensifying climate events at local, regional, national, and global levels are a growing concern. Experts estimate that there is a high incidence of mild symptoms from waterborne pathogens and a relatively small, but not negligible, mortality burden.

Research Highlights

There is a clear association between increases in precipitation and outbreaks of waterborne disease, both domestically and globally. Climate change is expected to produce more frequent and severe, as well as extreme precipitation events worldwide. In the United States from 1948 to 1994, heavy rainfall correlated with more than half of the outbreaks of waterborne diseases. Some of the largest outbreaks of waterborne disease in North America, particularly in the Great Lakes region, resulted after extreme rainfall events. For example, in May 2000, heavy rainfall in Walkerton, Ontario resulted in approximately 2,300 illnesses and seven deaths after the town's drinking water became contaminated with *E. coli* O157:H7 and *Campylobacter jejuni*. There are combined sewage and wastewater systems in and around the Great Lakes, with an estimated discharge of 850 billion gallons of untreated overflow water. Using a suite of seven climate change models to project extreme precipitation events in the Great Lakes region, scientists have been able to estimate the potential impact of climate change on waterborne disease rates. Their models predict more than 2.5 inches of rain in a single day will cause a combined sewer overflow into Lake Michigan, resulting in 100 percent more waterborne disease outbreaks in the region per year. Considering that the Great Lakes serves as the primary water source for over 40 million people and is surrounded by a number of large cities, both past events and these projections indicate a serious threat to public health in this region due to climate change alterations in the frequency of extreme precipitation. Globally, the impact of waterborne diarrheal disease is high and expected to climb with climate change. Improving domestic surveillance is a high priority, as this would enhance the epidemiologic characterization of the drivers of epidemic disease. In particular, weather- and climate-related drivers are not well understood. Waterborne disease outbreaks are highly correlated with extreme precipitation events, but this correlation is based on limited research and needs further investigation and confirmation. Prevention and treatment strategies for waterborne disease are well established throughout the developed world; climate change is not likely to greatly impact the efficacy of these strategies in the United States. However, climate change is very likely to increase global diarrheal disease incidence, and changes in the hydrologic cycle, including increases in the frequency and intensity of extreme weather events, and droughts may greatly complicate already inadequate prevention efforts. Enhanced understanding and reinvigorated global prevention efforts are very important.

Ocean-related diseases are those associated with direct contact with marine waters (aerosolized in some cases) or sediments (including beach sands), ingestion of contaminated seafood, or exposure to zoonotics. Pathogenic microorganisms (bacteria, viruses, protozoa, and fungi) that may occur naturally in the ocean, coastal, and Great Lakes waters, or as a result of sewage pollution and runoff, are the primary etiologic agents. Human exposure to these agents may result in a variety of infectious diseases, including serious wound and skin infections, diarrhea, respiratory effects, and others. Research has concluded that antibiotic-methicillin-resistant *Staphylococcus aureus* (MRSA) is persistent in both fresh and seawater and could become waterborne if released into these waters in sufficient quantities. While this has yet to emerge as a significant public-health concern, the potential for recreational exposure is significant, as people make nearly one billion trips to the beach annually in the United States alone. In contrast to diarrheal disease, there are few effective preventive strategies for marine-based environmental exposures beyond closing beaches to the public, and these areas need immediate additional research.

The effects of climate changes on the distribution and bioaccumulation of chemical contaminants in marine food webs are poorly understood and may be significant for vulnerable populations of humans and animals. The U.S. Climate Change Science Program (CCSP) reported a likely increase in the spread of waterborne pathogens based on the pathogens' survival, persistence, habitat range, and transmission in a changing environment. In one specific example, the CCSP noted the strong association between sea surface temperature and proliferation of many *Vibrio* species and suggested that rising temperatures would likely lead to increased occurrence of enteric disease associated with *Vibrio* bacteria (*V. cholerae, V. vulnificus,* and *V. parahaemolyticus*) in the United States, including the potential for the occurrence of cholera and wound infections. Further, the findings demonstrate that pathogens that can pose disease risks to humans occur widely in marine vertebrates and regularly contaminate shellfish and aquaculture finfish.

Section 37.2
Climate Impacts and Health Risk

This section includes text excerpted from "A Human Health Perspective on Climate Change," National Institute of Environmental Health Sciences (NIEHS), April 22, 2010. Reviewed March 2020.

Impacts on Risk

Climate directly impacts the incidence of waterborne disease through effects on water temperature and precipitation frequency and intensity. These effects are pathogen- and pollutant-specific, and risks for human disease are markedly affected by local conditions, including regional water- and sewage-treatment capacities and practices. Domestic water-treatment plants may be susceptible to climate change leading to human health risks. For example, droughts may cause problems with increased concentrations of effluent pathogens and overwhelm water-treatment plants; aging water-treatment plants are particularly at risk. Urbanization of coastal regions may lead to additional nutrient, chemical, and pathogen loading in the runoff. Public-health understanding of weather and climate impacts on specific pathogens is incomplete. Climate also indirectly impacts waterborne disease through changes in ocean and coastal ecosystems, including changes in pH, nutrient and contaminant runoff, salinity, and water security.

These indirect impacts are likely to result in the degradation of freshwater available for drinking, washing food, cooking, and irrigation, particularly in developing and emerging economies where much of the population still use untreated surface water from rivers, streams, and other open sources for these needs. Even in countries that treat water, climate-induced changes in the frequency and intensity of extreme weather events could lead to damage or flooding of water- and sewage-treatment facilities, increasing the risk of waterborne diseases. Severe outbreaks of cholera, in particular, have been directly associated with flooding in Africa and India. A rise in sea level, combined with increasingly severe weather events, is likely to make flooding events commonplace worldwide. A 40 centimeter (nearly 16-inch) rise in sea level is expected to increase the average annual numbers of people affected by coastal storm surges from less than 50 million at present to nearly 250 million by 2080. Several secondary impacts are also a concern. Ecosystem degradation from climate change will likely result in pressure on agricultural productivity, crop failure, malnutrition, starvation, increasing population displacement, and resource conflict, all of which are predisposing factors for increased human susceptibility and increased risk of waterborne disease transmission due to surface water contamination with human waste and increased contact with 292,293 such waters through washing and consumption. Climate change may also affect the distribution and concentrations of chemical contaminants in coastal and ocean waters, for example through the release of chemical contaminants previously bound up in polar ice sheets or sediments, through changes in volume and composition of runoff from coastal and watershed development, or through changes in coastal and ocean goods and services. Both naturally occurring and pollution-related ocean health threats will likely be exacerbated by climate change. Other climate-related environmental changes, may impact marine food webs as well, such as pesticide runoff, leaching of arsenic, fluoride, and nitrates from fertilizers, and lead contamination of drinking and recreational waters through excess rainfall and flooding.

Section 37.3

Mitigation and Adaptation for Waterborne Illness

This section includes text excerpted from "A Human Health Perspective on Climate Change," National Institute of Environmental Health Sciences (NIEHS), April 22, 2010. Reviewed March 2020.

Mitigation and Adaptation

Alternative energy production, carbon sequestration, and water reuse and recycling are some of the mitigation and adaptation options that could have the greatest implications for human health.

As with all technologies, the costs and benefits of each will need to be carefully considered and the most beneficial implemented. The potential impacts of different mitigation strategies for waterborne illness depend on the strategy. For instance, increased hydroelectric-power generation will have significant impacts on local ecologies where dams are built, often resulting in increased or decreased incidence of waterborne disease, as was the case with schistosomiasis (increase) and haematobium infection (decrease) after construction of the Aswan Dam in Egypt. Other modes of electric-power generation, including nuclear, consume large quantities of water and have the potential for substantial environmental impacts ranging from increased water scarcity to discharge of warmed effluent into local surface water bodies. Shifting to wind and solar power, however, will reduce demand on surface waters and, therefore, limit impacts on local water ecosystems and potentially reduce risks of waterborne diseases. The impacts on waterborne-pathogen ecology of other geo-engineering mitigation strategies, such as carbon sequestration, have the potential to be substantial but are largely unknown. Thorough health impact and environmental impact assessments are necessary prior to implementation and widespread adoption of any novel mitigation technology. There is also significant potential for adaptation activities to impact the ecology of waterborne infectious disease. Certain adaptation strategies are likely to have a beneficial impact on water quality; for instance, protecting wetlands to reduce damage from severe storms. Under drought conditions, water reuse or the use of water sources that may be of lower quality is likely to increase. Local water recycling and so-called grey-water reuse, as well as urban design strategies to increase green space and reduce runoff, may result in slower rates of water-table depletion and reduce the impact of extreme precipitation events in urban areas where runoff is concentrated. Other adaptation efforts may have both positive and negative effects. For instance, if the response to increasingly frequent and severe heat waves is widespread, adoption of air conditioning and its associated increase in electricity demand will require additional power, which in turn could impact water availability and regional water ecology.

In parts of the developing world, changing weather patterns and decreased food availability could lead to increased desertification or at least the need for more above-ground irrigation. If such projects are implemented in areas where parasitic diseases such as schistosomiasis are prevalent without close attention to potential ecosystem impacts, there may be changes in regional parasite transport and associated increases or decreases in human exposure. Climate-induced changes to coastal ecosystems are poorly understood, especially with regard to ecosystem goods and services related to human health and well being, and ocean and coastal disease threats. Interactions among climate change factors, such as rising temperatures, extreme weather events, inundation, ocean acidification, and changes in precipitation and runoff with coastal development, aquaculture practices, and other water-use issues need to be studied.

Section 37.4
Research Needs

This section includes text excerpted from "A Human Health Perspective on Climate Change," National Institute of Environmental Health Sciences (NIEHS), April 22, 2010. Reviewed March 2020.

The extent to which the United States is vulnerable to increased risk of waterborne diseases and ocean-related illness due to climate change has not been adequately addressed. Research need includes:

- Understanding the likelihood and potential magnitude of waterborne disease outbreaks due to climate change, including increases in the frequency and intensity of precipitation, temperature changes, extreme weather events, and storm surges

- Researching the vulnerability of water systems to sewer overflow or flooding caused by extreme weather events, especially in water systems where there is already considerable water reuse; and examining the impacts of other water reuse and recycling strategies

- Understanding how toxins, pathogens, and chemicals in land-based runoff and water overflow interact synergistically and with marine species, especially those important for human consumption, and the potential health risks of changing water quality

- Developing means of identifying sentinel species for waterborne disease and understanding of how they may provide early warning of human health threats

- Developing or improving vaccines, antibiotics, and other preventive strategies to prevent and reduce the health consequences of the waterborne disease on a global basis

- Improving understanding of harmful algal blooms, including their initiation, development, and termination, as well as the exact nature of the toxins associated with them conducting epidemiologic studies on the occurrence and severity of ocean-related diseases among humans, especially high-risk populations, in relation to climate change

- Evaluating and monitoring exposures and health risks of chemical contaminants likely to be increasingly released and mobilized due to climate change
- Improving methods to detect, quantify, and forecast ocean-related health threats, including improved surveillance and monitoring of disease-causing agents in coastal waters; in marine organisms (especially seafood), aerosols, and sediments; and in exposed human populations
- Assessing the capacity of the nation's public-health infrastructure to detect and respond to increased waterborne disease incidence, and developing training and evaluation tools to address identified gaps

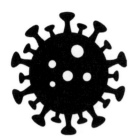

CHAPTER 38
Vaccine Development to Minimize Infectious Disease Burden in the 21st Century

Chapter Contents

Understanding How Vaccines Work

This section includes text excerpted from
"Understanding How Vaccines Work," Centers for
Disease Control and Prevention (CDC), July 2018.

Vaccines prevent diseases that can be dangerous, or even deadly. Vaccines greatly reduce the risk of infection by working with the body's natural defenses to safely develop immunity to disease. This section explains how the body fights infection and how vaccines work to protect people by producing immunity.

The Immune System—
the Body's Defense against Infection

To understand how vaccines work, it helps to first look at how the body fights illness. When germs, such as bacteria or viruses, invade the body, they attack and multiply. This invasion, called an "infection," is what causes illness. The immune system uses several tools to fight infection. Blood contains red blood cells, for carrying oxygen to tissues and organs, and white or immune cells, for fighting infection. These white cells consist primarily of macrophages, B-lymphocytes and T-lymphocytes:

- **Macrophages** are white blood cells that swallow up and digest germs, plus dead or dying cells. The macrophages leave behind parts of the invading germs called "antigens." The body identifies antigens as dangerous and stimulates antibodies to attack them.

- **B-lymphocytes** are defensive white blood cells. They produce antibodies that attack the antigens left behind by the macrophages.

- **T-lymphocytes** are another type of defensive white blood cell. They attack cells in the body that have already been infected. The first time the body encounters a germ, it can take several days to make and use all the germ-fighting tools needed to get over the infection. After

587

the infection, the immune system remembers what it learned about how to protect the body against that disease. The body keeps a few T-lymphocytes, called "memory cells," that go into action quickly if the body encounters the same germ again. When the familiar antigens are detected, B-lymphocytes produce antibodies to attack them.

How Vaccines Work

Vaccines help people develop immunity by imitating an infection. This type of infection, however, almost never causes illness, but it does cause the immune system to produce T-lymphocytes and antibodies. Sometimes, after getting a vaccine, the imitation infection can cause minor symptoms, such as fever. Such minor symptoms are normal and should be expected as the body builds immunity.

Once the imitation infection goes away, the body is left with a supply of "memory" T-lymphocytes, as well as B-lymphocytes that will remember how to fight that disease in the future. However, it typically takes a few weeks for the body to produce T-lymphocytes and B-lymphocytes after vaccination. Therefore, it is possible that a person infected with a disease just before or just after vaccination could develop symptoms and get a disease, because the vaccine has not had enough time to provide protection.

Types of Vaccines

Scientists take many approaches to developing vaccines. These approaches are based on information about the infections (caused by viruses or bacteria) the vaccine will prevent, such as how germs infect cells and how the immune system responds to the infection. Practical considerations, such as regions of the world where the vaccine would be used, are also important because the strain of a virus and environmental conditions, such as temperature and risk of exposure, may be different across the globe. The vaccine-delivery options available may also differ geographically. There are five main types of vaccines that infants and young children commonly receive in the United States:

- **Live, attenuated vaccines** fight viruses and bacteria. These vaccines contain a version of the living virus or bacteria that has been weakened so that it does not cause serious disease in people with healthy immune systems. Because live, attenuated vaccines are the closest thing to a natural infection, they are good teachers for the immune system. Examples of live, attenuated vaccines include measles, mumps, and rubella vaccine (MMR) and varicella (chickenpox) vaccine. Even though they are very effective, not everyone can receive these vaccines. Children with weakened immune systems—for example, those who are undergoing chemotherapy— cannot get live vaccines.

- **Inactivated vaccines** also fight viruses and bacteria. These vaccines are made by inactivating, or killing, the germ during the process of making the vaccine. The inactivated polio vaccine is an example of this type of vaccine. Inactivated vaccines produce immune responses in different ways than live, attenuated vaccines. Often, multiple doses are necessary to build up and/or maintain immunity.

- **Toxoid vaccines** prevent diseases caused by bacteria that produce toxins (poisons) in the body. In the process of making these vaccines, the toxins are weakened so they cannot cause illness. Weakened toxins are called "toxoids." When the immune system receives a vaccine containing a toxoid, it learns how to fight off the natural toxin. The DTaP vaccine contains diphtheria and tetanus toxoids.

- **Subunit vaccines** include only parts of the virus or bacteria, or subunits, instead of the entire germ. Because these vaccines contain only the essential antigens and not all the other molecules that make up the germ, side effects are less common. The pertussis (whooping cough) component of the DTaP vaccine is an example of a subunit vaccine.

- **Conjugate vaccines** fight a different type of bacteria. These bacteria have antigens with an outer coating of sugar-like substances called "polysaccharides." This type of coating disguises the antigen, making it hard for a young child's immature immune system to recognize it and respond to it. Conjugate vaccines are effective for these types of bacteria because they connect (or conjugate) the polysaccharides to antigens that the immune system responds to very well. This linkage helps the immature immune system react to the coating and develop an immune response. An example of this type of vaccine is the *Haemophilus influenzae* type B (Hib) vaccine.

Vaccines Require More than One Dose

There are four reasons that babies—and even teens or adults—who receive a vaccine for the first time may need more than one dose:

- For some vaccines (primarily inactivated vaccines), the first dose does not provide as much immunity as possible. So, more than one dose is needed to build more complete immunity. The vaccine that protects against the bacteria Hib, which causes meningitis, is a good example.
- For some vaccines, after a while, immunity begins to wear off. At that point, a "booster" dose is needed to bring immunity levels back up. This booster dose usually occurs several years after the initial series of vaccine doses is given. For example, in the case of the DTaP vaccine, which protects against diphtheria, tetanus, and pertussis, the initial series of four shots that children receive as part of their infant immunizations helps build immunity. But, a booster dose is needed when the child is 4 to 6 years old. Another booster against these diseases is needed between 11 and 12 years of age. This booster for older children—and teens and adults, too—is called "Tdap."
- For some vaccines (primarily live vaccines), studies have shown that more than one dose is needed for everyone to develop the best immune response. For example, after one dose of the MMR vaccine, some people may not develop enough antibodies to fight off infection. The second dose helps make sure that almost everyone is protected.
- Finally, in the case of flu vaccines, adults and children (6 months and older) need to get a dose every year. Children between 6 months and 8 years of age who have never gotten a flu vaccine in the past or have only gotten one dose in past years need two doses when they are vaccinated. Then, an annual flu vaccine is needed because the flu viruses causing disease may be different from season to season. Every year, flu vaccines are made to protect against the viruses that research suggests will be most common. Also, the immunity a child gets from a flu vaccination wears off over time. Getting a flu vaccine every year

helps keep a child protected, even if the vaccine viruses do not change from one season to the next.

Some people believe that naturally acquired immunity—immunity from having the disease itself—is better than the immunity provided by vaccines. However, natural infections can cause severe complications and be deadly. This is true even for diseases that many people consider mild, such as chickenpox. It is impossible to predict who will get serious infections that may lead to hospitalization. Vaccines, like any medication, can cause side effects. The most common side effects are mild. However, many vaccine-preventable disease symptoms can be serious, or even deadly. Although many of these diseases are rare in this country, they do circulate around the world and can be brought into the United States, putting unvaccinated children at risk. Even with advances in healthcare, the diseases that vaccines prevent can still be very serious—and vaccination is the best way to prevent them.

Section 38.2
Current Status of Vaccine Development

This section includes text excerpted from "Encouraging Vaccine Innovation: Promoting the Development of Vaccines That Minimize the Burden of Infectious Diseases in the 21st Century," U.S. Department of Health and Human Services (HHS), December 2017.

Vaccines have an inherent societal benefit. They protect individuals and communities against serious infectious diseases and dramatically reduce the burden associated with such infectious diseases including hospitalizations, deaths, and healthcare costs in the United States. With further innovation and continued development, new and improved vaccines may have an even greater benefit to society.

The U.S. government (USG) is one of many key stakeholders involved in the U.S. Vaccine and Immunization Enterprise, a network of industrial, government, academic, nonprofit, and private partners engaged in infectious-disease surveillance, basic and applied research, product development, regulatory evaluation and licensure, recommendations for introduction and use, and vaccine uptake. The USG works with diverse partners to shepherd potential vaccine candidates through the staged development process. Once a vaccine is licensed by the U.S. Food and Drug Administration (FDA) for use, many stakeholders—such as patients, providers, payers, and public-health officials—become involved in the immunization-delivery system.

Pursuing the development of vaccines is a long, expensive, and high-risk endeavor. It begins with initial product interest, informed by existing and available information on disease burden and technical feasibility. Once the decision to pursue vaccine development is made, at least a decade of investment is typically needed to advance potential candidates from basic and applied research to licensure, production, and delivery into the immunization-delivery system.

Numerous candidates are tested in preclinical and early-stage clinical trials, but not all have the technical feasibility and potential product interest to move forward through the pipeline. As candidates move forward through the various stages of clinical trials, time and resource investments increase significantly. Data from clinical studies serve as the basis for licensure; it can take several years for a sponsor (i.e., the company, organization, or individual that sponsors the investigational new drug application (IND) for the conduct of clinical trials or biologics license application (BLA) for licensure) to demonstrate that the vaccine candidate meets the necessary FDA standards for vaccine safety and effectiveness. As a vaccine candidate progresses toward licensure, further investments are needed to demonstrate the ability to make the vaccine candidate at large scale and in the intended commercial production facility. Overall, the time and financial investments necessary to develop a single safe, effective, FDA-licensed vaccine are high.

These costs are even greater when considering the high-risk environment for investment, in which most vaccine candidates do not make it to FDA licensure and the costs of failed products must also be absorbed. The riskiness of the decision to invest in vaccine development takes into account the generally smaller markets for vaccines, which are usually administered once. This is in contrast to therapeutic products, which may be given several times or for a long duration throughout a patient's lifetime. The success of currently licensed vaccines in the immunization-delivery system and the anticipated markets for potential new vaccines also contribute to the risk of development. Factors that decrease the cost or risk of development, such as USG policies or actions, may help foster innovation and development.

Networks

This section focuses on the U.S. network of industry, nonprofit, foundation, government, and academic partners engaged in vaccine research and development (R&D). This network is responsible for developing the majority of new vaccines available worldwide since World War II, the number of which is a reflection of the current network's success in innovation. Cooperation and collaboration among these major partners are necessary to advance vaccine candidates through the development pipeline.

Industry plays a central role in this collaboration. The number of companies involved in the vaccine enterprise has evolved over the years with a significant decrease in the number of large manufacturers that produce vaccines. Currently, the vaccine industry consists of numerous small biotechnology companies and four large manufacturers: GlaxoSmithKline, Merck and Co., Inc., Pfizer, and Sanofi Pasteur. In addition to industry, organizations such as nonprofits and foundations support efforts to decrease costs and accelerate the pace of vaccine R&D and optimization (e.g., Global Health Vaccine Center of Innovation, Hilleman Laboratories, Coalition for Epidemic Preparedness Innovations).

Academic partners play a key role in the generation of new ideas and technologies. Both large and small companies bridge academic research and commercial development by supporting basic laboratory research for vaccine candidates and by conducting Phase 1, 2, 3, and 4 clinical trials. Phase 1 clinical trials evaluate early safety and immune responses to the vaccine candidate. Phase 2 clinical trials involve dose-ranging and more comprehensive safety and immunogenicity studies. Phase 3 clinical trials are pivotal and require large-scale studies of safety and effectiveness. Phase 4 clinical trials are conducted postlicensure and may be performed to fulfill postmarketing requirements and to provide additional assessments of less common and rare adverse events or information on the duration of vaccine-induced immunity. During Phase 1 and 2 studies, the vaccine manufacturing process is also developed and refined to ensure consistency and high quality. Due to limitations in capacity and funding, small companies often stop development at Phase 2 and large companies shepherd promising vaccine candidates through the later, costlier stages of clinical trials, licensure, and commercial production.

Vaccine development is also a global enterprise. Depending on the specific vaccine candidate in development, a manufacturer may seek licensure in multiple countries, and face varying regulatory requirements. Extensive resources are required to engage in a global market, which can be a key factor in deciding which vaccine candidates to support in development programs. Efforts to expand regulatory convergence across countries are ongoing.

The success of the vaccine industry in bringing FDA-licensed vaccines to the public is dependent on an environment shaped, in part, by government actions and policies. The USG has a general interest in supporting the development, licensure, and introduction and use of vaccines that protect the public against infectious disease threats. More broadly, the USG has an interest in innovation—bringing new ideas and technologies to fruition—that may further improve public health and address and/ or prevent emerging infectious diseases. Innovation can occur across the vaccine development spectrum, including with manufacturing processes (e.g., cell-based and recombinant influenza vaccines) and new delivery systems (e.g., a patch instead of a needle), as well as novel candidates and improvements to existing vaccines (e.g., use of new and improved platforms or adjuvants).

Section 38.3

Vaccine Research and Development

This section includes text excerpted from "Encouraging Vaccine Innovation: Promoting the Development of Vaccines That Minimize the Burden of Infectious Diseases in the 21st Century," U.S. Department of Health and Human Services (HHS), December 2017.

Currently, more than 120 vaccine candidates are under development for the prevention of more than 40 infectious disease targets as reported on the Pharmaceutical Research and Manufacturers Association of America (PhRMA) website. Additional sources that track vaccine development programs are the World Health Organization (WHO) and the United States government. The WHO Vaccine Pipeline Tracker lists vaccine candidates currently under clinical development. The United States government's (USG) ClinicalTrials.gov is the largest U.S. clinical trials database. While not an exhaustive list, these sources represent the vast majority of active development programs.

Vaccine development is at a turning point for three primary reasons: (1) the prevailing business model prioritizes vaccine candidates with large markets, yet market sizes are likely smaller for many remaining targets which focus on subsets of the population; (2) substantial investment is needed to address the scientific complexity of remaining targets, which may also require further investment in novel approaches to demonstrate safety and effectiveness; and (3) uncertainty of the public-health priority and demand for some targets may be unclear, which increases the uncertainty of the potential return on investment (ROI) and, therefore, constitutes an investment risk. Some vaccines currently under development are expected to receive a recommendation for administration to a subset of the population rather than a universal recommendation for a broad cohort of individuals. For example, vaccines that most benefit subpopulations—such as pregnant women or people undergoing elective surgery—may only receive recommendations for use among those populations. This presents several challenges, especially for small companies. The market for these products may be smaller and more difficult to estimate because of uncertainty about the population for whom the vaccine might be recommended and the expected level of utilization. Additionally, new vaccine targets are more scientifically complex and challenging. The challenges presented may require substantial investment in new tools, standards, analysis methods, and other novel approaches to demonstrate safety and effectiveness. Public-health priorities have historically been evident to stakeholders due to the clear disease burden of many infectious agents (e.g., measles, polio) and the public-health demand for vaccines. The development of certain vaccines—for example, universal influenza vaccines and respiratory syncytial virus (RSV) vaccines for infants—is considered a high priority as reflected in the number of companies working on these vaccine targets. However, the public-health priority for some vaccine targets is less clear. In order to support an enabling environment for continued innovation the following factors are important: having a shared understanding of market size, making investments in science and development programs, and knowing which vaccines are public-health priorities within the vaccine enterprise.

Small and Large Companies

While the U.S. government (USG) provides the majority of support for basic and applied research in the academic setting, most vaccine candidates are developed by small companies that drive innovation in early-stage development. Many of these companies rely on funding from multiple sources, including the USG and venture capital, until late-stage development when products with a potential ROI attract large companies for investment. The handful of large companies with the resources and expertise to support manufacturing, licensure, and commercial production may face vaccine development constraints in several ways. First, there are only a few companies to potentially shepard a vaccine through to licensure. Second, vaccine manufacturers are generally part of large pharmaceutical parent companies. Therefore, vaccines often compete with other pharmaceutical products—that can have a higher ROI and lower risks—for limited development resources. Third, vaccine manufacturers typically have capacity constraints, in that manufacturers plan for the global market. This requires navigating multiple regulatory authorities and immunization policies, which may vary from country to country. Reaching regulatory convergence across countries is a continued opportunity to improve efficient use of limited resources. Often, only products anticipated to have a global market provide sufficient incentive for large and risky investments. Investments in emerging priorities may also have opportunity costs. For example, supporting development of an Ebola virus vaccine (with an uncertain market) may require a company to shift resources from other development programs. Essentially, research and development (R&D) investment in new or improved vaccines depends on projected costs and ROI.

Role of Federal Agencies

The U.S. Department of Health and Human Services (HHS) has a far-reaching mission to protect and promote public health and respond to urgent and emerging disease threats. Within the HHS, the major federal agencies and offices in the vaccine enterprise working on vaccine development include the National Institutes of Health (NIH), the U.S. Food and Drug Administration (FDA), the Centers for Disease Control and Prevention (CDC), the Biomedical Advanced Research and Development Authority (BARDA), (within the HHS Office of the Assistant Secretary for Preparedness and Response (ASPR)), and the National Vaccine Program Office (NVPO). Outside of HHS, the Department of Defense (DoD) and the U.S. Agency for International Development (USAID) also make investments in vaccine development. Federal agencies and offices work in tandem with a broad range of stakeholders to optimize vaccine development. For example, the HHS plays a key role in ensuring timely development and production of well-matched seasonal influenza vaccines, and is leading and coordinating efforts to improve these vaccines. Because influenza viruses are constantly changing, seasonal influenza vaccines must be updated annually in order to match the vaccine with currently circulating virus strains. The yearly influenza vaccine strain selection, vaccine production, and licensure is a highly coordinated process that is based on global influenza data collected from health partners around the world, particularly the WHO. For more than 10 years, the Pandemic and Seasonal Influenza Risk Management Meeting has served as a senior-level forum for decision-makers from stakeholder agencies. Leadership from the BARDA, the CDC, the FDA, the NIH, the NVPO, and others regularly meet to identify and address risk-management issues related to the development, acquisition, deployment, and utilization of medical and public-health countermeasures for pandemic and seasonal influenza. Additionally, the HHS agencies and offices actively partner with the scientific community through workshops or other means to determine how to close the gap between vaccine discovery and delivery. The role of the HHS agencies and offices is described below.

National Institutes of Health

The National Institutes of Health (NIH) supports and conducts basic and applied research, translational research, and clinical evaluation focused on identifying vaccine targets and advancing novel candidates through the vaccine-development pipeline for a broad array of infectious diseases. The NIH works closely and collaboratively with partners in academia, industry, and other federal agencies to facilitate vaccine innovation and development. It also supports the training of research investigators and fosters communication of medical and health-sciences information. In addition, the NIH directly supports vaccine development through its intramural program. For example, the NIH Vaccine Research Center (VRC), is dedicated to improving global human health through the rigorous pursuit of effective vaccines, and is developing and evaluating vaccines for HIV/AIDS, influenza, Zika, and Respiratory Syncytial Virus, among other diseases. The NIH collaborates with multiple partners to facilitate the development of vaccine platform technologies that will enhance the USG's ability to respond to emerging-disease threats and accelerate vaccine development during public-health emergencies.

Basic Research

An initial critical component for vaccine development is the advancement of basic research aimed at understanding how pathogens cause disease and, in turn, how the immune system responds to infection. The NIH supports basic research on more than 300 pathogens to elucidate pathogen biology; examine interactions among pathogens, hosts, and the environment; and determine the ways that microbes survive and multiply. Historically, the NIH researchers have laid the groundwork for development of numerous vaccines by developing reliable animal models, identifying and characterizing multiple vaccine targets, defining the mode of transmission for such targets, and identifying critical components that trigger an immune response. In addition, the NIH supports programs to more fully understand the mechanisms involved in the immune responses to infection and vaccination, such as the Human Immunology Project Consortium (HIPC). The HIPC is a large, collaborative research effort that focuses on studying vaccine responses of well-characterized human cohorts to better understand the immune system, its regulation, and the differences between immune systems that do and do not respond to vaccination. Data from this effort will be used to develop and evaluate new vaccines and immunization strategies that work in a greater diversity of individuals and help identify those potentially at risk for an adverse event.

Translational Research

Advances in basic research lead to targets and strategies for the development of new and improved vaccines. The NIH supports translational research to turn concepts into products and provides services to researchers to facilitate vaccine development. The NIH Partnerships Program for Translational Research is a long-standing initiative that encourages new research collaborations among experts from different disciplines of academia and industry and ensures that basic research findings and technologies are translated into new product-development approaches. Recent Partnerships initiatives have focused on structure-based design of novel immunogens for vaccine development and the development of vaccines targeting antimicrobial-resistant bacteria. In addition, the NIH offers comprehensive preclinical services to industry partners and academic researchers that seek to fill the gap between discoveries made at the basic research stage and the development of clinical products, including evaluation of vaccine candidates, assay development, safety and toxicity testing, product optimization, and pilot lot manufacturing. Modern vaccines often require the addition of adjuvants, which are molecules that trigger the initial activation of the immune system. NIH adjuvant discovery and development efforts are critical to the development of new and improved vaccines against infectious diseases. The NIH conducts preclinical evaluation of novel adjuvants in combination with infectious-disease vaccine candidates. Together, these programs provide a tool box for vaccine developers looking to produce novel vaccines, such as vaccines with increased efficacy or vaccines for specific age groups.

Clinical Evaluation

To help turn basic research and translational discoveries into products that impact public health, the NIH has made a significant investment in establishing state-of-the-art clinical-trial networks for vaccine development and evaluation. This includes early clinical trials of novel vaccine candidates to evaluate safety and immunogenicity, efficacy trials, and postlicensure studies of vaccines that can help inform clinical practice. One of the key programs the NIH utilizes to evaluate promising vaccine candidates is the Vaccine and Treatment Evaluation Units (VTEUs), a network of sites that provides a ready resource for conducting clinical trials. The NIH frequently serves as the Investigational New Drug Application (IND) sponsor for vaccine candidates, and interacts with the FDA throughout the entire product lifecycle to ensure that all regulatory requirements are being met and that the vaccine candidate is on the right path for licensure.

U.S. Food and Drug Administration

The U.S. Food and Drug Administration (FDA) has a central role in vaccine development, as it is the federal agency charged with ensuring that vaccines undergo a rigorous and extensive development program to determine and ensure the safety, purity, and potency of these products. After a vaccine is FDA licensed, the FDA continues to monitor its safety, purity, and potency. Vaccine development programs include studies conducted by manufacturers according to FDA standards to evaluate safety and effectiveness in the target population. Clinical trials are conducted according to plans that reflect the FDA's expertise in clinical trial design. The FDA guides development of vaccines from pre-Phase 1 through Phase 4. Through meetings between medical and scientific experts from the FDA and the manufacturer, often early in the development of a vaccine candidate, and at critical later times, the sponsor (i.e., the company, organization, or individual that sponsors the IND for the conduct of clinical trials) gains valuable advice about planned clinical trials, development milestones, and data requirements.

Vaccine Review and Licensing

Thanks to staffing increases that are supported by industry user fees, the FDA has been able to further optimize its vaccine review and licensing process to encourage the development of new vaccines and make vaccines available for use sooner, without lowering the FDA's standard for safety and effectiveness. This is achieved by implementing available innovative, flexible regulatory mechanisms and pathways. Expedited development pathways (e.g., Fast-Track Designation, Priority Review, Accelerated Approval) and innovative regulatory mechanisms (e.g., use of the animal rule and adaptive trial designs) applicable to vaccine candidates are outlined. The FDA has worked effectively to implement these flexible regulatory pathways and review practices. This flexibility has translated into a high proportion of vaccine approvals on the first regulatory review cycle, thereby increasing predictability for vaccine developers.

Regulatory Science and Innovation

Research is fundamental to the FDA's ability to provide effective scientific and regulatory evaluation of vaccine candidates. The FDA conducts its research activities in conjunction with its regulatory activities, which provides the agency a unique perspective on both fronts. A wide variety of rapidly evolving technical and scientific issues concerning the safety and effectiveness of vaccine candidates requires knowledge of new developments in basic research in the relevant biological disciplines. For this reason, FDA scientists conduct research in a variety of areas, including evaluating new techniques and tools for regulatory testing of product safety and effectiveness, as well as developing strategies for new product development.

International Collaboration

The development, manufacturing, clinical evaluation, and regulatory review of vaccine candidates are a global enterprise. The FDA continually engages with its international regulatory counterparts to work toward harmonizing scientific standards and approaches for developing vaccine candidates, evaluating their safety and effectiveness, and overseeing their manufacturing and quality. For example, the FDA has been a Pan American Health Organization (PAHO) and WHO Collaborating Centers for Biological Standardization participant since 1998. As such, the FDA is a key participant to develop and revise specific recommendations for the production and quality control of vaccine candidates of major international public-health importance. In the hope that more vaccine candidates can be licensed and available to multiple regions of the world, the FDA also works with the WHO, other National Regulatory Authorities (NRAs), and with industry to encourage international convergence, more efficient product development, and development of the scientific and regulatory standards for safety and effectiveness that will help achieve these goals.

Postlicensure Manufacturing and Safety Monitoring

The FDA continues to intensively oversee vaccine production after the vaccine candidate and its manufacturing processes are approved in order to ensure continued safety and effectiveness. Furthermore, the FDA may also require, at or after the time of approval, manufacturers to conduct additional postmarket studies to evaluate known or potential serious risks. The FDA evaluates safety signals that may arise, and takes appropriate steps, such as communicating vaccine safety information to the public and healthcare providers or requiring manufacturers to change the prescribing information (i.e., vaccine labeling), as needed. The FDA monitors the Vaccine Adverse Event Reporting System (VAERS), a nationwide joint effort with the CDC to conduct postmarketing passive surveillance and collect information about adverse events reported to have occurred after the administration of licensed vaccines. In addition to VAERS, the Sentinel Initiative is the FDA's national electronic surveillance system for the postmarket safety monitoring of medical products. The Sentinel System was implemented as an Active Post Market Risk Identification and Analysis program in response to section 905 of the Food and Drug Administration Amendments Act of 2007. The Post Licensure Rapid Immunization Safety Monitoring (PRISM) System, the vaccine safety portion of the Sentinel system, was initiated in 2009 as one of several national vaccine-safety surveillance systems deployed during the H1N1 influenza pandemic. The PRISM database covers more than 190 million individuals in several data partner organizations. PRISM, which has capabilities for broad-based signal detection as well as for evaluating safety signals that may be identified, is used by the FDA to evaluate vaccine safety in the postlicensure setting.

Centers for Disease Control and Prevention

The CDC leads the U.S. immunization program, which defines disease burden and implements and evaluates national immunization policies and programs. The CDC identifies, controls, and prevents infectious diseases through public-health surveillance, epidemiologic studies, vaccine-use recommendations, vaccine purchasing and service delivery, health communications, and postmarketing vaccine safety, vaccine effectiveness, and vaccine impact studies. The CDC provides domestic and international leadership in laboratory technologies and techniques to detect and characterize vaccine-preventable and emerging diseases. The CDC collaborates with both domestic and global partners to maximize the effectiveness of immunization policies and programs.

Disease Surveillance

In the United States, laws and regulations mandate reporting cases of specified infectious and noninfectious conditions to local, state, and territorial health departments. Health departments work with healthcare providers, laboratories, hospitals, and other partners to obtain the information needed to monitor, control, and prevent the occurrence and spread of these health conditions. Health departments notify the CDC about the occurrence of certain conditions, and the CDC receives, secures, processes, and disseminates nationally notifiable infectious-diseases data. Through networks of state health departments, academic institutions, and other collaborators, the CDC is able to address important issues in infectious diseases and identify new problems as they arise.

Infectious Disease Detection and Response

It is critical to detect emergent, new diseases through domestic and international surveillance programs that characterize and track these diseases and identify potential targets for vaccine development. Through epidemiologic studies, diseases patterns are described and at-risk populations are identified. Etiologic agents are isolated and characterized in CDC laboratories, often in collaboration with networks of scientists across the United States and internationally. CDC laboratories also may develop vaccine candidates for emerging diseases. Before a vaccine is FDA-licensed, CDC subject-matter experts meet with pharmaceutical companies to share insights into the epidemiology and possible effectiveness of vaccines in development. The CDC also conducts modeling and analysis to predict the potential impact of vaccines and economic analyses to establish the value proposition of vaccines.

National Immunization Policy

Once a vaccine is licensed by the FDA, the CDC sets U.S. child and adult immunization schedules based on recommendations from the Advisory Committee on Immunization Practices (ACIP). The ACIP is a federal advisory committee that provides advice to the CDC director regarding the most appropriate use of licensed vaccines and related agents for control of vaccine-preventable diseases in the civilian population of the United States. In setting immunization schedules, the CDC establishes the standards of medical practice for immunization for the nation. In addition to inviting input from the ACIP, the CDC works with nongovernmental professional organizations or other public-health service advisory committees. The CDC and the ACIP work with professional organizations, including the American Academy of Pediatrics (AAP) and the American Academy of Family Physicians (AAFP), to harmonize the pediatric immunization schedule, and with the American College of Physicians (ACP), the AAFP, and the American College of Obstetricians and Gynecologists (ACOG) to harmonize the adult immunization schedule. Unique to the ACIP is its role in determining the vaccines included in the Vaccines for Children (VFC) program. Nongrandfathered private health plans, health plans offered through state and federal health insurance exchanges, and Medicaid expansion programs are required to provide first-dollar coverage (i.e., with no cost-sharing to the patient) for the vaccines included in the CDC immunization schedules. The CDC immunization recommendations provide an estimated potential market size for the vaccine manufacturer.

National Immunization Program

The CDC supports the nation's public-health infrastructure, which includes public-health experts and systems critical to the success of the nation's immunization program. This public-health infrastructure promotes immunization recommendations across the lifespan; fosters convenient access to recommended vaccinations; provides a safety net for those who cannot otherwise access immunization services; manages vaccine shortages; monitors the safety and effectiveness of vaccines and vaccine policies; prevents disease outbreaks and responds early and rapidly should they occur; and prepares to respond quickly and comprehensively to other urgent vaccine emergencies, such as pandemics.

In collaboration with the Centers for Medicare and Medicaid Services (CMS), the CDC implements the federal VFC program. Through this program, the CDC provides vaccines at no cost to eligible children from birth through 18 years of age. Through its federal contracts and centralized distribution system, the CDC purchases and distributes vaccines to a network of more than 44,000 enrolled provider sites each year. The nationwide VFC program is responsible for vaccinating more than half of

United States children annually. The CDC also provides vaccines to 64 immunization program awardees for vaccinating uninsured, poor adults, and for use in outbreak responses.

The CDC conducts communications research and develops evidence-based tools, training, and resources about immunization for the public and healthcare providers. The CDC's health communications work is focused on describing the benefits of vaccines and risks of vaccine-preventable diseases, and responding to frequently asked questions about vaccines. The CDC also implements a robust provider education program on topics ranging from how to make a recommendation to answering questions about vaccine safety.

Through the National Immunization Survey, the National Health Information Survey, and the Behavioral Risk-Factor Surveillance System, the CDC measures childhood, adolescent, and adult immunization coverage. The CDC uses these data to inform program decisions and to reduce disparities in immunization coverage.

Postmarketing Vaccine Safety and Effectiveness

Following introduction of a new or improved vaccine recommendation, the CDC and the FDA collaborate on conducting studies to monitor the impact of the vaccine in the community setting. This work includes monitoring vaccine safety through VAERS in collaboration with the FDA, and conducting vaccine-safety studies through the Vaccines Safety Datalink (VSD) network and the Clinical Immunization Safety Assessment (CISA) network.

The CDC also conducts postmarketing studies to evaluate the effectiveness of vaccines. These studies help characterize the performance of vaccines when used routinely among the recommended population. The findings from these studies are used by vaccine manufacturers and the FDA in making decisions to revise the license; and by the ACIP and the CDC in making decisions on recommendations for the use of vaccines, such as number of doses, time intervals, and recommended populations.

Biomedical Advanced Research and Development Authority (BARDA), Office of the Assistant Secretary for Preparedness and Response

The Biomedical Advanced Research and Development Authority's (BARDA) mission is to develop and procure needed medical countermeasures (MCMs), including vaccines against chemical, biological, radiological, and nuclear (CBRN) agents; emerging infectious diseases; and pandemic influenza, whether natural or intentional in origin. BARDA funding bridges the "valley of death."—the critical juncture between R&D and late stages of product development where funding requirements significantly increase and many development programs are forced to stop due to lack of funding. The BARDA provides nondilutive funds for the late-stage development of new product technologies toward approval, clearance, or licensure of MCMs. Many such MCMs lack meaningful commercial markets and, without USG support, would be unlikely candidates for development.

National Vaccine Program Office

Created in 1987 to provide leadership and coordination among federal and nonfederal stakeholders on vaccine-related activities, the NVPO works to ensure activities are carried out in an efficient, consistent, and timely manner.

Section 38.4

Developing New and Improved Vaccines

This section contains text excerpted from the following sources: Text in this section begins with excerpts from "2010 National Vaccine Plan," U.S. Department of Health and Human Services (HHS), 2010. Reviewed March 2020; Text under the heading "National Vaccine Plan: Develop New and Improved Vaccines" is excerpted from "Develop New and Improved Vaccines," U.S. Department of Health and Human Services (HHS), June 24, 2016. Reviewed March 2020.

The 20th century could be considered the century of vaccines. The life spans of Americans increased by more than thirty years in large part because of vaccines, and mortality from infectious diseases in the United States decreased 14-fold. Death or disability from many once-common diseases is now rare in the United States. A child born in the United States can now be protected against 17 serious diseases and conditions through immunization. The widespread use of vaccines has helped to eradicate smallpox worldwide and eliminate polio, measles, and rubella in the United States. Globally, vaccination saves 2 to 3 million lives per year. Vaccines have the unique quality of protecting both individuals and communities. However, they have been so effective for many years in preventing and eliminating a number of serious infectious diseases that the significant contributions that vaccines make to the society and its health may have faded from public consciousness. Before the development and widespread use of safe and effective vaccines, infectious diseases threatened the lives of millions of children and adults in this country and abroad. What were once referred to as the "common diseases of childhood" are now vaccine-preventable diseases (VPDs). In the United States, children are no longer crippled by polio nor killed by infections such as diphtheria or *Haemophilus influenzae type b* (Hib). Vaccines also help prevent cancers caused by human papillomavirus (HPV) and hepatitis B virus (HBV).

The 2010 National Vaccine Plan provides a vision for the United States vaccine and immunization enterprise for the next decade. The Plan articulates a comprehensive strategy to enhance all aspects of vaccines and vaccination, including research and development, supply, financing, distribution, safety, informed decision making by consumers and healthcare providers, VPD surveillance, vaccine effectiveness and use monitoring, and global cooperation. The actions contained in the strategies of the Plan are conditional and are subject to the availability of resources. The scope of the Plan is broad and addresses vaccines and key vaccine-related issues for the United States and its global partners. It provides a strategic approach for preventing infectious diseases and improving the public's health through vaccination for the coming decade. Although vaccines are being developed to treat diseases and conditions (therapeutic vaccines) and for noninfectious diseases, the focus of this Plan is on vaccines for the prevention of infectious diseases as guided by the law that established the National Vaccine Program (NVP).

The Plan has five broad goals:

- **Goal 1:** Develop new and improved vaccines.
- **Goal 2:** Enhance the vaccine-safety system.
- **Goal 3:** Support communications to enhance informed vaccine decision-making.
- **Goal 4:** Ensure a stable supply of, access to, and better use of recommended vaccines in the United States.
- **Goal 5:** Increase global prevention of death and disease through safe and effective vaccination.

Existing national and global vaccine-related initiatives such as improvements in regulatory science, the development of medical countermeasures for emergencies, and global health partnerships are embedded within the Plan. Strategies of this Plan will also be coordinated with those developed through other federal efforts. One example is the National Prevention, Health Promotion and Public Health Council, established in the 2010 Affordable Care Act (ACA). The Council coordinates federal prevention, wellness, and public-health activities, and develops a national strategy to improve the nation's health.

In conjunction with other federal efforts, such as the National Prevention and Health Promotion Strategy, Healthy People (HP) 2020, and the Public Health Emergency Medical Countermeasures Enterprise Review, the 2010 National Vaccine Plan provides the strategic guidance to build a stronger preventive health system. It also helps bridge disparities in the use of, and access to vaccines, and provides innovative strategies to guide the nation's vaccine enterprise across the next decade and beyond.

National Vaccine Plan: Develop New and Improved Vaccines

The greatest and most rapid changes in health occurred during the last century, primarily attributed to a higher standard of living, improved public-health measures, and the application of science-based medicine. In addition to clean water, sanitation, and the use of antibiotics, vaccines are an essential part of these public-health achievements. Vaccine research and development, as well as the implementation of effective vaccine-delivery programs, has led to the eradication and elimination of several once-common serious infectious diseases.

Discovery begins with the recognition of an infectious-disease burden and the opportunity to prevent it through immunization. Basic scientific research brings ideas forward into the product-development pathway toward the ultimate goal of translating these ideas into safe and effective medical products. Safety and efficacy testing are conducted at every step of this product-development pathway. Both basic and targeted research is the basis for the development of vaccine candidates and new vaccine platforms that offer greater flexibility in vaccine development and production. New tools, such as efficient antigen-identification techniques, coupled with a profoundly greater understanding of the immune response are, available to define basic mechanisms of disease to support design and development of novel and improved vaccines. Determining "proof of concept" regarding immunogenicity and safety follows—initially in preclinical studies in animals and then in humans to further evaluate safety and efficacy. Finally, researchers conduct scientific characterization of the vaccine and the process for producing it, including scaling the manufacturing process to commercial levels before vaccines are moved into human testing.

Vaccines are developed through public–private partnerships—including researchers, government, manufacturers, purchasers, and policymakers—who have been successful at bringing new vaccines to licensure for broad use. These partnerships are central to the success of vaccine innovations. Through targeted investments in science and technology, such partnerships have led to the development of hundreds of vaccine candidates at various stages of maturity in the development pipeline. The Global HIV Enterprise is an example of unprecedented collaboration among organizations worldwide, including the National Institutes of Health (NIH), the International AIDS Vaccine Initiative, USAID, the Bill and Melinda Gates Foundation, and many others working together to accelerate the development of a preventive HIV vaccine.

Because vaccine development is time- and resource-intensive, establishing and understanding priorities for development and encouraging collaboration between stakeholders is essential in addressing the challenges of developing new and improved vaccines. Fostering continued investment from all sectors is critical as technological approaches and disease threats expand amid increasing costs to develop, license, and deliver vaccines.

The aim of Goal 1 is to develop new and improved vaccines and to address the upstream research and development aspects of vaccines for domestic and global health priorities. The research needs of other aspects of the vaccine enterprise (e.g., program implementation, distribution logistics, communication) are included within other goals in the Plan.

Objectives

- Prioritize new vaccine targets of domestic and global public-health importance.
- Support research to develop and manufacture new vaccine candidates and improve current vaccines to prevent infectious diseases.
- Support research on novel and improved vaccine-delivery methods.
- Increase understanding of the host immune system.

- Support product development, evaluation, and production techniques of vaccine candidates and the scientific tools needed for their evaluation.
- Improve the tools, standards, and approaches to assess the safety, efficacy, and quality of vaccines.

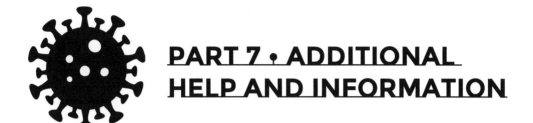

PART 7 • ADDITIONAL HELP AND INFORMATION

CHAPTER 39

Directory of Organizations Researching and Providing Support to People Who Acquire Diseases and Illnesses from Animals, Insects, and Contaminated Food and Water

Government Agencies That Provide Information about Illnesses and Diseases

Center for Food Safety and Applied Nutrition (CFSAN)
U.S. Food and Drug Administration (FDA)
5001 Campus Dr., HFS-009
College Park, MD 20740-3835
Toll-Free: 888-SAFEFOOD
(888-723-3366)
Website: www.fda.gov/
about-fda/center-food-safety-
and-applied-nutrition-cfsan/
contact-cfsan

Center for Nutrition Policy and Promotion (CNPP)
3101 Park Center Dr.
10th Fl.
Alexandria, VA 22302-1594
Toll-Free: 866-632-9992
Phone: 703-305-3300
Fax: 703-305-3300
Website: www.cnpp.usda.gov

Resources in this chapter were compiled from several sources deemed reliable; all contact information was verified and updated in March 2020.

615

Centers for Disease Control and Prevention (CDC)

1600 Clifton Rd.
Atlanta, GA 30329-4027
Toll-Free: 800-CDC-INFO
(800-232-4636)
Phone: 404-639-3311
Toll-Free TTY: 888-232-6348
Website: www.cdc.gov
E-mail: cdcinfo@cdc.gov

Division of Foodborne, Waterborne, and Environmental Diseases (DFWED)

Centers for Disease Control and
Prevention (CDC)
Website: www.cdc.gov/ncezid/
dfwed/waterborne/index.html

FoodSafety.gov

U.S. Department of Health
and Human Services, Web
Communications and New Media
Division
200 Independence Ave., S.W.
Washington, DC 20201
Website: www.foodsafety.gov

healthfinder.gov

Office of Disease Prevention and
Health Promotion (ODPHP)
200 Independence Ave.
Washington, DC 20201
Website: www.healthfinder.gov
E-mail: healthfinder@hhs.gov

National Health Information Center (NHIC)

U.S. Department of Health and
Human Services (HHS)
1101 Wootton Pkwy.
Ste. LL100
Rockville, MD 20852
Fax: 240-453-8281
Website: www.health.gov/nhic
E-mail: nhic@hhs.gov

National Institute of Allergy and Infectious Diseases (NIAID)

Office of Communications and
Government Relations (OCGR)
5601 Fishers Ln.
MSC 9806
Bethesda, MD 20892-9806
Toll-Free: 866-284-4107
Phone: 301-496-5717
Toll-Free TDD: 800-877-8339
Fax: 301-402-3573
Website: www.niaid.nih.gov
E-mail: ocpostoffice@niaid.nih. gov

National Institute of Environmental Health Sciences (NIEHS)

P.O. Box 12233
MD K3-16
Research Triangle Park, NC 27709
Phone: 919-541-3345
Fax: 919-541-4395
Website: www.niehs.nih.gov
E-mail: webcenter@niehs.nih.gov

National Oceanic and Atmospheric Administration (NOAA)

1401 Constitution Ave., N.W.
Rm. 5128
Washington, DC 20230
Website: www.noaa.gov
E-mail: webmaster@noaa.gov

The National Science Foundation (NSF)

2415 Eisenhower Ave.
Alexandria, VA 22314
Toll-Free: 800-877-8339
Phone: 703-292-5111
TDD: 703-292-5090
Toll-Free TDD: 800-281-8749
Website: www.nsf.gov
E-mail: info@nsf.gov

The United States Agency for International Development (USAID)

Phone: 202-712-0000
Website: www.usaid.gov

U.S. Department of Agriculture (USDA)

1400 Independence Ave., S.W.
Washington, DC 20250
Phone: 202-720-2791
Website: www.usda.gov
E-mail: feedback@oc.usda.gov

U.S. Department of Health and Human Services (HHS)

200 Independence Ave., S.W.
Washington, DC 20201
Toll-Free: 877-696-6775
Website: www.hhs.gov

U.S. Environmental Protection Agency (EPA)

1200 Pennsylvania Ave., N.W.
Washington, DC 20460
Phone: 202-564-4700
Fax: 202-501-1450
Website: www.epa.gov

U.S. Food and Drug Administration (FDA)
10903 New Hampshire Ave.
Silver Spring, MD 20993-0002
Toll-Free: 888-INFO-FDA
(888-463-6332)
Website: www.fda.gov

The U.S. Global Change Research Program (USGCRP)
1800 G St., N.W.
Ste. 9100
Washington, DC 20006
Phone: 202-223-6262
Fax: 202-223-3065
Website: www.globalchange.gov

Private Agencies That Provide Information about Illnesses and Diseases

Academy of Nutrition and Dietetics
eat right®
120 S. Riverside Plaza
Ste. 2190
Chicago, IL 60606-6995
Toll-Free: 800-877-1600
Phone: 312-899-0040
Website: www.eatright.org

American Academy of Family Physicians (AAFP)
11400 Tomahawk Creek Pkwy.
Leawood, KS 66211-2680
Toll-Free: 800-274-2237
Phone: 913-906-6000
Fax: 913-906-6075
Website: www.aafp.org
E-mail: aafp@aafp.org

Allen County Department of Health
200 E. Berry St.
Ste. 360
Fort Wayne, IN 46802
Phone: 260-449-7561
Fax: 260-427-1391
Website: www.allencountyhealth.com
E-mail: info@allencountyhealth.com

The American Mosquito Control Association (AMCA)
One Capitol Mall
Ste. 800
Sacramento, CA 95814
Toll-Free: 888-626-0630
Fax: 916-444-7462
Website: www.mosquito.org
E-mail: amca@mosquito.org

American Society of Tropical Medicine and Hygiene (ASTMH)
241 18th St., S.
Ste. 501
Arlington, VA 22202
Phone: 571-351-5409
Fax: 571-351-5422
Website: www.astmh.org
E-mail: info@astmh.org

American Veterinary Medical Association (AVMA)
1931 N. Meacham Rd.
Ste. 100
Schaumburg, IL 60173-4360
Toll-Free: 800-248-2862
Fax: 847-925-1329
Website: www.avma.org

Animal Welfare Institute (AWI)
900 Pennsylvania Ave., S.E.
Washington, DC 20003
Phone: 202-337-2332
Website: awionline.org
E-mail: awi@awionline.org

Association of Public Health Laboratories (APHL)
8515 Georgia Ave.
Ste. 700
Silver Spring, MD 20910
Phone: 240-485-2745
Fax: 240-485-2700
Website: www.aphl.org
E-mail: info@aphl.org

The Association of State and Territorial Health Officials (ASTHO)
National Headquarters
2231 Crystal Dr.
Ste. 450
Arlington, VA 22202
Phone: 202-371-9090
Fax: 571-527-3189
Website: www.astho.org

Born Free USA
8737 Colesville Rd.
Ste. 715
Silver Spring, MD 20910
Phone: 301-448-1407
Website: www.bornfreeusa.org
E-mail: info@bornfreeusa.org

Center for Food Safety (CFS)

660 Pennsylvania Ave., S.E.
Ste. 402
Washington, DC 20003
Phone: 202-547-9359
Fax: 202-547-9429
Website: www.centerforfoodsafety.org
E-mail: office@centerforfoodsafety.org

Center for Science in the Public Interest (CSPI)

1220 L St., N.W.
Ste. 300
Washington, DC 20005
Toll-Free: 866-293-CSPI (866-293-2774)
Phone: 202-332-9110
Fax: 202-265-4954
Website: cspinet.org

Clean Water Fund

1444 I St., N.W.
Ste. 400
Washington, DC 20005
Phone: 202-895-0420
Fax: 202-895-0438
Website: www.cleanwaterfund.org
E-mail: cwa@cleanwater.org

Entomological Society of America (ESA)

Three Park Pl.
Ste. 307
Annapolis, MD 21401-3722
Phone: 301-731-4535
Website: www.entsoc.org
E-mail: esa@entsoc.org

Evidence Action

1101 K St., N.W.
Ninth Fl.
Washington, DC 20005
Phone: 202-888-9886
Website: www.evidenceaction.org
E-mail: info@evidenceaction.org

Food Allergy Research and Education (FARE)

7901 Jones Branch Dr., Ste. 240
McLean, VA 22102
Toll-Free: 800-929-4040
Phone: 703-691-3179
Fax: 703-691-2713
Website: www.fare.foodallergy.org

Food and Health Communications, Inc (FHC)

3739 Balboa St.
Unit #5015
San Francisco, CA 94121
Toll-Free: 800-462-2352
Toll-Free Fax: 800-433-7435
Website: foodandhealth.com

Heifer International

One World Ave.
Little Rock, AR 72202
Toll-Free: 855-9HUNGER
(855-948-6437)
Fax: 501-907-2902
Website: www.heifer.org
E-mail: info@heifer.org

Institute of Food Technologists (IFT)

525 W. Van Buren St., Ste. 1000
Chicago, IL 60607
Toll-Free: 800-IFT-FOOD
(800-438-3663)
Phone: 312-782-8424
Website: www.ift.org
E-mail: info@ift.org

International Food Information Council (IFIC) Foundation

Website: foodinsight.org
E-mail: info@foodinsight.org

International Food Protection Training Institute (IFPTI)

5220 Lovers Ln.
Ste. LL-130
Portage, MI 49002
Phone: 269-488-3489
Fax: 269-488-3939
Website: ifpti.org

Lifewater International

2972 S. Higuera St.
San Luis Obispo, CA 93401
Phone: 805-541-6634
Website: lifewater.org
E-mail: info@lifewater.org

National Eating Disorders Association (NEDA)

1500 Bdwy.
Ste. 1101
New York, NY 10036
Toll-Free: 800-931-2237
Phone: 212-575-6200
Fax: 212-575-1650
Website: www.nationaleatingdisorders.org
E-mail: info@NationalEatingDisorders.org

Partnership for Food Safety Education

2345 Crystal Dr.
Ste. 800
Arlington, VA 22202
Phone: 202-220-0651
Website: www.fightbac.org
E-mail: info@fightbac.org

Stop Foodborne illness

4809 N. Ravenswood
Ste. 214
Chicago, IL 60640
Phone: 773-269-6555
Fax: 773-883-3098
Website: stopfoodborneillness.org
E-mail: info@stopfoodborneillness.org

Unite For Sight, Inc

International Headquarters
234 Church St.
15th Fl.
New Haven, CT 06510
Phone: 203-404-4900
Website: www.uniteforsight.org
E-mail: ufs@uniteforsight.org

U.S. Right to Know (USRTK)

4096 Piedmont Ave.
Ste. 963
Oakland, CA 94611-5221
Website: usrtk.org

World Health Organization (WHO)

20 Ave., Appia
1211 Geneva
Switzerland
Phone: +41-22-7912111
Fax: 41-22-791-4857
Website: www.who.int

Zoetis

Head Office
10 Sylvan Way
Parsippany, NJ 07054
Toll-Free: 888-963-8471
Website: www.zoetisus.com